W9-AAK-661

Living With Childhood Cancer

Living With Childhood Cancer

A Practical Guide to Help Families Cope

By Leigh A. Woznick and Carol D. Goodheart

APA
LifeTools

American Psychological Association
Washington, DC

Fifth Printing July 2010

Published by
American Psychological Association
750 First Street, NE
Washington, DC 20002
www.apa.org

To order
APA Order Department
P.O. Box 92984
Washington, DC 20090-2984
Tel: (800) 374-2721, Direct: (202) 336-5510
Fax: (202) 336-5502, TDD/TTY: (202) 336-6123
Online: www.apa.org/books/
Email: order@apa.org

In the U.K., Europe, Africa, and the Middle East, copies may be ordered from
American Psychological Association
3 Henrietta Street
Covent Garden, London
WC2E 8LU England

Typeset in Garamond by EPS Group Inc., Easton, MD
Printer: Edwards Brothers Inc.
Cover designer: NiDesign, Baltimore, MD
Technical/Production Editor: Amy J. Clarke and Catherine Hudson

Library of Congress Cataloging-in-Publication Data
Woznick, Leigh A.
Living with childhood cancer : a practical guide to help families cope / by Leigh A. Woznick and Carol D. Goodheart.—1st ed.
p. cm.
Includes bibliographical references and index.
ISBN 1-55798-872-2 (cb : acid-free paper)
1. Cancer in children—Popular works. 2. Adjustment (Psychology)—Popular works. I. Goodheart, Carol D. II. Title.
RC281.C4 W69 2001
362.1′9892994—dc21

2001040187

British Library Cataloguing-in-Publication Data
A CIP record is available from the British Library.

Printed in the United States of America
First Edition

For each and all in our family,
with love, strength, ties, resilience, gratitude, and everlasting hope

Hope is the thing with feathers
That perches in the soul,
And sings the tune without the words,
And never stops at all,

And sweetest in the gale is heard;
And sore must be the storm
That could abash the little bird
That kept so many warm.

I've heard it in the chillest land,
And on the strangest sea;
Yet, never, in extremity,
It asked a crumb of me.

—Emily Dickinson

Contents

Acknowledgments

We would like to thank the people who helped and inspired us, parents, survivors, professionals, colleagues:

Christine Aney; Kathleen Barry; Terry Doyle Beck; Prentice Beckett; Laura Bedrossian; David Beele, LCSW; Natalie Billings; Jennifer Boyd, RN; Barbara Bradley; Jocelyne Brent; Chris Brown, MS, CCLS; Susan Buckhold, MSW; Karen Busch; Melanie Callender, PhD; Debora Caron; Janine Chapin; Cathy Chavez, RN, CPON; Mark Chesler, PhD; Mary Choroszy, RN, CPNP; Lisa Ciarrocca, CCLS; Deb Clemente; Ruth Collins, RN; Barbara Cook; Donna Copeland, PhD; Lenore Cortina; the Critellas; Ruth Daller, PNP; Jamie D'Amico; Niki Daubach; Dennis DeMott; Cindy Dick; Debbie and Roland Doll; Terri Douglas; Andrew Downes; Daniel and Abbe Effron; Regina Ellis; Consuela Feinman; Patricia Feist; Joan Fleitas; Bernadette Foley, MSW; Julia Frank-McNeil; Jude Freeman; Jane Furst; Lisa Gagen, MSW; Polly Georgiou; Linda Gillick; Tom Golden, LCSW; Joel Goldwein, MD; Hugh Goodheart; Roxie Glaze; Jennifer Greene; Sheryl Guterl; Lisa Hacking; Joyce Hall; Nancy Hammer; Sue Heiney, RN, CSPN; Connie Herron; Janet and John Hoehl; Judy Hoffman; Ruth Hoffman; Jenna Honig, RN; Mary Hubbell; Margie Huhner; Emy Hyans, MSW; Darlene Jones; Tommie Lou Judson; Ernest Katz, PhD; Nancy Keene; Terri Kluey; Gerald Koocher, PhD; Missy Layfield; Pamela Lee; Steve and Kelly Lee; Carol Levin; Cynthia Levitt; Allison Levitt; George Linzenbold; Debra Lobato, PhD; Gerri Long; Rebecca Louie; Todd and Cheryl Matters; Beth McQuin; Anna Meadows, MD; Kim Mehalick; Donald Meyer; Cyndi Miller; Vickie Moffatt, CCLS; Steven Moskowitz, MD; Lisa Nehmer; Jim Newton; Christine Nickle; Colleen O'Brien; Andrea Patenaude, PhD; Laura Pierce; Marla and Gregg Pembleton; Beverly Phipps; Jeffrey Pusar, PsyD; Laura Randall; Jamie L. Reich; Janet Ruffin; Patricia Ruiz, PNP; Nancy Sacks, RD; Sirgay Sanger, MD; Thomas Santisi, RPH, CCN; Juliette Schlucter; Lisa Sciotto; Elaine Sciotto; Mark Schumann; Gerry and Debbie Sims; Dorothy Sims; Howard Snyder, MD; Michael Solomon, MD; Dane Sommer MDiv; Linda Spanos; Anne Spurgeon; Debra Stern; Cynthia Stutzer, RN; Cindy Tate, RN; Glenda

Thompson, RN, PNP; Frances Verter, PhD; Joel Vine; Elaine Vizena; Carolyn Walker, CPON, PhD; Kathryn Weidener; Pam Westmoreland; Jan Williamson; Richard Womer, MD; David Woods; Richard Woznick, Jr.; Richard and Jane Woznick; Linda Goettina Zame, D.M.H.; Susan Zappa, RN, CPON; the women of W2W; the staff of the Pediatric Center; the staff of Children's Hospital of Philadelphia; members of the Family Advisory Council; and many others who wish to remain unnamed.

Living With Childhood Cancer

Introduction: The Big Picture

May you live all the days of your life.
—*Jonathan Swift,* Polite Conversation

An (Un)Natural Disaster

You are leading a normal life, riding its ups and downs like everyone else. Then, over a few days or weeks, your child seems tired or out-of-sorts . . . bruises easily . . . has an unexplained fever . . . a droopy eye that starts to swell . . . a skin-tag that might be getting larger . . . a sharp bellyache . . . a minor sports injury . . . a lump in the cheek. A fault line begins to form deep beneath the surface of your world. Concerned but not alarmed, you consult your pediatrician. Together, you try to treat whatever minor issue is going on. When the problem doesn't go away, a voice nags at the back of your mind, like Miss Clavel from the *Madeline* storybooks: "Something is not right." The tectonic plates begin to shift. When you finally get an answer, it isn't the one you expected. It isn't mono, a virus, a blocked tear duct, a skin tag, constipation, a twisted ankle, or an abscessed tooth. It is cancer. And the earth buckles and heaves under you.—*Leigh and Carol*

Cancer, like an earthquake, is a disaster of nature. It upends your world, collapsing the life you had built, weakening your once-solid foundations, shattering the windows that looked into your future, unearthing deeply buried fears, and looting your sense of security. You never saw it coming, and your life is transformed. *But you are not alone.* You can assess the damage, fight the fires, prepare for the aftershocks, and rebuild with the help of a team of experts and loved ones.

Help is real. You *can* build a life during the shocks of cancer and in its aftermath. We did, and so have many other families. Homes and towns are rebuilt after a disaster levels them. Families, too, can be aided, repaired, and reinforced. The landscape may be altered; you might not have chosen these changes. But in facing the realities of cancer, the rebuilding process works. We want to give you the materials to mobilize and rebuild your family's life after the earthquake.

Our Story

We are the mother and grandmother of a child who had cancer. In April 1994, Leigh's younger daughter was diagnosed with rhabdomyosarcoma, a soft-tissue cancer. Our whole family was thrown into the cancer world with a shock. This was an entirely new and terrifying obstacle. Knowledge and action seemed our most valuable weapons. Every member of the family adjusted quickly to battle mode. Leigh stretched her editorial research skills to find out everything she could about the illness and treatment. Carol used her professional knowledge and connections as a psychologist to get the best services and strategies to help us all cope, prevent and solve problems, and lessen the trauma. She also rearranged her professional schedule to be there for every aspect of her granddaughter's treatment, allowing Leigh's husband to focus on the needs of their other child and maintain his career as well. Generous loved ones, thankfully, kept the rest of our world turning. We counted ourselves enormously fortunate to possess these resources.

We saw for ourselves that cancer is not choosy. It strikes families from all paths of life, all races and religions, all ethnic and economic backgrounds, the educated and the uneducated, those with good support systems and those without, and those with good coping skills and those who have trouble coping. All these families deserve help, but precious few receive *all* the help that could be available. Above all, what struck us hardest was that so much pain, both emotional and physical, could be diminished or avoided if only people knew how.

Looking around the hospital unit one afternoon, Carol said to Leigh, "These children look like trauma victims in a war zone. We could be in Belfast or Bosnia. . . . Look at the expressions on their faces; look at the body language . . . the parents, too. When we get through this ourselves, we have to find ways to help." From very early on, we started talking to other parents, gathering stories and practical coping ideas. Leigh became involved in programs to help other families. From their experiences and our own, she found that families encounter significant emotional effects, as well as physical, that come with treatment and survivorship. Over and over again, people told us that the missing piece is emotional help. Carol was amazed that the practical help that she had been offering in her clinical practice as a psychologist for 20 years was not routinely offered to families in the medical setting, except in extreme cases. Self-help books for parents did a great job explaining medical issues but only scratched the surface of the emotional ones. We knew we could begin to fill that void.

What Cancer Families Need and Deserve

Thanks to medical advances, cancer is now commonly managed as a chronic disease. We rearrange priorities and expectations and schedules, as well as hopes and dreams, to accommodate the long-term possibilities for our children.

Surviving

A diagnosis of cancer is *not* the death sentence it once was. Out of 12,000 children newly diagnosed in the United States each year, roughly 75% will survive. There are more than 250,000 survivors of childhood cancer in the United States, and that number is rising steadily as medical treatments improve. These advances are truly something to shout about. The next logical step for professionals and families is to make sure we have not won a Pyrrhic victory, in which losses are so great that there's little joy left in the win.

Thriving

Our children not only need to survive, they need to thrive. As parents, we have a strong need to live well with a child who has cancer, from diagnosis to coping to survival to positive growth and a fruitful life, *no matter how long or short the life.*

We want psychologically healthy youngsters. We want our children to cope better, to achieve successes, to focus on parts of life other than cancer, to recover from the frightening experiences, and to master new skills. We want them to grow, to experience themselves fully and not be limited to views of themselves based on cancer. We want them to grow into adults capable of work and love, give and take, and balancing independence and dependence well. We want the same things for our other children and for ourselves. Advances in medicine and psychology bring those goals within our reach.

Practical Support

You cannot be expected to know how to cope, alone, with potentially overwhelming medical information, frequent invasive procedures, heavy financial burdens, and crippling emotional stress. Yet practical support for cancer families lags behind the medical advances. Psychological cancer expertise is not as well integrated or widely available as medical expertise is, at least not yet. The immediate focus for the medical staff is, of course, survival, so special supportive services (provided by psychologists, social workers, child life specialists, as well as nutritionists and physical and occupational therapists) are commonly put off until a problem arises. This is unfortunate, because using them earlier can have a major positive impact on physical effects.

There is no advanced training program for cancer. Like that age-old nightmare, you've shown up for a final exam having never been to class or cracked the textbook, except this time your child's life is on the line. Even life's *A+* students feel ill equipped to deal with the trauma of treatment and its long-term effects. Cancer puts such a strain on you and your child that it is unrealistic to expect anyone to function at his or her best. You don't have to be perfect! But you do need special strategies tailored to your needs. Key information, applied early enough, can boost coping, lessen the trauma, and forestall serious long-lasting emotional consequences. Our book offers this kind of practical support.

How This Book Can Help

The book is a coping guide and resource for cancer families and their support teams. Regardless of which treatment your child receives or what effects you encounter, you will have feelings, you will need to deal with your unique situation. In recognizing the ways to cope, you can feel better and function better. Some skills or ways of looking at things may be new, but some of it will seem quite familiar and practical. Our intent is to build on hope, to give you our hard-won personal and professional expertise about how to live better with and after childhood cancer.

Handy tips and suggestions—gentle reminders—can be referred to easily, even when you don't feel much like reading. You will find them in boxes and bulleted lists throughout the book. These tips include "tricks of the trade" and practical strategies for relieving anxiety and boosting coping. All of the recommendations are based on sound psychological research and principles.

The topics are illustrated with stories from families like yours—insights and practical ideas from our own family and more than 100 members of the childhood cancer community who were interviewed. Our story alone would be limited: These diverse families add many different views and experiences. Their candor, eloquence, and astute insights are invaluable. For the stories and quotations from families, names have been changed and identifying details have been disguised to protect their privacy and the privacy of the children.

Professionals of many stripes and shadings were interviewed, and their writings are incorporated. We are consistently awed by the caliber of people who make childhood cancer their life's work. Their level of caring, their sense of community, and their creativity in finding new ways to make the journey easier for our children are amazing.

Under the title of each chapter and throughout the book are other snippets—quotes, song lyrics, and sayings—whose messages resonate for cancer families. We hope that you will find them as relevant and encouraging as we did.

Resources, including organizations, books, and Web sites, that may be especially useful to you are listed in the last chapter. There is also a bibliography for professionals and others interested in the underpinning of psychological research for the book's tips, strategies, and suggestions.

Although cancer is a medical subject, this book does not offer medical information or advice. We do not list side effects of particular drugs or give detailed explanations of what is involved in various testing procedures or treatments. Many of the resources at the end of this book provide that information.

We offer this book from our family to yours. As one mom described it, cancer is the "we" disease ("we got chemo today," "we go back for a scan next week"), and its ripples extend far beyond the sick child. Yet each family member may respond to that distress in a different style. A child with cancer who is frightened and clingy one week may act like a superhero the next, a brother may have repeated tummyaches, a sister may act sullen, a mother may have sleepless nights, a father may talk endlessly about money worries, and a grandparent may question long-held faith. Each family member's personal reactions, emotions, and needs deserve to be addressed.

Families are diverse. Your family may resemble a traditional nuclear family; a single-parent family; a blended family with a stepparent and stepsiblings; or a multigenerational, multiethnic, multireligious family. Your family may include close partners who do not have any marriage or blood kinship ties. Any combination of people who functions as a family is a family in our definition.

Childhood cancer's impact ripples out, reaching beyond the immediate family to extended family members; friends and neighbors; child care providers; classmates and teachers; and the medical and psychosocial system of physicians, nurses, psychologists, social workers, and child life specialists. We hope that they, too, can learn from the stories and strategies presented here.

Dip into the book according to your interests and needs. Not every piece will apply to your circumstances. A book is a linear thing, but what happens to you does not follow a straight line. Read the parts that make sense to you for the moment.

CHAPTER 1

Navigating the Emotional Terrain

In a dark time, the eye begins to see.
—*Theodore Roethke,* In a Dark Time (1964)

When we got the diagnosis of Wilms' tumor, my initial gut reaction was to want to let the "specialist" take care of things. I didn't know anything about cancer, so I just wanted the people who did "know" to tell me exactly what to do. But that's not how it works. It's kind of like calling 911 when someone is choking and having the operator tell you, "The person is choking. If you do nothing, he will die. Here are some options you could try, and here is some information on why some people like and dislike each option. And these are the side effects of each option." All I really wanted to hear at that time was, "This needs to be done. This is what you have to do."—*Diane*

The mother who told us this story is not unusual. No one is ready to deal with the first shock of cancer. No one imagines that one's own child will have cancer. The coping skills needed to handle the emergency are not in place yet. Old ways of facing life's stresses may feel woefully insufficient when you are confronted with the high-stakes, multilayered, long-term stresses of cancer.

In a cancer journey, there are many transitions; each involves new adjustments. In this chapter, we discuss the demands and hallmarks of these transitions and the accompanying shift in perspective that occurs. Each phase requires understanding and acknowledging the changes and adjusting to the new landscape.

Diagnosis

Diagnosis catapults you and your family into a period of shock. This transition is sudden and devastating. Many parents wonder if they can cope, if their child can cope, if they can ever be happy and feel safe again. Your key task at this point is to regroup from the shock and make the necessary decisions to begin treatment, using whatever methods and means of support that can help you to do that. It is the process of getting this information, getting the support, making the decisions, and taking the first steps that allow you to regroup.

> Diagnosis was a life-altering weekend. I was in a tunnel, and there was no light ahead. It took a long time to see a glimmer of light at the end, that maybe we will actually come through this and be okay.—*Gina*

* * *

> The first week in the hospital after diagnosis was the worst. I hung in there as best I could, but I do remember a couple of times when someone would be there to stay with Liam, and I'd go sit outside the hospital by the fountain until I could pull myself together.—*Sharon*

Making Big Decisions

During the initial period of extreme emotional turmoil, you are under pressure to make a lot of important decisions very quickly. Decisions associated with cancer treatment can be complicated matters, with risks and uncertainty. No answer is definitive. There are benefits and drawbacks for most alternatives. Treatments change as new and better methods are discovered. Even the experts do not always agree on the best course of action. It is easy to get caught wavering between options that sound equally good and equally bad. You may not be prepared for how often you need to use your own judgment along the way.

When all is said and done, there can be only one major guideline for the decision-making process. You have to be able to live with your treatment choices for your child without remorse or regret. Whether your child lives for 5 months, 5 years, or 50 years, you must know that you did your best for your child but that you cannot control the outcome. Your need is to have some sense of peace and security that no matter what happens; you made the best possible decisions under the circumstances. If you need help with a particular decision, get it. This is no time for false pride.

> If decisions were a choice between alternatives, decisions would come easy. Decision is the selection and formulation of alternatives. Kenneth Burke, *Toward a Better Life* (1932)

Gentle Reminders for Making Decisions

- Obtain information from a variety of expert childhood cancer sources: oncologists, medical literature, reputable cancer organizations, and so forth (see the Resources at the end of this book).
- Get second and third medical opinions.
- Have more than one person at each meeting. Take notes or tape record meetings so you can refer back to them and not just rely on your memory afterward.
- Make sure a knowledgeable pathologist is making the diagnosis. A pathologist usually can be found at major cancer research centers; you can ask the oncologist to see that a tissue sample is forwarded.
- Talk to people you trust. Remember, opinions from family and friends can be misinformed or emotionally charged.
- Consider long-range goals, rather than short term difficulties.
- Do not get bogged down or distressed by statistics. Your child is not a number, and statistics are frequently misleading.

It is comforting when the people most important to you (your spouse, other family members, or trusted advisors) arrive at the same choices you do. Sometimes there is no choice in a matter, and therefore no decision has to be made. While having no other options can be worrisome, it can also be a relief. If there is only one chance for your child, you take it.

> After our baby daughter was diagnosed, we spent about five days getting consultations and trying to find the best treatment and facility for her. We visited two local hospitals, a famous cancer center, and a top-notch children's hospital. My husband and I asked my mother to join us for all of the consultations, to have an extra pair of ears as well as a competent and knowledgeable advocate. The protocol was pretty much the same at all of them; the doctors were all competent. But all three of us responded strongly to the children's hospital. It had the most ongoing experience with her type of cancer, both an outpatient clinic and an inpatient onco unit, and aggressive but not inhumane recommendations for treatment. The atmosphere was warm and friendly, the support staff phenomenal. Most of all, the team of doctors who met with us that day looked us in the eye and *connected.* They gave us hope.—*Marta*

The great decisions of human life have as a rule far more to do with the instincts and other mysterious unconscious factors than with conscious will and well-meaning reasonableness. The shoe that fits one person pinches another; there is no recipe for living that suits all cases. Carl Gustav Jung, *Contributions to Analytical Psychology* (1928)

You may find yourself too numb to take in any more information, you may detach yourself and intellectualize about what is happening, or you may have waves of intense emotion. Do not be afraid of these initial reactions, because they are typical, and you will regain your footing as you go forward. These early reactions are defenses against feeling overwhelmed or are signs that you have become temporarily swamped and your defenses are not working well. With information and support you will gain confidence and function better.

For suggestions on choosing a doctor or hospital, see chapter 2, about working with the team. Following are some of the other decisions you may have to make and suggestions from parents on what to take into account in making those decisions.

Treatment options

Most often, treatment is set by a standardized *protocol*—a treatment guideline with proven effectiveness—used in all the major cancer centers. Yet sometimes within that "roadmap" there are nuances and choices offered to you. There may or may not be a clearly favored choice. If you obtain second opinions, be prepared for each of them to give a different answer. Despite good collaboration, physicians do not always arrive at the same decision for the same problem, unless there is clear evidence that one treatment works and another does not. With cancer, there are few final answers yet.

If you are offered a choice, ask your child's doctors about

- their experience level with each option
- success rates
- possible and probable side effects or risks (short and long term) and methods available to prevent, lessen, or cope with them
- comparisons to other options
- what makes an option effective or preferable
- what the latest studies show
- where and how the treatment will be done, such as inpatient, outpatient, or in a different facility
- how long the treatment will take
- who will be in charge of your child's case
- how your child will be monitored for effects.

Weigh the benefits and risks of each option, and choose what is right for your child.

Participation in clinical trials

Trials are scientific attempts to gain better survival rates or lessen effects. They may simply "tweak" the standard treatment with slight changes or involve the use of promising new drugs and treatments. Many parents are frightened at the prospect of doing something "experimental," and insurance companies may balk at paying for the treatment. Do not allow yourself to be pressured into something that is not right for your child, but do remember that evidence from clinical trials developed the standard treatments for your child's cancer in the first place. An ethical oncologist will not let any child remain on a trial that is not working for that child. To make a truly informed decision, get all the information first, from your child's doctor and the national cancer organizations (see the Resources at the end of this book). You are entitled to a full copy of your child's entire protocol. Know that this document is highly technical and includes clinical details and every possible effect. Not everyone feels comfortable with all of that information.

> The doctors were saying we could do a, b, or c, and it was up to us to decide quickly. Sam qualified for the experimental chemotherapy protocol for leukemia. Looking back now, the down side of our choice was that when we got on to the maintenance phase, we discovered that they had changed the whole protocol again. We went through one round of delayed intensification, and now the standard procedure is for two rounds. That scares us terribly, because they made this decision that every kid should get double, and we've only done it once. What does that mean? We don't know. Yet what they've doubled is the most horrible, caustic, toxic, chemo drug. It's a double-edged sword. In retrospect, [choosing the experimental] was a fairly good decision, because the new protocol now includes the substitute drug he received. I feel very good about that.—*Barbara*

Gene testing

When a child develops cancer, some people wish to know if cancer "runs in the family" and if their other children are at risk for developing cancer, too. This may complicate a couple's decision to expand their family later on. The technology exists now for testing DNA to learn whether there is an identifiable genetic risk for certain types of cancer in your family. Examples of childhood cancers with predictive gene markers are retinoblastoma, familial Wilms' tumor, and Li-Fraumeni syndrome.

The decision to pursue genetic testing is a highly personal matter. The decision to test any and all family members should be undertaken only with genetic counseling, which will help you understand the limits of the information and its potential impact. Statistics and risk information can be misleading. The National Institutes of Health publicizes that most cancers are not inherited: Despite the fact that cancer arises from gene mutations (mistakes), most of these mutations occur during a person's lifetime and only in the cell that becomes a tumor (see the Bibliography). Also not all people with a positive gene test result develop cancer. Instead, the information offers only probabilities, not certainties.

The prospect of gene testing can be a divisive issue for some families. People can have very strong reactions, pro and con, to both the testing and the implications of the results.

I had a conversation with my grandmother that was upsetting. She voiced the opinion that we should take permanent precautions against having more kids. I told her I wasn't prepared to do that. She said, "Even though you are carriers for genetic cancer, you'd still consider having another child and putting them through all that? How could you do that?" She went on to say that it would be more appropriate if Larry got a vasectomy, implying that genetically I'm ok but Larry is not, since he had the same cancer as a child. Larry doesn't and shouldn't feel guilty about hereditary aspects, because it's nothing he can control. I found it disturbing that one of my relatives openly displayed an attitude that we should be sterilized so as not to pass the genes on.—*Diane*

The benefit of testing is that the knowledge can provide relief if the result is negative (no marker found) and the forewarning to make informed decisions for screening and health choices in the future if the result is positive. The risk of testing lies in the psychological impact and the impact on family relationships. Be especially careful about getting children tested; they may think that a positive result means they will definitely get cancer, or a negative result may trigger guilt for being the one who is spared. Another testing concern is the lack of guaranteed privacy of information. Currently there are no uniform U.S. laws to protect your family from insurance or employer discrimination if test results are revealed. When considering gene testing, select a comprehensive, reputable testing center that offers both confidentiality and the services of genetic counselors who are trained to help you understand your results. The National Cancer Institute's Cancer Information Service has an informative booklet, *Understanding Gene Testing*, which you may find helpful (see the Resources at the end of this book).

Sperm banking/egg preservation

This is an issue that you may need to bring up with your child's oncologist. Sperm banking is an option for young men who have already reached puberty. It may seem to be a delicate subject to broach, but some teenagers are aware of and concerned with the issue of becoming parents themselves in the future. The process involves some time and more than one collection, which may be difficult for a teenager who is really sick. If your hospital does not have the knowledge or facilities, seek out area fertility experts. Unfortunately, at this time, the collection process makes it rarely feasible to bank reproductive eggs for young women who are receiving cancer treatment.

This is such an awkward subject for teen boys. We had to address it right after diagnosis and, for us at least, the topic gave us some much needed laughs. Just last month, as we were leaving the lab, David looked over at the area where they do the fertility testing and sperm collections and commented, "Maybe I should go see the kids?"—*Lucille*

* * *

> We were approached about [sperm-banking]. Our son was 16. We had to make the decision as parents. When we met with the oncologists at the outset, they told us about sterilizing side effects of his treatment, and they mentioned this as an option. I told my wife, if he were a little older, I would talk to him about it. He's got enough on his mind. Later, when he relapsed, he told us that if he had to undergo the heavy chemo, he wanted to do it. But it was too late. Which made us feel like maybe we should have done it the first time. —*Martin*

Nonmedical decisions

In the whirlwind of diagnosis, there are also many domestic decisions that can affect the family. Arrangements need to be made for child care, for both the sick child and his or her siblings, for daily and emergency situations. Day care, with its high germ traffic, may be an unattractive option now. Taking into account the effect on the family's finances, child care availability, and the question of insurance coverage, you may have to decide whether or not you should keep working. Big decisions that were already in the works may be put on hold or decided differently, for example, home buying or remodeling, vacations, adding to the family, and major purchases. Following through on plans may be an affirmation of life, a toehold on normalcy. On the other hand, it may compound the stress level, be financially impossible, or be medically inadvisable.

Explaining to the Children

An important issue at the time of diagnosis is how to explain everything to your child or children. Pediatric cancer psychologist Andrea Patenaude tells us that it is rarely possible to hide a serious diagnosis like cancer in a family member from children and that secrecy has harmful effects on them. However, you need tact, emotional control, and an understanding of how children think about illness to present it to them.

> I explained it to him matter-of-factly. It was something like, you have a lump in your stomach. It is cancer. They will give you special medicine, and it's really strong medicine and it might make you feel crummy. This will not be gone in a week. This could go on for a couple of years. My mother sat there listening. When I was through she told me that I did a really good job and I was a good mother, and that really meant a lot. It really made me feel good.—*Maggie*

* * *

> A few days before Lloyd's first chemo treatment, Rob and I told him he had something called "cancer" and that he was going to have to take a lot of medicine for a long time to make sure that no other cancer bumps ever, ever came back anywhere on his body. We all cried, and then we told him he could ask for a "family hug" anytime he needed one, and

> then we did a family hug. It was very emotional but also a relief that we finally told him. But until he went through it, Lloyd really had no idea what was coming, despite us telling him.—*Sandy*

You do not have to do all of the explaining yourself.

> Daniel (age 10) wanted to know every detail—"how many milligrams of medicine are you giving me, how are you going to do this?" When Dr. L. would sit and explain stuff to me, he would sit and explain it to Daniel. Sometimes we discussed it afterwards. This made things easier for Daniel and for me. I didn't always have to be the bearer of bad news. The doctor took that job from me. I could just pick up the pieces afterward, which is more what you want to do, as a mom.—*Sarah*

Ask your child's doctor, nurse, child life specialist, or social worker to provide a simple description of your child's particular cancer and treatment to you or directly to your child. Children usually respond to familiar images and words.

> He got the concept of leukemia very well. He was very into the Power Rangers. We told him the way the Power Rangers fight the bad guys, there are good cells trying to fight the bad cells inside your body. The medicine is going to help fight the bad cells. As simplistic as that is, he understood. One day he said, "Mom, I can feel it, they're in my leg." I'm thinking, what now? I asked, "What's in your leg?" He said "I can feel them fighting. The bad cells are putting up a fight, but the good cells are winning. They're right over my knee." —*Gina*

Remarkably, most children expand their vocabularies to include a host of medical terms, but even some of the simplest words can be frightening. Many sources advise against using negative or pain-associated words for young children. Yet the cancer world is a painful one, and parents find it nearly impossible to avoid these terms completely. Often, children and families come up with their own more comfortable terms and nicknames for frequent procedures. Some words have associations outside the cancer world that make them easy for a child to misinterpret. Soften their impact by explaining these words with less threatening or confusing words. Here are a few examples.

Commonly heard	**Parents or kids might say**
Shot, stick, poke, injection, needle, pain	Pinch, owie, medicine under the skin, boo-boo
Put to sleep, anesthesia, deaden	Sleepy medicine, "Anastasia," numby stuff
Test	Find out how "X" is working
Incision, cut, surgery	Opening to see inside, make you better
Scalpel, knife	Tool
Bug	Germ, something that makes you sick

Dye, contrast	Coloring so we can see things better
Damage	Hurt
X-ray, CAT scan	Picture
Straps, restraints	Seatbelts
Ultrasound	Jelly-roll picture
Drug	Medicine, medication

Think about the words you use, and remember that to children *induction* means the army, *nuclear* has more to do with weapons than medicine, *blasts* are for rocket ships, *mutations* are video-game monsters, and *mets* are a baseball team.

The following guidelines give suggestions for how to explain cancer to a child or a sibling in nonthreatening, easy-to-understand terms. The information is a combination of the authors' suggestions and those of Debra J. Lobato, a clinical psychologist and professor who specializes in chronic childhood illnesses and development disabilities (see Bibliography).

Guidelines for Explaining Cancer to Children

- *Offer brief, ongoing, age-appropriate discussions in simple terms.* Everything cannot be covered in one conversation. Allow time to process the information. Young children don't need to know the long-term implications right away but do need honesty and truth about what is happening to them.
- *Allow for and encourage questions.* Admit it if you do not know the answer, and suggest sources you can go to together for answers. Answer just the question asked; sometimes the simplest answer is best. Teenagers may need to ask other adults and not just their parents.
- *Explain that there are many forms of cancer and that this kind may be different from ones you have heard about.* Many people are afraid of the word *cancer,* because they think people always die from it. But that is not true. Some people die from cancer, but doctors and nurses can make some kinds go away. It means spending a lot of time going to doctors and hospitals, getting very special medicines and treatments.
- *Explain that cancer means something inside the body is growing wrong or out of control.* You can't always see it. State which body parts or systems are involved and what symptoms or effects were caused by the disease. Practice with the experts (a nurse or doctor), so they can tell you if you are accurate, and you can be comfortable with the new words yourself.
- *Use all the terms the child might encounter* (such as leukemia, lymphoma, cancer, tumor, bump, mass, growth, malignancy, Hodgkin's, Wilms', lymphoma, neuroblastoma, sarcoma, blast, carcinoma, abbreviations like AML and ALL). This will help the child not to be surprised or frightened when people use another term.
- *Do not be afraid to use the real words.* However, understand that these are easily misunderstood by young children and require explanation in simpler and more familiar terms.

Box continues next page

Continued

- *Differentiate between ordinary "sick" and cancer* (especially for siblings, who might panic at ordinary bumps, bruises, or fever). Cancer does not go away as quickly or on its own.
- *Reassure the child that cancer is not contagious.*
- *Tell them over and over again that they did NOT cause the cancer by any means.*
- *Talk about the very special medicines for cancer, which are not like regular medicines.* The medicines will make the child feel sick, throw up, be tired, lose hair, lose or gain weight, make other changes in appearance, and so forth. None of this is the child's fault, and these symptoms are only temporary.
- *Reassure young children that you are not abandoning them.* Tell this to the sick child and his or her siblings.
- *Talk about what the child will and will not be able to do.* Temporarily, he or she might not be able to ride a bike, swim, or attend school. Stress that he or she will still like the same music, cartoon characters, television shows, Internet sites, or books and can still do some activities. The child is still the same person. Focus on the continued strengths and abilities of the individual child.
- *Make an optimistic statement that the family and the doctors are doing everything possible to make the child better.* Give the child hope but not falsehoods. Children need to know that treating the cancer will be difficult but that you will stick together to get through it.
- *Give a time frame.* Explain that treatment will take _____ number of months or years and that there may be delays.
- *It is realistic to admit that you are scared sometimes, too, and do not have all the answers, but do not burden your children with the task of taking care of you.* Turn to others for your own support.

The main message to convey to a child with cancer is that we do not know why some children get cancer, but everyone is going to work hard together to make the child better. Siblings need special explanations, too. For example, it is helpful to convey that children cannot go for treatment alone, so mom and dad will spend a lot of time at the hospital. Siblings need to hear that they will still be taken care of and loved.

Being on Treatment

Being on treatment is a long, drawn-out period that requires many adjustments. Treatment may last anywhere from months to years. Your family must accustom themselves to unexpected events, delays, setbacks, and cancellations. The hallmark of this phase is the necessity for making cancer treatment the dominant, consuming focus of life. Other priorities and life tasks tend to fall away for the duration.

Family members' lives are disrupted. Adjusting to life in the hospital means being sleep deprived, watching or participating in putting your child through painful procedures, communicating with staff, and getting along with roommates. If one parent is working and not at the hospital most of the time, the separation of duties between caretaker and breadwinner can bring its own strains. If the caretaker has to continue working, the strains are even bigger. Siblings resent the lack of attention for themselves and the constant focus on the sick child. The emotional toll is heavy. Alterations in lifestyle abound. The physical condition of your sick child is difficult for you and other family members to witness.

> At the beginning, his physical appearance was hard on everybody. I took pictures of Anthony, just as he was coming into the intense phase of treatment. My sister said not only did he physically look bad, but he looked so sad. My mother was upset, too. She asked how I could have taken them when he didn't look good. But I couldn't just put away my camera for three years. I couldn't only take pictures of the other two. At first, when I looked at these pictures, I would think, my baby, look at what's happened. But now, I find those pictures empowering, because we've come so far.—*Lynn*

* * *

> I was getting scared. He just couldn't eat, couldn't keep anything down. I don't think he even wanted to try. His clothes were just hanging on him. One time, we walked up five flights of steps to the clinic. He said, "Wait Dad, I gotta rest." Here's this 15-year-old kid who was an athlete, and here's the 45-year-old dad, and I had to wait for him. That hit home. In between chemo sessions, I came home from work one night, and he's sitting up on the couch downstairs. He said "I had two bowls of soup and some crackers," and it was such a big deal. He was so proud that he could say that to me, and it was really heart-wrenching. I was glad, but also thinking, this is what we've come to?—*Al*

Gentle Reminders for Coping With Treatment

- Let go of unnecessary routines, chores, and obligations.
- Create an information update system on your answering machine, via newsletter, or on a Web site. You might assign someone else to be in charge of updating it, with you supplying accurate information.
- Take pictures. This experience is a part of your child's and your family's life. You do not have to ever look at the photographs, but if you do not take them, you will never have that option. They may also help your child process the experience later.
- Get a Medicalert bracelet for your child. The company's database holds information about your child's latest treatments and can be accessed by most emergency room personnel (see the Resources at the end of this book).

Box continues next page

Continued

- Use an eye mask or ear plugs for sleeping in the hospital. Bring a flashlight or book light to read by after your child is asleep, or listen to books on tape with headphones. Bring a generic remote control for the TV (hospital remotes often get lost).
- Wear comfortable shoes with good support; hard hospital floors are bad for your feet, legs, and back.
- Some tips for coping with the central line (the tubing sutured into a blood vessel, usually from the upper chest or back, for the purpose of giving chemotherapy, blood transfusions, or other medicines) are keeping clothespins on top of each room's doorway to clamp off a central line in case the child cuts it or somehow gets the lumen off; tucking the line in the pants or pinning it (making a tab of tape around the tube first) to the shirt instead of taping it to a child's irritated skin; making or buying clothes with Velcro at the shoulder or side seam so that staff can access the line without undressing the child; and tucking the line into the neck of a bib when bathing a baby or toddler.
- Keep a nightlight or flashlight in child's room at home to check on pumps.
- Place a baby monitor beside the child's bed at home to keep tabs on your child.
- Outline to medical residents any special rules that are important to you. Request one to come in and report back to others; do not allow them to wake a sleeping child or examine child in your absence.
- Use a dry-erase board in the hospital room or on the door to post messages to staff.
- Bring your child's own pajamas and sheets (bring extras and be willing to change them daily or even more often) and other personal items to make the hospital room seem homier.
- Pack all your stuff in a travel suitcase or backpack on wheels.
- Plead a bad back, if necessary, to get a bed or cot for sleeping in your child's room.
- Bring your own food. Order from restaurants, if your child has no dietary restrictions.
- Use the hospital swimming pool or gym.
- Get up, get dressed, and open the blinds; follow your regular routines for meals and baths. Develop new routines for injections and dressing changes.
- Develop ground rules with roommates: Follow the golden rule and be willing to compromise. Ask if they have special needs or requests, then politely describe

Box continues next page

Continued

yours, including your routines, typical bedtime, and so forth. Be considerate and ask the roommate to do the same. Turn off lights, the TV, and noisy games if the other child is trying to sleep. Monitor visitors' behavior; take them for a walk or to the playroom. Make no late-night phone calls. If your take-out dinner makes the other child nauseated, eat it elsewhere. Keep "baby-sitting" requests to a minimum. Be alert to cues; some families do not want to share stories, so don't intrude. If you have a problem with an uncooperative roommate, ask the hospital floor manager to move you.

- Whenever you leave your child with a baby-sitter, at school, or at day care, leave a signed permission-to-treat letter along with an updated list of latest treatments and medications in case of emergency. Your child's doctor can help you write one. (This should be done for siblings, too.)
- Look into wish fulfillment organizations; your child does not have to be terminal to get a wish.
- Start a journal. Some people choose to write about feelings, some about medical information, and some a combination.

Maintenance

Not every child has a maintenance phase of treatment, but it is usually one part of the regimen for children with leukemia who have gone into remission. We mention this one because this is a step that many parents describe as noticeably easier. The hallmark of this phase is relief. You get to be home more, visits to the hospital are less frequent, and your child might not get quite so sick and may be able to return to some activities and his or her hair may start to grow back. You get more time to recover in between treatments. This is a drawn-out transition between being on and coming off treatment, with some of the advantages and disadvantages of both. Maintenance can last a long time, and there are still infections, steroid effects, and other surprises to deal with. Still, there is a sense that treatments are actively working.

> The turning point came when Anthony started maintenance. Once I knew we had gotten through the "hard part," the extra weight from medications was coming off, he wanted to get off the couch and go outside and play, that was when I knew that we would come through this. When his hair came back, it was platinum blond. It was spectacular to look at. As his hair came back, and he got thinner and could move more, we were outside all the time, and we weren't at the hospital. It was a physical change in him. He was coming back. We were going to get our little boy back again, the one that we recognized.—*Lynn*

* * *

David finally started maintenance. He's feeling good, other than the steroid effects. He has been exercising and reading. We moved out of our apartment that we leased while we were at the hospital. Part of me is a little nervous having given it up (is this a jinx?). The other part is thrilled to be moving on. I have gone back to work half-time, so I still have time to go to clinic every 2 weeks. I'm trying to work into this "back to normal" thing, but am finding it harder than expected. After spending 10 months in a constant "crisis" mode, coming out of warp drive is hard. I have found some helpful habits from the last year though, like being able to pack in under 5 minutes and never letting the gas tank fall below half-full. Other things are less useful, like knowing the daytime TV schedule and what pizza the hospital cafeteria serves on Tuesday.—*Lucille*

Transplant

Bone marrow or peripheral blood stem cell transplant is a treatment option for some cancers. Very few children with cancer will go through this, but for some, it is their best chance of survival (at the time of this writing). Some children require more than one transplant. This is one of the most difficult of treatments. Long- and short-term side effects are amplified; risks multiply. Parents describe it as bringing a child to the brink of death to save the child's life. The hallmark of this phase is described by Sue Heiney, a psychiatric nurse and researcher in pediatric oncology: "Take the normal stresses of treatment, and multiply by five."

There is a large emotional investment in this harsh but potentially life-saving treatment. One mother described the transfusion procedure as a "big let-down . . . with all the hooplah, and then a little bag of blood, dripping in. That's supposed to save my child?" Other parents viewed it as a miracle, in which every drop was life.

Family member donors (adults or children) often feel a great sense of honor, pride, and gratitude that they can provide the healthy marrow, although very young sibling donors might be confused or frightened by the process if not appropriately informed. Pride can turn to guilt and despair if the procedure is unsuccessful. In that case, the donor (adult or child) needs extra reassurance that it is not his or her fault and would benefit from counseling to help cope with those feelings. Families may grapple with cloudy ethical questions, such as having a baby who might match as a donor, using donated umbilical cord blood, and gauging how much or how little of a marrow type match is acceptable. Unrelated donors have a special place in the hearts of parents. Although a one-year (or longer) waiting period is often required before the identities of families and donors are shared (with some donors requesting absolute anonymity), many parents ultimately welcome these benefactors into the family, exchanging letters, photographs, and visits.

Transplant involves a necessary period of isolation, sometimes quite lengthy, to prevent exposure to infection. The isolation takes its toll on the family's social life, support system, and patience. During the time while the child is still hospitalized, the child may be too sick to need much entertaining. However, after the child goes home and starts to feel better, boredom may set in. If the transplant must be done at another hospital, especially one far away from home, that change may contribute further to the experience of isolation. It may be a hardship to travel a long distance to a major cancer center, live away from family and support, and get used to a new staff and differing hospital policies. The exorbitant expenses and question of whether the procedure will be covered by insurance adds to the stress. There are sources of help and support, both informational and emotional, found in the Resources at the end of this book.

> The transplant hospital was so different from the friendly atmosphere we were used to at our clinic, where he was assigned a child life specialist and a social worker. After they had done the chemo, Daniel sat on the edge of the bed, looked at me, and said, "I'm getting out of here. I hate this place. I hate the nurses. Pack my bag, we're out of here." I said, "Honey, you have no bone marrow, we can't go anywhere." He said, "Then find somebody else to take care of me." I knew we needed to do something. The social worker would promise to play a game with him, then wouldn't show up. We ended up connecting with the pain management doctor. He spent a lot of time with Daniel.—*Sarah*

Gentle Reminders for Coping With Transplants

- Be prepared. Ask the medical team: what will happen, who's in charge, what to expect, how long isolation must be, time frame for effects, how to alleviate and cope with side effects, necessary care and precautions, accessibility of the transplant center, pain management guidelines, psychosocial support, amenities (such as room size, visitor policies, and computer access), infection control rules, and local resources.
- Educate, prepare, and support the donor (through written, verbal, or video information and talking, encouraging questions and expressions of hopes and fears), especially if the donor is a sibling.
- Parents and siblings need breaks, time away; take turns with care.
- Patients need diversions. Be creative but sensitive to child's low energy level. Some useful pastimes (to be used with discretion) are marathon Monopoly or other board games, jigsaw puzzles in roll-up carriers, videos, and computer games. Stockpile disinfected toys, games, and other distractions.
- Make use of all your resources, including financial, emotional, spiritual, and practical support. This is no time to try to "go it alone."

Box continues next page

Continued

- Find alternate means of support and human connection (such as telephone calls, Internet chat rooms, e-mail, and hospital support groups).
- If your child is frustrated by an inability to talk because of breathing tubes or mouth sores, use paper and pen, a code system (blinking eyes or squeezing hands once for yes, twice for no, or a number of times to correspond with letters of the alphabet), or nonverbal communication (patting, stroking, or massaging feet) to reassure your child, depending on his or her level of energy and alertness.
- Practice infection control. Practice good and frequent handwashing (20 seconds vigorous rubbing with soap and warm water); stock up on antibacterial soap, disinfectant, and bleach; and avoid home remodeling, contact with animal feces, crowds, and public places. Hospital or home care should help you prepare your home before the child is ready to be discharged.
- Celebrate the anniversary of transplant day as a new "birthday."
- Reimmunize your child when the doctor deems it safe to do so.

Coming Off Treatment

The end of treatment is described by parents as both wonderful and frightening. The hallmark of this phase is the presence of mixed feelings. It can come as a surprise to experience anxiety and let down, when only relief was expected. Mood swings are not uncommon. On the one hand, you are ecstatic that your child has remained in remission, grateful that he or she is alive, the ordeal of treatment is over, there are no more toxic drugs, you can go back home to your life, and you do not have to be at the hospital so often. On the other hand, you are terrified of not doing anything actively to fight the cancer. Fears of relapse are kick-started. Signs of illness and limitation remain. Vivid dreams and nightmares can surprise children and adults.

When you walk to the edge of all the light you have, and take that first step into the darkness of the unknown, you must believe that one of two things will happen: there will be something solid for you to stand upon, or, you will be taught how to fly. Patrick Overton, *The Leaning Tree* (1975), *Rebuilding the Front Porch of America* (1997)

> I am extremely anxious about him stopping his treatment. As excited as I am that our three years are coming to an end, I am petrified because this medicine made it go away and made it stay away. And we're going to stop it. Then what? Every time something's wrong, I can tell already that I'm going to be very anxious and scared.—*Toni*

All through treatment, you have hoped that when it was over, you would be finished with doctors and hospitals and sickness. When you get there, you find that it is not entirely true. Symptoms do not immediately disappear. Blood counts can take months to come back to normal. Some chemotherapy drugs produce withdrawal symptoms when they are stopped. Hospital or clinic checkups are frequent, and you may now need additional specialists to deal with effects or complications. Your child may have more trouble with blood tests, because the central line has been removed. It's not over when it's over.

> I am so glad to know that it's "normal" to experience this excitement and fear all at once when treatment comes to an end. I thought I was nuts because I was so scared that his treatment was done! And of course our families wanted us to just "get on with life, cancer is over" and that made me feel even more strange. In a way, ending treatment was also a grieving process. When your whole life is focused on treatment and then one day it's just done, it's weird. The security of knowing that the staff is keeping track of your child, the friends you've made in the hospital, the familiarity of the routine, being around people that are experiencing the same issues.—*Iris*

Some children are anxious to jump back into their old lives. Other, especially younger, children may be uncomfortable returning to or starting school and having to catch up, acknowledge limitations, or redefine themselves. The child misses the attention and may wish to still be sick or may not know anymore how to be "well." This does not mean the child cannot reintegrate into life, it just means he or she needs a period of adjustment.

The hospital staff sends you on your way with good wishes but perhaps with little preparation for the fears and emotions that arise. You and your child miss the support of the hospital or clinic team. Parents sometimes feel as though the staff has abandoned them. They are no longer a priority, as the doctors are busy saving other children's lives, but the parents still want the attention and connection. This produces a combination of gratitude and guilt. A relationship with staff was forged in a time of adversity, making it very powerful. An abrupt cutoff makes the relationship seem less personal. It can be a distressing ending. In addition, many doctors seem to focus on your child as a success story and may not be as attentive to your observations of late effects as you would want.

> The doctors say, "Hurray, hurray your child's alive," and send you on your way. They take it as a criticism when you say, "My kid doesn't walk right anymore," or "My kid can't learn anymore." It is really hard to say, "Yes, it is a wonderful thing this child is alive, but we

> have to deal with these problems assertively." It gets better. You don't hold your breath for as long a period of time, as you see it isn't coming back.—*Liz*

The support networks created since diagnosis are dismantled when treatment ends. People unrealistically expect you to get right back to normal. By being at the hospital less frequently, you lose not only the treatment team but also the support of other cancer families. This is a period in which many parents seek out a support group or counseling. Now that the ordeal is over and your time and energy are not put wholly into caring for your child, you can deal with the emotional aftermath.

> I've noticed a shift in how others view our relationship, mother and son. While he was ill and I was with him at the hospital, it seemed that I was viewed as a supportive, caring mother, almost in the martyr category. As he became stronger and approached departure for college, I noticed a preponderance of comments regarding how hard it would be for me to "let him go," as if I had been the one holding him back. People appeared to think that we had grown unusually close and that would make his departure for college that much more difficult. For the record, my husband and I are thrilled that he has the opportunity to go to college. A good part of the pain of relapse was that he had come so close to his dream and had it snatched away. Maybe we've become so close that, now, we more closely identify with his feelings, rather than ours as parents, which might normally be a feeling of loss. While we miss him, we feel that he is living his dream, how can we be sad about that? —*Lucille*

* * *

> [Joining] Candlelighters' was really helpful for us because we could be with other families whose kids were getting off treatment. That's the point at which you have the time and energy. You're at a crossroads, you can choose to ignore it, forget it, let it go, or to try and do something.—*Trish*

Many hospitals have established late-effects or follow-up clinics. The staffs typically include specialists qualified to deal with specific problems, such as cardiologists and neuropsychologists. Contact with other long-term survivors and their families is an encouraging and powerful resource. Transition usually occurs 2–4 years after treatment ends. You might not work with the same oncologist or nurses you have known throughout treatment, but the new team is likely to be on the same page you are: looking toward the future and watching for effects. Some families mark the end of treatment with a party or similar celebration. Others are too cautious to do so. Some parents cannot wait to throw away the supplies, others feel the need to hang on to them. Many feel the urge to say thank you to the staff or institution that treated their child with a small token of their gratitude. One mother calligraphed a poem that had personal meaning and gave it to her child's oncologist.

Lon (age 5) wanted to get all the medical junk out of sight as soon as possible! He wasn't one of those kids who wanted to keep his central line catheter after treatment. After it was removed and we were on our way out the door, Lon checked the trash can to make sure it was there! We had so much fun watching him flush all that expensive, awful medicine down the toilet one by one—"Goodbye Peridex! Goodbye stool softeners!" Wish we had pictures of us all crowded in the bathroom, cheering our heads off! Weirdly, I was still too antsy to throw away the sterile saline, bandages, and tape, though. Let's just say that Lon's soccer team had the best stocked first aid kit in town.—*Jeanne*

Gentle Reminders for Coming Off Treatment

- Insist on a "coming off treatment" meeting with the medical staff. Ask the doctor about the schedule for scans or tests both for relapse and effects. Who will monitor the child's case? How long before the child feels better, counts come up, body functions return to normal, and the central line is removed? Are there effects from discontinuation of any of the child's medications? Are there any medications that need to continue, and for how long? What are the signs of relapse or side effects you need to watch for and the time frame they might be expected? How likely is relapse, and what options remain in the event?
- Get any necessary baseline exams (such as neuropsychology, hearing, cardiology, thyroid, endocrine, liver function, and kidney function).
- Add new services as needed, such as physical therapy.
- Join a support group, and talk to other parents.
- Continue to practice coping techniques (see chapters 3 and 9) for your child during follow-up procedures.
- For back-to-school issues, get an individualized education plan in place, and educate teachers and classmates (see chapter 2).
- Do something to mark the occasion—have a party, take a trip, or give or throw away medical supplies. Donate leftover (unopened) supplies to the hospital or a cancer organization (see the Resources at the end of the book).
- Buy hair gel, bows, and bands; donate hats to other kids who need them.
- Take the child swimming once the central line is removed and counts are back to normal.
- Hire a baby-sitter, and go out dancing or to the movies.
- Spend some special time with the child's siblings.
- Donate a cookie platter for staff, toys for the hospital playroom, or linens for the Ronald McDonald House; donate blood or platelets or join the bone marrow registry.

Box continues next page

Continued

- Organize a record of treatment, so when the child is grown, he or she will have a resource to refer to. Get copies of medical records.
- Get involved in parental support or advocacy programs, volunteer for the PTA or PTO, or become a scout leader, things you may have put off during treatment.
- Don't overdo it. There is still a lot going on, and you are all "in recovery," which is a long process.

Relapse

Many families do not encounter this phase, because their child does not relapse during or after treatment. But for those who do, it is a painful time. The longer the remission, the harder a relapse is to bear. There is an overwhelming sense of disappointment and injustice, whether the relapse occurs immediately or years later.

One grandparent made the analogy that relapse is like childbirth: When you have done it once, you know what to expect. It is frightening, because you know your child will be very sick again, and the cancer seems so strong. The next step in treatment may be harsher chemotherapy, a bone marrow transplant, radiation, or a brand new treatment. Parents worry that their children are "maxed out" on acceptable maximum doses of effective cancer-fighting medications and that long-term side effects from additional or new treatment will be more significant. "What ifs" and "If onlys" may throw previous decisions into question, paralyzing the current decision-making process. Throughout the first treatment, it was easier to be buoyed by the reassurance that the treatment regimen was working. At relapse, the family comes to terms with the possibility that their child may die. The hallmark of this phase is stated well by Carolyn Walker, a nursing professor and pediatric oncology nurse:

> The biggest issue that arises after relapse or recurrence is that the "best" treatment option has failed, so the family is terribly afraid that the next course of therapy may not work either. The reality that their child may not make it is very real and very frightening. The family needs support in every way possible.

Relapse does mean that further treatment is necessary, but it does not always mean the child will die. Many children do not. The anxiety surrounding this period is intense. Strong feelings are aroused for all of the family members, perhaps even more so than at initial diagnosis. You may find strength in that because you have battled this before, you can handle it again. Fall back on routines and coping mechanisms that worked, and change the ones that did not. The second time around, you might feel more confident in asking questions, asserting yourself, and communicating your needs to staff.

> Mike's learned to speak up for himself. He was starting to feel like a guinea pig, with the residents asking his medical history. He said, "I really don't feel like talking about this anymore, why don't you go read the chart and come back." —*Fred*

* * *

> When he relapsed I finally realized that cancer was here to stay. I poured myself into restarting a Candlelighters group here. —*Iris*

* * *

> When we finished treatment, I believed we were through the worst of it. I had worries about relapse, but I vowed that they would not consume me. I looked for the bright lights, the happiness in our lives, and made a conscious decision not to dwell on the fear. When my son relapsed, I felt fear and panic and anger. It's hard to adequately describe the cauldron of emotions of those days. Once again, we had to decide how to deal with this. I feared having to look back and say our last months together were spent in fear and anger. We know what we are facing, but we have chosen to look toward the light instead of the darkness in our lives. It's not always easy, and it is a conscious decision of ours, which needs constant renewal. The struggle to cope with the fear is one of the hardest things we'll ever do. —*Lucille*

Gentle Reminders for Coping With Relapse

- Regroup your support network. Renew old contacts and helpers and add new ones.
- Redouble information-gathering efforts for treatment options (such as what worked before, standard options, clinical trials, new drugs and treatments, experimentals, and second opinions).
- Prepare for new treatments and their effects. Talk to staff and other experienced parents.
- Talk to someone about your feelings and fears, other parents or a therapist.
- Encourage your child and his or her siblings to express feelings and fears.
- Continue keeping a journal.

Even if relapse occurs and another round of treatment follows, a significant number of children will be survivors and go on to lead normal lives as adults (see chapter 13).

CHAPTER 2

Creating and Working With the Team: Doctors, Nurses, Health Insurers, Teachers, and Others

The first and great commandment is, Don't let them scare you.
—*Elmer Davis,* But We Were Born Free (1954)

When choosing up sides against the toughest possible opponent—cancer—you need to pick positive, capable players for your team. Choose those who can work in harmony and play a thinking game. Obviously, fighting cancer is no game, but if you think of all those involved in your child's life and care as team members, you realize that they each play a different position. Replacements and substitutions are available, and each player is important to the ultimate outcome. It is up to you to recognize and use the unique capabilities of each member to the best advantage.

Putting together this team will be an ongoing process. Your needs and the composition of your team will shift over time. Think of yourself as the bridge to all of the other team members.

The Parent as the General Manager

You are your child's best advocate. You are with him or her more often than anyone else, your child trusts you, and you have a life investment in him or her. No one knows your child as well as you do.

This is not a simple job, nor one that parents are really prepared for. The resistance met; the time, energy, and organizational skills required; and the ongoing nature of the job can contribute to parents' burnout. With patience and fortitude you can do it and at a level at which you feel comfortable.

Gentle Reminders for Managing Your Child's Illness

- Understand your child's illness and treatment. Speak up for his or her needs.
- Write down and ask questions. Let the staff know how you and your child want to receive information (such as verbally, written, demonstration, and video) and what level of detail you feel comfortable with. Ask for clarification of anything you do not understand.
- Find out who is responsible for what so you can address the proper authority.
- Enlist a staff member (a nurse or a social worker) as your advocate, translator, and go-between.
- Collaborate with staff in a reciprocal relationship: Be understanding and respectful of each other.
- Recognize that staff is *not* all-knowing or all-powerful.
- Present a calm, informed, united front to staff.
- Be "information central" for the medical team, other staff, and the family at home.
- Help perform your child's medical care at home.
- Report truthfully about food, fluid, or medication intake and symptoms and effects.
- Be an early-warning system: How is your child doing?
- Bring up problems and concerns to staff immediately.
- Troubleshoot by making your child's allergies, idiosyncrasies, and preferences known to staff.
- Support and comfort your child.
- Monitor your child's emotions, and foster his or her coping skills.
- Buffer your child from pain, unnecessary intrusions, stress, and extraneous people.
- Provide ongoing education for your child about the disease and follow-up care.

Box continues next page

Continued

- Keep tracks of schedules and records.
- Manage financial and insurance issues.
- Research and pursue additional services.

The Health Team

Choosing a Hospital and Doctor

No hospital or doctor can guarantee the future, but you need to feel comfortable in your working relationship. For some is "only one game in town" offering the necessary expertise. For others, treatment starts in such a hurry there isn't time to look around. Others have more options. In any case, you may need to choose a new hospital or physician for further treatment; to deal with long-term effects; or in the event that you relocate, your child's doctor retires or moves, your insurance changes, or you are unsatisfied. If you need another specialist, your pediatrician or oncologist can refer you to one, or your insurance company may dictate your options. Seeking additional opinions is perfectly appropriate and actively encouraged by many parents and professionals.

> We had several options for where to do his BMT [bone marrow transplant]. The first thing the transplant doctor at one hospital told us was some scary statistics. Also, he wasn't warm to kids, and that facility recommended a longer isolation afterwards. We ultimately chose another hospital. Our oncologist had left our local cancer center to go there, and we'd had a good relationship with him. They had a shorter isolation period, and the BMT guy was incredible. It was closer to home. Our family could commute there to visit. Noah needed family and friends, and for us, it was the best choice.—*Andrea*

Rank these criteria for doctors and hospitals. Determine which are most important to you and choose accordingly.

- Cancer center or community hospital (expert opinion strongly recommends a facility with at least three trained pediatric oncologists and a staff dedicated to treating children)
- Teaching hospital (best teachers and doctors mixed in with students and residents)
- Proximity to home and family; travel time; accessibility to airports, trains, and parking

- Atmosphere (collaboration and attention); Child friendly
- Reputation and experience; what is the success rate in treating your child's particular cancer (some numbers can be slanted, depending on the criteria the facility uses to accept patients for a study)? How many cases of your child's particular cancer do they treat a year?
- Acceptable or reasonable treatment regimen (follows national protocols, agrees with other opinions, is aggressive or conservative, offers outpatient treatment)
- Clinical trials (new treatments); criteria for acceptance
- Availability of other pediatric medical specialists: pediatric oncology nurses, radiologists, cardiologists, neurologists, anesthesiologists, and orthopedists, for example
- Extent of psychosocial services: social workers, child life therapists, psychologists, neuropsychologists, and psychiatrists
- Acceptance of parents as partners and decision makers for the child's care
- Willingness to accommodate your career, cultural, dietary, or religious needs
- Peer companionship; support groups
- Insurance coverage; financial counseling
- Facilities for families; visitor policies and amenities
- Accreditation (official sanction based on meeting specific standards) by a national hospital, physician, or cancer organizations
- Competent, helpful support staff
- Pain management policies.

A positive doctor–patient relationship

Parents and patients value a doctor who will talk to them and answer their questions patiently and honestly. Compassion, respect, good communication skills, thoroughness, approachability, availability, and a good rapport with the child and the parents are all high on a wish list of physicians' qualifications. A physician who is open to collaboration with colleagues and is creative in finding solutions to fit an individual is the cream of the crop.

> Those doctors who are true experts are absolutely delighted to be able to share their research interests and the diverse considerations that go into treatment planning. As a general rule of thumb, a good doctor will have a positive reaction to a request for more explanations.
> —*Rona*

* * *

> I look upon the relationship with the family as a partnership. There are some things, like treatment schedules and chemo doses, that are fairly inflexible. But there are a lot of other things that are flexible. No matter what you're dealing with, you have to make the treatment

> work for the family. What I've tended to do is let the family know what I'm thinking, and make a recommendation, and to solicit what the family thinks and then make the decision together, instead of just me making all the decisions. That way it really is a partnership. I think that's the core to a good relationship between family and doctor.—*Richard Womer, MD*

Many parents and patients feel a deep respect and gratitude toward their doctor. It is a wonderful bonus when a relationship with a physician goes smoothly and positively.

> If you're a warm, friendly, giving person who obviously cares about the child, you win. If you're someone who can examine a child without having to grab, if you have the sense and the nuance to look at a child and figure out what's a good moment, or a good question, asking the child's permission, as in, "I need to push on your tummy right now, let me know if that hurts," that sort of thing. Our best resident was wonderful at these things. After treatment was over, I opened up the newspaper and saw her name. She'd been hired by the clinic as a pediatrician. I picked up the phone and asked if she was taking new patients. So she's now our pediatrician. She is incredible.—*Liz*

* * *

> I found a friend in my doctor. The best man alive. I have a relationship with him that is very unique. I trust him and feel comfortable talking to him about things other than health-related issues. I go to him for advice and sometimes just to talk. He is a great person and has definitely made a difference in my life.—*Francine, a long-term survivor*

Be careful, however, of drifting into hero worship. Doctors are human beings, with faults, limitations, personal and job-related stresses, personality quirks, prejudices, and defense mechanisms, just like you. Respect is appropriate for their knowledge, training, and experience. Reverence demands more than any doctor can possibly give you. Putting a physician on a pedestal makes for uneven dialogue, too. For the sake of your child's health, you must not be hesitant to ask questions, request explanations, demand pain medication, call in the middle of the night, or report problems because you think you might be bothering the doctor, wasting his or her time, or insulting his or her expertise. The doctor is the center of your team but can't pitch a no-hitter without input from you.

Working With Nurses

Nurses are a pivotal part of the medical team. Nurses do the bulk of in-patient care, assess a family's educational level and style, teach medical information and skills to patients and parents, help prepare for and perform procedures, assess pain, pass on "tricks of the trade" to parents, do emotional "pulse-taking," act as liaisons between physicians and families, and advocate for their patients.

> Learn the names and faces of the doctors and nurses, and call them by name. Help your child learn the names, also. We had a mom who sometimes asked for outrageous things, but when she would call out, "Hey, there's Miss Susan, how are you, can you help us? Look T., it's Miss Susan." I'd just melt and do whatever she needed.—*Susan Zappa, a pediatric oncology nurse*

The wealth of hands-on knowledge of an experienced oncology nurse is immeasurably helpful. The nurse is usually the first one you approach when you need something or have a problem. Advanced practice nurses, such as clinical nurse specialists or pediatric nurse practitioners, can diagnose and treat acute minor illness and stable chronic illness. Rather than focusing solely on disease, they also treat the patient's response to the illness and assess and address family situations as well. Of course, as with doctors, some nurses will function better than others, and not all of them will fit your or your child's style. You can approach the hospital floor manager if you have a personality clash or significant complaint. Some parents reported relief in relying on nursing staff to temporarily take over jobs like central line care, tube placement and feedings, and shots while the child was in the hospital. Numerous parents we spoke with suggested requesting a primary nurse, one who will oversee and take care of your child consistently throughout treatment, in the interests of continuity.

> There is little that can be done about IV alarms going off during the night and nurses entering your room to change meds. As a mother, I appreciate nurses who make an effort to move quietly and carry a flashlight. I worship nurses who make note of when the IV will need changing and get there before the alarm rings.—*Sonal*

Interacting With Related Staff

During an average short-term hospital stay, your family can interact with up to 50 or 60 hospital staff members. Over the course of cancer treatment, that number grows exponentially. All those interactions contribute to the flavor of the experience. The same relationship principles outlined previously apply as additional members join your team.

The crucial roles of the pain management team members; nutritionists; physical, occupational, and speech therapists; and other service providers are touched on where appropriate throughout the book. Many hospitals also provide financial consultants, legal advocates, family relations staff, clergy, home care consultants, tutors, and volunteers to support families' other needs. With a long-term illness, you also come to know admissions or billing clerks, receptionists, phlebotomists, lab or radiology technicians, food service staff, and housekeepers. Information exchange, patience, courtesy, and an understanding of their assigned functions and limitations are the keys to constructive interactions. Getting to know them and letting them get to know you can not only smooth your way but also can lead to positive exchanges.

My daughter wants to be a phlebotomist (blood-taker) when she grows up, like her favorite person at the hospital, Pat. She gives Pat a big hug and talks and smiles through the blood draw. She says Pat does it the best and gives her extra stickers and prizes. She cries when anyone else does it.—*Charlean*

* * *

All the kids on the floor loved Abraham, the guy who came to clean the floors. He told jokes, listened to them, talked about movies or Nintendo or whatever, and remembered little things they liked or said. They could tell he cared. Another mom told me if you were nice to the cleaning staff they might do a better job, but I think it was more important that he was a friend who made them happy.—*Winnie*

Communicating With Staff

> One man's simple is another man's "huh"? David Stone, *Omni Magazine* (May 1979)

The communication and relationship strategies introduced in chapter 5 are useful for fostering relationships with your medical team. Still, there are some special considerations in communicating with staff. Medical personnel have a language all their own—a melding of verbal shorthand, abbreviations, and Latin that can zoom right over a parent's head.

At first, you may be intimidated and embarrassed to ask questions or for something to be repeated. Without medical training and experience, you cannot be expected to know and understand everything. The average person takes in only a fraction of what he or she hears, even in a normal conversation. When that conversation is distressing and complex, even less of it gets through. That's why it is a good idea to have at least one other adult present in consultations with the doctors, so that another pair of ears might hear and remember what you missed. It is also helpful to take notes or tape record consultations (with permission); ask for clarification; and ask more than one person to get multiple opinions, angles, and confirmation. Request copies of printed information, blood counts, surgical notes, and progress reports to study at home. As you get more comfortable with the medical atmosphere and accustomed to the language and routine, you will feel more able to assert yourself.

Talking with staff can be a bit like talking to a person from another culture. Although you speak a similar language, not everything translates precisely the same. Both staff and family attribute motives, rationalizations, and reasonings from their own perspective to the other. Before you jump to conclusions about what a person is telling you, ask for clarification. Avoid assumptions on the part of staff by clarifying what you're saying or asking and why. In these relations diplomacy is a great asset. Putting staff on the defensive stops communication cold. If you are informed, calm, rational, but firm, you come across as an equal, deserving of respect, attention, and answers. You are more likely to get what you need. Some parents swear by the old adage, "You catch more flies with honey than you do with vinegar." On the other hand, politeness is not the same as submission. Those same parents also live by another truism, "The squeaky wheel gets the grease." Don't be afraid to stand up for yourself and your child.

> The bottom line is that you have to watch out for your kid's well-being. I said to our doctors on many occasions, "You have hundreds of patients to care for, but I only have one." They seemed to understand me when I said that.—*Roger*

* * *

> During the first few months of treatment, every trip to the emergency room included a medical student asking questions, starting with, "When did you first notice something was wrong?" Finally I realized they were just practicing taking histories, and I stopped cooperating. I felt I had already done my share to educate the future pediatricians of America. —*Ginny*

* * *

> When Scott had a porta-cath put in, they told him he could have EMLA cream, so it wouldn't hurt when he got stuck. One night, they weren't going to use the cream, because it takes an hour to take effect and somebody wanted to go home. I insisted they use it, because they had promised him; I didn't care if somebody had to stay late. And that's what they did. But you've got to speak up, or they'll just do what's convenient for them.—*Maggie*

Health care professionals are taught to remain at an appropriate distance. They try to remain emotionally neutral and to have a relationship with you that is "therapeutic." This may seem insensitive or cold, but they are not able to do their jobs and make the best decisions if they get too emotionally involved with patients and family members. This is their own human coping mechanism for a job that is emotionally stressful. Remember that staff members also have private lives that affect their moods. A staff member who is distracted, frowning, or seems sad may not be indicating bad news for your child but maybe had an argument with a spouse or has a kid at home with the flu.

Doctors and nurses are not robots and will gravitate naturally to the patients and parents they like. These professionals also struggle with their own negative reactions.

> There was a mother who was really witchy, and no one wanted to take care of her. I spent some time with her and realized we staff don't always know what the parents give up. She said, "I lost my job; I lost my mortgage; I can't move and get a house. I worked eight years as an accountant to get a comfortable place to live, have a healthy child, and all of that has been taken from me." I've been an oncology nurse for nine years, and we really do become immune. What kind of nurse would I be if I cried every day because your child was sick? But I really got to look at things in a whole new light talking to that woman.—*Dottie, a nurse*

Many parents believed that staff made assumptions about them, what they were capable of and how much they needed to know. A few parents felt that they were discriminated against, because they had less education or fewer economic resources, because they were working parents, or because of race or class distinctions. One mother did all she could to combat these kinds of power differences:

> As a parent, you don't feel like you're on equal footing. I made an effort to pack my best dresses and slacks for hospital stays. I never wore sweats or jeans, because it was obvious that you were gauged on how intelligent and together you seemed. There were mornings I didn't really feel like combing my hair, or putting on makeup. But I did it. You didn't know who was going to come in the door next. I learned to throw around the vocabulary, too. Knowing enough, being comfortable enough in that environment, asking the right questions, to be taken seriously. You have to show how rational and calm you are.—*Krista*

Overall, parents tend to develop good working relationships with most medical and nursing staff. They appreciate the efforts made on their children's behalf. Try to express appreciation for a job well done or for that staff member who goes out of the way to make your child's experience easier. Say thank you, share a hug, or give a pat on the back. If you have time and energy, send a card, write a letter to the supervisor, or nominate them for a staff award.

Unfortunately, almost all parents also reported instances of one or more distressing conflicts or breakdowns in communication. This is not surprising, because the stakes are high, and both parents and staff are under pressure.

> I was a bit miffed at the oncologist, feeling that because Zachary was off treatment, he wasn't important anymore, and I was uninformed and left out of his plan of care. I wrote a letter about my feelings and took it in with me to Zachary's appointment. This 15-minute appointment turned into 2 hours. The oncologist did a wonderful job of reassuring me and letting me help with a long-term care plan. Express your concerns to the doctors. Try to back up your concerns with examples.—*Iris*

If a conflict arises with hospital staff that cannot be worked out individually, you can turn to the department head, family relations staff, family liaison, ombudsman, legal or ethics staff, or hospital administrator for help in resolving an issue. Put your complaints in writing. Succinctly state the problem, what you want done about it, and what you are willing to do to help provide a solution. Try to focus on one problem at a time. Keep a copy for your own records.

> When he had a central venous access line put in, the recovery room nurses didn't know how to flush a pediatric catheter. Plus, they didn't have needles small enough. Afterwards I was flipping out, and they sent a rep from the hospital to meet with me. I said, since you do have the pediatric oncology center here, all the staff should be trained in flushing catheters,

and the proper-sized needles should be available. If a nurse doesn't know how to do that, someone from pediatrics should be called down instead of making the child suffer. They implemented my suggestions.—*Tracy*

Mistakes happen that range from inconvenient to life-threatening. When mistakes happen, you will naturally get upset. It's okay to let people see that you are hurting; it's okay to have expectations of them. However, the most useful course is to find a constructive way to channel your anger. Consider what is the effect or damage? What can be done about it? Where is your energy best applied? Present a calm, collected front to the proper authorities, if necessary, and put it in writing. Unfortunately, the child is usually the one who has to suffer the consequences. What parents want most is an acknowledgment, an apology, the least intrusive remedy as compensation (being placed first on a surgical schedule, for example), and measures taken to avoid similar occurrences. These are all reasonable expectations.

Choosing Psychological Help

> The purpose of psychology is to give us a completely different idea of the things we know best. Paul Valery, *Tel Quel* (1943)

Many families are reluctant to ask for emotional help, thinking it means they are weak or mentally ill. Having a child with cancer does not make you mentally ill, and we are not suggesting that cancer families need psychotherapy. As any other cancer parent will tell you, you are a normal person in an abnormal situation. Psychological skills and strategies are simply another important element of the arsenal available to you in fighting childhood cancer. If you feel stable, comforted, and supported, you can deal with whatever happens and take better care of your child. And if your child is coping well, you will not feel so crazed. Psychology's techniques are as effective for the mind as medical techniques are for the body.

Psychology's function is not as well known as oncology's or nursing's, for example. Since this is our focus and area of expertise, we will explain it a bit. Psychology provides a sound basis for understanding how and why people behave, think, feel, react, and relate to others. Anyone can improve coping abilities with the use of key strategies.

Psychological techniques can help you to

- Make decisions
- Reduce symptoms such as pain, anticipatory nausea, and panic attacks
- Manage stress
- Recognize and address fears, anxiety, and depression
- Channel, express, and handle emotions

- Improve crucial relationship skills
- Build support networks
- Improve self-esteem and self-image
- Create buffer zones to maintain physical and mental equilibrium
- Acquire information or decrease information overload
- Identify personality or temperament style and use strengths of family members
- Adapt to altered circumstances such as changed roles and limitations
- Increase motivation for adhering to a difficult or long regimen
- Enhance ability to soothe and be soothed
- Set, maintain, and reassess priorities, limits, and boundaries
- Solve problems and ease roadblocks to progress
- Find personal meaning in the cancer experiences
- Ask for treatment for troubled family members.

Psychological counseling and therapies involve a partnership between a person, couple, or family and the professional. The purpose is to explore and understand the difficulty and then to integrate changes that will relieve or lessen the difficulty. Sometimes that means adding new understanding, ideas, behaviors, and scripts to your daily living patterns; sometimes it means working to overcome thoughts, feelings, and behaviors that are working against your best interests.

> My older son, Mark [not the one with cancer], has had a lot of problems sleeping, but he can't articulate why. We took him to a psychotherapist. She asked us each to draw a picture of what we could change if we could. Mark drew himself and Sam, saying, "I wish I wasn't fighting with my brother." My husband drew a picture of the family at the dinner table, saying he wishes he could be home more. And I drew a picture of a kid in bed with the universal sign through it, saying no more illness. Mark was focusing on his relationship with his brother. Jim was drawing the whole family. I was focusing on Sam. [Mark and the therapist] played all sorts of games where he would express feelings, tell stories. Mark really liked it. He asked to go back again. He felt this was for him alone.—*Barbara*

You have a choice from among professionals trained in different fields. All of these fields have practitioners who offer clinical expertise and therapeutic tips that can be helpful to you. The service offered might be called counseling, psychotherapy, or just plain therapy, but often it is not called anything. It may be introduced as just another "consult" or meeting. In some cancer centers the consult is routinely integrated into cancer care. In other settings, it may not be mentioned unless you ask. Examples of psychological service fields are social work, psychiatry, and psychology. The basic distinctions and overlaps are

- *Social workers* address the social and psychological needs of individuals and families by providing access to information and financial and supportive resources within the hospital and community and by counseling to improve coping. For the most part, social workers are master's-level (MSW) professionals, although some have doctoral (DSW) or bachelor's degrees (BA or BS).

- *Psychiatrists* are physicians (MD) and thus are able to prescribe and monitor medications for problems such as depression or serious mental illnesses. Some limit their practices to psychopharmacology (drugs), but many also offer nondrug psychotherapy or a combination of medication and psychotherapy.
- *Psychologists* are doctoral level (PhD, PsyD, or EdD) professionals who assess and treat people with emotional and behavioral concerns. They teach new patterns for relating to others and solving problems and new patterns for your own and your family's understanding and adaptation. Some specialize in health, cancer, and medical issues. Some practicing psychologists are also researchers. Neuropsychologists specialize in recognizing and evaluating cognitive delays or learning disabilities and developing practical recommendations to help your child learn and reach his or her potential.

The social worker is likely to be the first of these professionals you have access to. At most hospitals, your family would be assigned to one who will remain part of your team. As with doctors and nurses, you may or may not get a good match. Some parents complained that they rarely saw their social worker or that the person "only tried to cheer me up." Other parents reported long-lasting, fruitful relationships with a social worker who was attuned to their needs and could be counted on. A competent, caring social worker can serve as a sounding board or a shoulder to cry on, a finder and coordinator of local resources, a problem solver, and a counselor. One social worker describes his job,

> A social worker addresses the family's concrete needs. I assess psychological, social, emotional, and financial needs, but also let a family know that there is help with regard to all those areas. I then help them access those resources. Talking to them, I encourage management of their inner and outer resources—because all people have those.—*David Beele, ACSW, LCSW*

You may need more in-depth help. There are a number of ways to find qualified, reputable professionals.

- Ask your medical team for a consultation with a psychologist or a psychiatrist within your clinic or hospital center.
- Contact community-based counseling agencies, cancer organizations, and local or state psychological associations (which often offer referrals by specialty, such as health, cancer, children, or family, as well as by geographic location).
- Call the American Psychological Association (APA) at 1-800-964-2000 for information on how to reach your state's psychology organization for referrals in your region. Additional helpful information can be found on the APA Web site,

www.apa.org. Contact information for other related professional organizations are found in the Resources at the end of this book.

- Other sources for referral recommendations include your child's school counselors, other cancer parents, trusted friends, and colleagues.

There are three important requirements in finding a professional:

- *Find a professional who is appropriately licensed (a social worker, psychiatrist, or psychologist).* Licensing guarantees that the person has met the standards of education, training, and supervision for his or her field. Call the state licensing board for the particular field.
- *Find a professional who can readily understand your circumstances.* He or she does not need to know the specific details of the medical treatment protocols but does need to know what you are facing, the implications, and the strategies for dealing with the circumstances effectively. For example, you might want someone to help you with anxiety, your child with pain relief or school adjustment, you and your partner with marital problems, or the entire family with adaptation to the strains of cancer.
- *Find a professional who is helpful from the outset.* Although there are differences among professionals' backgrounds and "theoretical" orientations, more important is your innate sense of whether you and the professional have a good fit. Most experienced clinicians are able to choose what is most applicable to you from among the strengths of the different orientations. Ethical therapists will tell you if your needs are outside of their capabilities and refer you to someone else.

I have members of my family who think a therapist is a cop-out, but I'll tell you what I've found. A third party, who isn't involved in your situation or related to you, can be a very objective listener. It doesn't matter what others think when you're in the room with this person. Therapists won't judge you. They help to sort through thoughts. Now, a therapist does have a personality, so if you go to one and don't feel like you're talking to someone on your side, don't feel bad about finding another. Another thing is they can also recognize when medication might be necessary.—*Perri*

A relatively new but growing field is that of child life. Child life specialists are usually bachelor's-level staff who are trained in child development theory. Through age-appropriate education, play, and recreation, they help children cope with their fears and anxieties about medical treatment. Child life techniques can minimize a child's stress, distress, and anxiety, as well as the potential for psychological trauma, by preparing the child for and supporting the child during painful procedures and medical routines. They also help the child maintain normal development and living. For more information on play therapy and a child life specialist's role, see chapter 3 and the special avenues for coping.

The Home Team

Medical Back-Up

Families seldom see much of their pediatrician while the child is on treatment, but it is helpful to maintain a relationship. Eventually, if all goes as planned, you will transfer your child's care back to this person. Have copies of your child's paperwork and progress reports sent to the pediatrician, so he or she is well informed and able to predict and address future needs. For example, pediatricians are knowledgeable about childhood development and may be able to pinpoint losses or delays. Several families reported that the pediatrician was more familiar with normal childhood illnesses and better able to spot and treat them. If you are in a managed care insurance plan, your pediatrician must give you referrals for treatment and follow-up care, so a good relationship is vital. If your primary physician gives you a hard time about referrals for tests or specialists you know are necessary, get another opinion, change doctors, ask your child's oncologist to explain and justify it, or appeal to the insurance company for help.

Other valuable assets to your home team include the pharmacist, home health care supply company, visiting nurses, and hospice care (in some states, hospice is not just for terminal cases, but can also provide much-needed breaks for caregivers). Usually, once you have established a good working relationship, you can rely on the person to go the extra step to give you what you need.

Community Resources

Help can come from formal or informal groups: neighbors; places of worship; firefighter or police associations; and philanthropic organizations such as the Elks, Kiwanis, Knights of Columbus, Lion's, or women's clubs. These groups take on tasks such as raising funds, conducting blood drives, or coordinating meals and transportation. One family we know received help from the local motorcycle riders' club, several have sent letters or articles seeking help to local newspapers, and another received regular blood donations from coworkers. There are also local, state, and national organizations that offer legal or financial assistance, information, services, and support (see the Resources at the end of this book).

Insurance Companies and Financial Issues

Medical insurance coverage is an important issue for families. Dealing with the insurance system is very stressful. The biggest concern most parents have is that the hospital will refuse to treat their child if they are in arrears. That is extremely unlikely. Out of necessity, your insurance coverage may color decisions about your child's treatment, but it should not be the only factor in choosing treatment options, unless you truly have no other alternatives. Before you conclude that you have no choices and are powerless to affect the system, educate yourself. Regulations and benefits vary from state to state, so check with local resources for specifics. Get information from your state insurance commission office, the U.S. Department of Labor, the Institute for Health Care Research and Policy at Georgetown University, legal advocates (Childhood Cancer Ombudsman Program or the local Bar Association, law school, or attorney general's office), accountants or credit counselors, the state's department of social services, hospital finance staff, or cancer support organizations. Other good sources of information are the Association of Cancer Online Resources Web site and Nancy Keene's books about childhood cancer (see the Resources at the end of this book).

Follow these hard-won parents' tips to increase your effectiveness and decrease your anxieties about reimbursement.

Gentle Reminders for Financial and Insurance Issues

- *Know your coverage.* Talk to your employer's benefits manager or human resources person; read the master policy. There are lots of "ifs, ands, or buts" in the small print. Be aware of the type of policy, covered services, deductibles, copayments, out-of-pocket expenses, and lifetime limits. Some plans will not pay for you to go out of state for treatment. Even if a professional or treatment center is on a preferred providers list, he or she may have dropped the plan or stopped accepting new patients on that plan. Teenagers' insurance coverage under a parent's policy may end at a certain age or if they are not enrolled as full-time students.
- *Get organized.* Create and maintain an orderly filing system. File claims by date of service, along with any explanations of benefits or denials of coverage. Make copies of everything. Keep a log of services, procedures, and hospital stays. If you have to fill out forms, write in basic information (such as name, address, ID numbers, employer) once and make copies. Record all associated costs (keep receipts) not covered by insurance, as they may be paid by a charitable organization or be tax-deductible.
- *Deal with your insurance company wisely.* Pay premiums on time. Request a case manager. Correspond in writing, via the postal service, return receipt requested. Document telephone conversations: the date, the name of the person you spoke with, and what was said. If certain claims are outsourced to another company, regularly check to see that the bills have been forwarded and received. Most

Box continues next page

Continued

billing is done electronically, including generating statements and forwarding to collection agencies: Do not take mistakes, messages, or threats personally. Mistakes are made all of the time. Go over everything with a fine-toothed comb to make sure you are not being charged more than your deductible or copays, for a previously paid bill, or for more than the discount fee your insurance company may have contracted for. If a claim is rejected, do not give up; make a formal appeal. Request that the insurer work out a contract with the out-of-network hospital, get your doctor to talk to the medical director, write a letter of medical necessity, or resubmit a claim with a different code that applies to the same service. Ask your company's benefits manager for help. If necessary, contact your U.S. senators and representative, "cc" all correspondence to your state insurance commissioner, threaten to go to the press, and get a lawyer. Call the local bar association or state insurance commission for a referral to an attorney with insurance litigation experience or a claims assistance professional.

- *If your insurance company's "reasonable and customary" fees are significantly lower than your providers', contact several other providers in the area and request a written fee list (with service codes) to send to your insurance company.* The insurance company's aim is to lower its "losses" (paying medical bills), and it will take diligence to get what you deserve. If you pay for something you are not responsible for or that you dispute, be aware you will probably never get reimbursed.
- *If you must pay, work out a payment plan or request that the provider "accept assignment" (take whatever the insurance company is willing to pay).* Either way, you must formally address (in writing) the person with the power to authorize it and get a written agreement. Keep copies of checks you send, as well as the cancelled checks. As long as you are sending the provider something regularly (however small), you are fulfilling your obligation. Do not panic if your bills are forwarded to a collection agency. Respond in writing: Detail the status of the bill, your contacts, and relevant information. If you do agree to pay part of a bill, pay directly to the hospital, indicating exactly which bill (date and service) you are paying. The collection agency is simply pursuing a lump sum and won't credit your payment accurately.
- *Seek out sources of financial assistance.* Talk to your social worker, state or county social services agency, public welfare department, or child or family services departments about applications for state insurance programs, medical services or catastrophic illness funds, Supplemental Security Income (through your local So-

Box continues next page

Continued

cial Security Administration office), or Medicaid (ask about a "Katie Beckett" waiver, which may allow you to get around income qualifications). Some hospitals have assistance funds. City, county, or state government agencies offer temporary aid to families who are needy due to adverse circumstances. Housing authorities may have emergency funds that will cover you for a month or two of rent. Utility companies and credit card companies, if notified early and in writing, may offer a reduced rate or a temporary reprieve; Consumer Credit Counseling Service is a free service that can intercede for you. Pharmaceutical companies have assistance programs to supply medications free of charge, but your doctor must apply for you. Many local and national cancer organizations offer financial assistance to families See the Resources at the end of this book for information on many of these programs.

- *Choose a new policy carefully.* It may be anxiety-provoking to change jobs because of the insurance issues. Study your options very carefully. Big companies with group policies are best, because they do not require medical exams or reject you or charge more for high-risk status. Individual plans and state high-risk pools are viable options but are expensive and limited. Federal laws like HIPAA (Health Insurance Portability and Accountability Act, which allows workers to change jobs and still get medical coverage, may eliminate waiting periods for coverage of pre-existing conditions and prevent you from having higher premiums than others within a group plan), COBRA (Comprehensive Omnibus Budget Reconciliation Act, which is an up to 18-month extension of your current benefits, with the premiums paid by you, but is applicable only if your new job does not offer you any coverage at all), and ERISA (Employee Retirement and Income Security Act, which keeps workers from being fired because of a child's medical history) help protect you from discrimination but *do not* guarantee good coverage. Do not assume anything; check with your state insurance commissioner for laws in your area *before* you make a change. Those of you who are self-employed who have at least two employees in the business may be able to apply for a group policy, or your local chamber of commerce may underwrite your company as a group. Your family may also be eligible for group insurance through alumni organizations, unions, and community or professional associations.

Emotional money issues

Cancer treatment is expensive, and not everything is covered by insurance. If parents need to resign or scale back their jobs, income is reduced. As the bills pile up, pressure mounts.

Parents may feel inadequate, ashamed, or frustrated if they cannot pay their bills and fearful that they will lose their house or other assets. Money is an issue that may be associated with personal and family conflict, even without a catastrophic illness. When necessity overrides pride, borrowing from family or taking out a second mortgage on your home may be wise or necessary. If that is the case, consider the impact on you and your relationships. Each person has a history and set of personal feelings about money matters. Will you be embarrassed or resentful if you owe money to a relative, or will you be relieved by the reprieve? Are monetary gifts or loans a source of jealousy in your family? Will you be able to pay a loan back? Fundraisers and charitable organizations, while more public, have fewer "strings" attached. Most parents we spoke with reported some guilt in accepting donations but knew they could not do it on their own and were grateful for the help—whether it was $8 from a girl scout troop, $50 a week from parents for housecleaning, or thousands from a community fundraiser toward hospital bills.

> Our social worker got an organization to buy us a few cases of PediaSure—they sent the money right to our pharmacy. I felt bad at first, because there must have been other families who were worse off than we were. But that saved me about $100 cash that I didn't have. —*Alice*

Your Child's School

When school staff is part of your team, everyone benefits. Teachers, school nurses, child study teams, guidance counselors, and administrators can be valuable allies both during and after treatment for cancer children and their siblings, too. One mother told us that the head of her son's nursery school arranged play dates and baby-sitting for him (the sibling). Many wonderful educators go out of their way to help keep a child involved when missing so much school time, to coordinate with hospital tutors on what the child is doing, and to educate classmates and maintain their contact with the student.

One stellar team consisting of teacher, nurse, and guidance counselor educated themselves and their students in preparation for a little girl with a brain tumor to come back to school. In a special meeting with the class, they encouraged discussion and questions, emphasizing that "she was still someone who could write and draw and could laugh." The team kept in touch with the family for progress reports, visited the child's home, coordinated with the hospital tutor, organized fundraisers, and sent cards and a video of a holiday play from classmates. The teacher said, "By the time she got here, I worked with her like I do anyone else, but gave her a lot of extra time. She left reading and writing, and I feel good about that." Children took turns staying in with her at lunch and recess, which was fun for them, as well as for the sick child. When the child died suddenly, the team called classmates' parents so they could prepare their children. Another discussion was held with the class and that of her older sister. For an hour and a half, as a rose sat on the child's desk, the class read a book about death, and the children expressed their memories verbally and through artwork, which was then bound and given to the child's parents. The guidance counselor completed a workbook with the sister, telling us, "That helped her, it gave a little structure, other than just 'tell me how you feel'." For the rest of the school year the girl's picture remained on her desk. At the end of the year, the class planted a tree by the playground and made a birdhouse in a memorial service.

Other parents describe their positive experiences:

> Sean's teacher had an old orange suitcase that she filled with papers and projects, whatever they were working on. If he felt up to it, he could do it in the classroom, or his brother would bring it home. We had a good hospital school, too: lots of personalized attention. That was a lot of fun. A couple of his buddies were also kindergartners, and they would sit around cutting and pasting and chatting and doing stuff out of this suitcase. He always felt like he was part of things.—*Bridget*

* * *

> A nurse from our hospital went to Mia's school both in first and second grade, while she was on treatment, to explain things. She made a big point that it is different from adult cancer, because so many kids may have known a grandparent who died, for example. Mia chose not to be there for the presentations. She felt more comfortable that way—everybody would know what was what without her having to answer questions or be stared at. —*Natalie*

Many parents and patients strive and succeed in keeping up with the child's school work; there are children on treatment who make the honor roll. This can be an effective way to cope, particularly for older children. Others forego school work, opting to avoid the extra stress and demands on the child's time and energy. Gauge your child's capacity.

> At first, we had a tutor at home for Anne. I was in a panic about her getting behind, but Anne found the tutor to be an invasion of her space. She said, "Mom I want the teacher to send the work home, and you and I will do it." So that's what we did. One of her teachers had a good point: "If we're doing five subtraction worksheets and she does fine on the first one, why should she do the rest? She was right, that's just extra pressure. I wanted Anne to be as normal as could be, but I guess that put some pressure on her.—*Pam*

Not everyone has a good experience. School nurses and teachers may be afraid they do not have the expertise to handle emergencies or worry about infection control. They have their own fears and misconceptions about cancer. Some school staff members will not bend rules or give extra help or may balk at the costs or inconveniences of your child's special needs.

Thanks to the Individuals with Disabilities Education Act (IDEA), children ages 2–21 have the legal right to an appropriate education, including special services tailored to meet unique needs. The school district must evaluate your child, design an individual education program (IEP), and include you in the decision making.

Formulating an individual education plan

Request an IEP *in writing* to the school's principal or the district special education coordinator. Having had cancer, your child is eligible as "other health impaired" but may also be eligible under other classifications. You will have a meeting with the school's Child Study Team, usually consisting of your child's teacher, a special education teacher, a case manager, an administrator, the school psychologist, a basic skills instructor, and possibly others who provide services such as speech or physical therapy. You may want to invite the child's tutor, psychologist, an education advocate or lawyer, or an education specialist from the hospital.

Initially, your child will be evaluated, and after that, update meetings should be held at least once a year. You need to supply letters, documents, and evaluations from all your child's doctors detailing medical history and deficits and be able to describe your child's difficulties. Your child will be observed in class and tested one-on-one to see if he or she is working at grade level. You may request other relevant evaluations for learning disabilities, gross and fine motor skills delays, speech and language problems, and hearing and vision deficits. You may prefer to have specific evaluations privately done (get a referral from your doctor); not all school districts will have these specific professionals available, nor are their experts always versed in the issues of cancer survivors.

The IEP states your child's present level of performance; effects on school performance; short-term objectives; annual goals; and any specific accommodations or services your child needs such as assistive technology, modifications for tests, alternative assignments, extra help or time to do tasks or grasp concepts, special seating arrangements, home instruction, small classes, extended school year services, aides, special transportation, adaptive gym, speech therapy, and physical or occupational therapy.

Deficits are often difficult to discern. If the child excels in some subjects or is not lagging behind significantly enough or if the deficits are not considered to affect school performance, the school district may decide that the child should not receive special services. If you do not agree with the school's results, notify the district in writing within 30 days and request an independent evaluation or have tests done privately. If the district is unable to accommodate your child, they can suggest an out-of-district program, or you can suggest placement in a private program (if you can prove that it can serve your child appropriately and your district can't). Mediation and due process hearings are formal ways to clear up disagreements.

An individualized transition program (ITP) serves high school students moving toward graduation, trade school, or college. It addresses graduation requirements, career or vocation plans, special instruction, and services available after graduation. Early intervention programs serve children under the age of three and can include physical, occupational, and speech therapy, as well as socialization skills. Contact your state department of education for written information on your parental rights and how to access any of these services.

The best you can do is know your rights, enlist help, be clear about your expectations, and push for what your child needs. This is not an easy or quick job. It can be a very frustrating, time-consuming, maddeningly slow, seemingly never-ending process. You may encounter resistance, subtle or direct. Ultimately, your child will be the beneficiary of your hard work.

Gentle Reminders for Working With Your Child's School

- Educate teachers, classmates, and other friends about your child's illness, anticipated effects, and changes in appearance and abilities. Use visuals: books, videos, and props from the hospital, library, or cancer organizations. Ask hospital staff to make the presentations if you are unable to do so.
- Distribute a letter to classmates and their families explaining your situation and requesting notification of chicken pox or other infectious diseases.
- Discuss issues such as attendance, participation in gym or recess, naps, snacks, and medications.
- Enlist the help of the school nurse; provide information, medical supplies, and strict instructions. Be respectful of district regulations and the nurse's limitations.
- Have a written emergency plan, and give copies to everybody.
- Share your attitude about homework.
- Take advantage of tutoring (at home, in the hospital). Coordinate with the school's curriculum.
- Send progress reports when your child is not in school.
- Contact local, county, and state government departments for information on special child health and education services.
- If you are so inclined, opt for home schooling, particularly for children who have difficulty in the standard school environment.

A comprehensive list of education resources for parents and teachers is given at the end of this book.

CHAPTER 3

Coping Successfully

Action is the antidote to despair.
—*Joan Baez,* Rolling Stone (1983)

They gave us a computer with Internet access during transplant. That was a lifesaver because you're stuck in a room; you can't go anywhere or do anything. There's only so much TV and reading you can do. I was constantly researching all kinds of stuff. Noah and I decided that he would pick a topic in the morning, like penguins, wildlife, Antarctica. The two of us would sit together and research facts. When my husband came in at night, he would get quizzed. It kept Noah's mind going and kept us both occupied.—*Libby*

Who should be the judge of whether someone is coping effectively or not? Most people say they cope well, which means they think they are doing as well as can be expected under the circumstances. They are keeping their heads above water. You know how well you are coping and how much you are floundering.

Some professionals see certain coping styles as negative because they are uncomfortable with them. For example, hospital staff might not like the intense, noisy, emotional release within a family's normal cultural background. Some staff might feel threatened by a parent who seems pushy and aggressive by asking many questions. Ethnic, religious, generational, or gender differences can lead to misinterpretations of coping styles, too, by family and friends, as well as by staff.

Do not assume that you are coping inadequately if you or your child becomes discouraged. Depression may occur around the time of diagnosis, relapse, or the end of life. At these times a pervasive sadness is expectable and understandable. They are times of re-evaluating possibilities and of making the transition to another phase of life. They are times of moving on to other ways of coping and understanding. Do remember, however, that depression can be treated effectively and lifted in most instances.

Do *not* feel pressured to change your basic personality style of coping. By the same token, don't pressure others to cope the way you do, either. Most of us have our preferred ways of thinking about tough situations and responding to them. Gathering medical information makes some people less anxious, others more so. Some people are naturally introverted, and some are naturally extroverted. Some people are more carefree naturally, and others are more prone to anxiety. Enduring personality styles are not likely to change, but every personality style can add new strategies to the mix. The only exceptions are people who were already fragile, rigid, fragmented, or brittle before the cancer struck. In those cases, extra support and psychological treatment are warranted.

Successful coping provides relief from both short- and long-term stress and leads to adjustment and adaptation. This chapter considers what has worked for others and gives suggestions about what you might like to use for your own situation. Make sure to read both the adult and child sections, because there are differences between the two. If you think you or another family member is having trouble coping, see chapter 8 for the "red flags" that signal a need for professional assistance.

"Once and Future" Effect on Coping

Previous life experiences can affect how you cope with the current crisis. If you have had a series of bad experiences, you may feel jinxed and stretched to your coping limit. Experiences with cancer in a parent or other close family member can particularly shade your reactions.

> A year before my son was diagnosed, I had lost my father to cancer. He had only fought it for one year. So my first thought was my son's going to die.—*Debra*

Before you had a sick child, you handled everyday stresses such as traffic, office politics, and the family's busy schedule and bigger ones such as money worries, divorce, the loss of a job, or caring for an ailing parent. Think about how you have handled stress in the past. What helped and what did not? You can use these experiences to gain perspective and apply that perspective now.

> There were some things Tommy didn't understand [about his brother's treatment] and things he was frightened of and jealous of. We talked to him more about his own birth, when we almost lost him. We talked to him about the weeks we spent in the hospital when he was little and what that was like. The needle pokes, and the different things . . . isn't this pulse oxygen machine cool; when you were a baby it was so sad they didn't have one and they had to poke you to find out about the oxygen. He would say "oh really!" It helped him relate a little and feel less left out.—*Liz*

* * *

Chuck's older brother Bobby was born with an intestinal problem and has had three surgeries to correct it. So we know all about having a sick kid. But cancer is different. It's not so fixable.—*Samantha*

* * *

Our first two children, twins, were born very prematurely. They died within 24 hours. We went through that whole emotional upheaval, where the world is no longer a safe place. Bad things happen, and you wonder if life will ever be good again, if you can ever be happy. Over the next five years, our two other daughters were born. We were pretty normal again. Then came the diagnosis of cancer in our youngest. At first, it felt unfair, like we'd already had our share of heartache. But I think we were able to mobilize ourselves quicker, because we weren't paralyzed. Okay, we already know life stinks, so what are we going to do to get through this?—*Leslie*

Hope is the ultimate optimism—and one thing a cancer family cannot live without. Hope enables you to endure the harshest treatment, overcome injuries to body and soul, and return to life. Even the smallest flicker of hope, the tiniest flame deep within you, can insulate you against the arctic winter of cancer. In the beginning, everyone hopes for a cure, for a healthy, whole child and a family returned to normal. Even those in our "club" who ostensibly achieve that goal acknowledge that the sense of "normal" is changed. So, most families begin to take it down a notch and hope for short-term, achievable goals: having good blood counts, receiving good test results, or avoiding a nasogastric tube. Later, we hope for a limit on disabilities, a smooth adjustment, continued remission, relief from pain, or a release from suffering.

Hope is fiercely guarded and should never be taken away from anyone. When you hit the inevitable setbacks or get overwhelmed, when things are not going as planned, or when people around you have negative attitudes, hope can take a beating. Without hope, you fall into despair and lose your way. You can fan the flame of hope by focusing on positive possibilities, surrounding yourself with positive people, reading hopeful stories, talking to survivors and their families, and turning to personal beliefs in spirituality or science or both.

Stresses and Resources

Your family, like every family, has its own perceptions of the impact of cancer, but there are some common triggers for crisis.

How are you, your child, and your family to handle it all, especially when the stresses seem overwhelming? One solution is to pare down and get rid of nonessential demands.

Stressors Faced by Parents and Children With Cancer

- Too little, too much information
- Decision making
- Confusing medical jargon
- Fear of the unknown
- Unfamiliar, distressing sights
- Emotional distress, anxiety, depresion, guilt
- Altered expectations
- Loss of normalcy
- Lack of privacy
- Lack of control
- Lack of independence
- Fear of losing child
- Pain and discomfort
- Performing home care
- Fears of death, mutilation
- Invasive procedures
- Disrupted sleep patterns
- Change in self-image, identity
- Starting, ending treatment
- Job, financial worries
- Reorganization of family roles
- Lack of support
- Misguided support attempts
- Marital strain
- Sibling needs
- Strained, lost relationships
- Boredom
- Unpredictability, unexpected events
- Waiting for scans, blood test results
- Isolation from family, friends
- Disruption of routines
- Extended family's upset
- Grief, sadness
- Spiritual distress
- Developmental, school delays
- Reverting to younger behavior
- Differences in coping styles
- Symptoms, side effects

Focus only on the most important or pressing coping tasks, and let go of or delegate the rest. The better you are able to manage, the stronger you and your child will be. In the box are some examples of stress that are typical in childhood cancer families.

When stresses pile up and coping is tough, mobilize your resources and draw strength from those assets you know you can count on. The resources might be tangibles, such as money, or intangibles, such as the strengths of different family and community members to contribute time, labor, problem-solving smarts, or connections. Think about the resources you possess, and take note of the tasks you're handling well, big or small. Do you have access to a major cancer treatment center? Are you good at research? Is your spouse willing to rearrange priorities? Does your family pull together in times of trouble? Can friends help care for the siblings and do your errands? Is there a nurse who lives next door who can help you with home care? Does your faith give you strength? Is your child resilient? Will someone do a fundraiser for you? Do you have good insurance coverage? Any of these positives can serve both as defense and offense, your protection and your weapons in the fight against cancer. You might surprise yourself by realizing tht you have more resources than you thought you did, besides recognizing where you need to ask for help. Being aware of what you're up against is half the battle.

Adults' Coping Strategies

No coping strategy is good or bad in and of itself. Common sense would tell you there are lots of ways to cope. In general, coping with cancer, or anything else, is a matter of both action and reaction.

> Don't get hung up on a snag in the stream, my dear. Snags alone are not so dangerous—it's the debris that clings to them that makes the trouble.
> Anne Shannon Monroe, *Singing in the Rain* (1926)

Action strategies focus on a concrete problem and are designed to change a situation. Here is what one mother did when she tired of answering questions from medical staff over and over again:

> I typed out a summary of my son's health and treatment. I included date of diagnosis, what meds he's had, when the last dose was, last echocardiogram, MRI, that sort of thing. It's been most helpful for admissions through the emergency room. The idea came to me after a 3 a.m. admission, when I really didn't have the patience to repeat myself and remain pleasant. If I'm feeling testy when I'm asked something they should know or could find in the chart, I'll say, "well, I'm sure it's in the chart, but I also have it right here." I update it about twice a month.—*Lucille*

Another mother tried to spare a son's distress in predictable emergencies:

> We tried to minimize the impact on Luke's brother Tommy. These stupid fevers would always show up on Saturday night, in the middle of the night. We learned halfway through, it didn't have to be an entire family ordeal with lights coming on and all four of us getting in the car. Tommy would cry. It's so hard to wake up and be frightened like that. I learned to pack a bag quietly, or even the night before. My husband would slip Luke and me into a taxi and off we would go to the ER. It was such a relief. You get to the point where even something this bizarre, you routinize it for your children. You give them some expectation so they're not totally freaked out.—*Liz*

Reaction strategies are used in situations that cannot be changed and focus on emotions. In those instances, you try to influence how you and your child perceive and deal with the stress internally. Examples are using self-talk to stay calm, distracting your child during a procedure, minimizing, distancing, and using positive imagery (these techniques are explained in chapter 6 on reducing stress).

A reaction strategy is not the same as a reaction. For example, your first reaction might be to panic. A reaction strategy is what you do deal with the panic and make it into something more constructive.

Maxie told us she was able to distance herself from her distress at her son's illness, releasing at other, "safer" times:

> I'm a very emotional person, but since Adam's illness, I can turn off the crying in the flip of a switch [when] I feel it welling. I always felt, for Adam and for the grandparents, too, I needed to be on an even keel, because if I was this emotional basket case up and down, they would be the same way. I needed to stay in control, emotionally. I've gotten very good at it. Am I burying it? Yes. Does it sometimes surface? Yes. Once, I passed nearby a bad accident, saw the skid marks, and I started to cry. I didn't even know the people.

Fred comforted himself and his teenage son by concentrating on the temporariness of treatment:

> Going through chemo wears on you mentally. I said, "Mike, I can sympathize with you, but I don't know how you feel. The one thing you can hang your hat on is you know you're getting better." It's working. It comforted me and his mother. I think he just put up with it. He just swallowed it. He took the attitude, "Let's get it over with, and I can get on with my life."

Maggie, a survivor herself, talked with her children about maintaining a positive outlook:

> Since we are both survivors, we talk about this stuff all the time. I tell him, "Look Scott, you know you always have to go for these checkups, and so do I, so it's just our lives." Today he was complaining, "I hate my life, I can't play sports, my pencil broke. . . ." I said, so let's think of some good things. He said "let's see"—this is out of his mouth—"I'm still alive." Yeah, you're still alive, and I'm still alive. And my daughter said, "We're all together"! Okay, I think we put this in perspective.—*Maggie, breast cancer survivor*

Tried-and-True Coping Strategies

Reliable ways to cope have been well identified over the past 25 years by families in circumstances like yours. They have all been strongly supported by psychological research, too. These coping strategies are used by children too, sometimes in different forms. As a basic rule, you want to buffer your child and your family from stress whenever possible and reduce stress when it cannot be warded off.

Communicating and expressing emotions

Communication and emotional expression are central to emotional well-being. Communicate your needs and expectations, and listen to those of others. As Bill Withers wrote in the song "Lean on Me," "No one can fill those of your needs that you won't let show." Very often, family members are afraid to talk about "It," the cancer. They may wish to protect each other from painful feelings or avoid being "negative." The conspiracy of silence is very isolating.

Each member of the family should be encouraged to express personal feelings without fear of being judged for them. Putting words to feelings demystifies them and helps you to process them. The sharing of feelings can bond a family together: Instead of each one suffering alone, you walk the difficult road side by side, helping each other when one of you stumbles. Getting fears and frustrations off your chest and out into the open strips them of some of their weight, making them press less heavily on your spirit. You will not transfer the burden to the shoulders of the listener, nor do they have to solve the problem for you —you just need a sounding board. Your sounding board can be a spouse or other family member, a friend, a member of the clergy, a social worker, or a counselor.

> A mistake I made was thinking that if I leaned on my husband, I would be sapping his energy, and he needed it himself. So I would lean on friends, without realizing that he's wondering why I'm cutting him out and why I'm going to them and not him, and he was strong enough to hear the things I needed to say, and I should have been talking to him. —*Margaret*

* * *

> My 4-year-old was having trouble. I couldn't get her to talk about anything. Then we showed her two videos about cancer. It was like a light went on. If it was okay for Mr. Rogers and Linus to talk about cancer, it was okay for her, too.—*Marta*

Using denial or distancing

Denial or distancing of bad news, at first glance, might seem to be a lack of coping, but it is a natural form of self-defense. It allows you to keep going rather than being stopped abruptly or paralyzed with anxiety. To protect themselves from a threat, all people are capable of denying the full extent of a reality or the worst possible outcome of a situation. This kind of distancing or denial allows you "breathing space," within your own mind, to absorb news little by little. Denial is adaptive to the extent that it allows you to live positively and with hope. It is a drain of your energy to focus on the possibility of a negative outcome day in and day out. Using denial and related ways of protecting yourself—partializing, minimizing, postponing, and just plain refusing to be daunted in the face of severe threat—is not a denial of the facts of a child's cancer. It is a form of relief.

> Rosiness is not a worse windowpane than gloomy gray when viewing the world.
> Grace Paley, *Enormous Changes at the Last Minute* (1960)

You do not have to practice denial or learn how to do it. It occurs spontaneously and automatically within you, when you need it. Be aware, however, that it can seem unsettling to you if you are not using denial about an issue but another family member is. For example, sometimes spouses argue, each blaming the other for having a false picture. Fortunately, it is usually a temporary situation. The only time that denial is not appropriate is when it interferes with responsible parenting for a sick child, in other words, when it interferes with positive coping. You and those close to you will know the difference.

Focusing on positive aspects

While no one goes through treatment "with a smile and a song," many families find positive changes can come about: bringing a family closer together, having better priorities in life, cementing old friendships and forging new ones, and—as the children usually point out—getting presents and meeting famous people. Focusing on the positive is the opposite of catastrophizing; saying to yourself, "I can handle this, I will not fall apart," is more effective than, "I can't bear this." Having a positive attitude will not cure cancer, but it will improve the quality of your life.

> We went to hell, but we met a lot of really nice people.—*Gwen*

* * *

> You still have to go on living: doing whatever you would have done if this had not happened; accepting the limitations of what this has brought, while continuing to do what you like. Don't let [treatment] get you down. That's the hardest piece of advice to follow. If you keep a good attitude that this will be over, this does have an end in sight, it's a whole lot easier to deal with on a daily basis.—*Gloria, long-term survivor*

* * *

> I found out that my job was going to be eliminated. Maybe a week later, I found out about Harry. The loss of a job is devastating, but it paled in comparison to what else was going on. He was my priority. I could always find work; I couldn't find another son. Since I was out of work, I was able to take him to all his treatments. God works in strange ways. —*Alan*

Managing information

Managing information is a valuable strategy. You may be a person who is comforted by gathering information, or you may be one who finds too much information distressing. You can choose how you want to regulate the flow.

Parent after parent describes information as power. Since they cannot control the cancer itself, many people find comfort in knowing about their child's illness and treatment, what to expect, and what to watch for. Information combats feelings of helplessness.

Some parents go to great lengths, searching out research protocols, studying medical text books, or contacting treatment centers or doctors all over the world. There have been instances of parents bringing to their oncologist's attention new information.

> When Anne was diagnosed, I felt a strong need to find the very best person for osteosarcoma . . . dig, dig, dig, until you find the person who has the experience your child needs.—*Pam*

For some parents, this represents a drive for vigilance, to do everything possible to cure the child. Information is part of their armory: Knowing the enemy helps to conquer it. Understanding that doctors and nurses are human and fallible, some parents take it upon themselves to know how to calculate every dose of chemotherapy and check for accuracy before anything is administered to their child. This is an active measure of control over a potential negative outcome. For others, knowledge can "level the field," making a parent feel on equal footing with the medical staff. Sometimes, a parent just feels an obligation to know what is happening to his or her child.

> I learned as much as I could, because I felt I should. If this is what's going to happen to my son, I want to know about it. But I can't say it made me feel any better. All we could do was take care of him and give him all the support we could.—*Alan*

Other families take comfort in trusting in the experts—reading the material that their child's doctor gives them to be informed but not being interested in "going to medical school." Instead of empowering or preparing them, the process of gathering information, deciphering it, and wading through remote possibilities just adds to their stress level. Extended research is an activity they feel would take them away from their job, which is being with and comforting their child.

> My wife read everything she could find, but I didn't want to do that. I don't want to know about it, I just want the doctor to fix it. Why worry in advance about what might happen? If something happens, then we read about it, then we ask the doctors. It's like you're looking for things to go wrong.—*Emmanuel*

* * *

> I hate reading. I didn't go out and read up on it at the library. I read the materials they gave me. If I need to know it, they'll tell me. I respect the [doctors]. They know what they're talking about. I trust them. I trust what they tell me, the medications they give me, because I know nothing about them.—*Elaine*

Information is equally important to children—both the children with cancer and their siblings. Young children engage in "magical" thinking and have an imperfect understanding of language and concepts. As a result, what they imagine is even worse than the truth. They will react to what you are not saying as much as what you are saying. You will not be able to hide much. It is better if they hear news from you than if Aunt Sophie blurts it out at the dinner table. Knowledge about the illness, the treatment, upcoming procedures, and events help a child prepare and cope with the difficult aspects of cancer. If left in the dark about what is going on, children's fears and misconceptions mount.

> A couple of months ago we were riding in the car. I asked her, Mia, were you scared when you had cancer? She said not really, because I knew my chemotherapy was working—that was a phrase we used a lot—and I knew if it wasn't working, you and Daddy would tell me so I could prepare to die. That statement meant so much to me, that she trusted that we were up front with her, and that if things weren't going well that we would tell her.
> —*Natalie*

Seeking support

Most veteran cancer parents warn that it is difficult to put aside guilt, sense of responsibility, and embarrassment, to accept help wherever and from whomever you can get it. They will also tell you to swallow your pride and do it anyway, because you and your child will be better off. This is one of the most valuable resources you can tap. You could probably "handle" things yourselves, but you would be under great strain, and your child would lose his or her best advocate and source of support.

Other cancer families can be excellent stabilizers. They provide practical tips, normalize your strong feelings, and are living examples of what to do or what not to do. As nurse clinician and researcher Sue Heiney told us,

> I believe that group support is critical, because you learn that you're not alone and you learn what other people are doing to deal with it. The most healing thing we can provide for people is to let them know they're not alone in what they're going through.

To contact a support group, create one, or just network with other families, see the Resources at the end of this book for some of the many organizations that will help you to get started. Also, ask at your child's treatment center. Although it is likely that major medical centers will have more resources than community hospitals, the social services departments in smaller hospitals and day treatment centers often will have referral contacts in your local community.

Creating a buffer zone

At times when you cannot afford to be totally overwhelmed, you put up a wall of glass, a moat, or a neutral space around yourself that protects you from stressful intrusions. When you need to be alert, focused, aware, and collected to get through a difficult event, you shelve your emotions for later release. It is a form of self-preservation.

> As our 14-month-old baby was going in for surgery, I handed her to the nurse, and turned to go. My husband tried to give me a hug, and I put up my hands and said, "Don't hug me now, or I'll lose it." I was afraid that if I let go, I wouldn't be able to get through the eight hours of surgery. I didn't want to deal with the emotional and life-altering implications yet. Of course, that night when we went to bed, I cried all night, and many nights afterward. I later felt badly about not accepting that hug, because I think my husband may have needed it.—*Marta*

Your hold on this buffer can become tenuous if you let it continue too long. One father said that he would cope with the major stuff, but something trivial, or an unexpected act of kindness, would break down the wall and send him over the edge.

Sometimes, creating a buffer zone takes a different form than shelving your emotions. To prevent yourself from being overwhelmed, turn off the telephone when you can't bear to talk any more, delegate the dirty dishes to others (or to permanent residence in the sink), take a nap, or latch onto any other practical way of calling it emotional quits for the day and temporarily saying no to the noise of the world.

Living one day at a time

If you have to, temporarily live one hour at a time. Set small, attainable goals. Don't weigh yourself down with trying to anticipate too far in the future.

> I can't remember really wanting anything specific, like a "Get out of Hell Free" card. You just trudge through it day-by-day, hour-by-hour, minute-by-minute.—*Edmund*

Searching for personal meaning

Searching for personal meaning is a way to integrate the experience into the wider frame of your life. Almost every parent questions "why my child" or "why me"? Through your own personal odyssey, you discover what the cancer means to you and to your child. What place does it have in your life?

Some parents reported a sense of destiny, or a "reason" why their particular child got cancer. Maggie said Scott was "picked" because he could understand it. Another parent believed that she had gotten through many hard tasks in life, so God put this in her life either because she could handle it or because she had handled past things too well. While most angrily reject the notion of a supreme being who would single out parents or children for this illness, this way of thinking could also be looked at as a mother's self-awareness and appreciation of her own or her child's positive coping abilities. Other families see the cancer experience as a "wake-up call" to pull the family together or rearrange priorities, as a call to duty, or as a learning experience that can be shared to help others.

Searching for meaning is not an assignment on your to-do list. It is a natural phenomenon, one that takes shape according to your needs and inclinations. Some people turn for help in their quest to philosophical or spiritual reading, nature, or their personal religious leaders. Many people find meaning and solace by talking to others within their own family.

Making comparisons to others

Making comparisons to others brings comfort by comparing your situation to people around you in similar circumstances. Your reference group shifts from neighborhood school children to children with cancer. It is the relativity that allows you to tolerate your own experience. If they can make it, so can we, or what happened to us is not as bad as what happened to them. Remember the old saying, "I cried because I had no shoes, until I saw the man who had no feet." Unfortunately, sometimes this makes you feel guilty if you feel you "got off easy" or angry if the situation is reversed.

Developing a sense of mastery or control

Lack of control is an ongoing issue for parents and children dealing with cancer. Choosing which arm gets the needle and when to take pills, using personal imagery to get through procedures and relaxation exercises to reduce stress, and altering diet to enhance body health all provide a modicum of control over treatment and side effects for the child. It is helpful, too, for you and any other caregivers who have taken action to seek out and teach new choices to the child.

Reappraising life

Reappraising life occurs in many families. They alter their expectations for the future, rearrange their priorities to put intangibles (such as family, love, and health) at the top of the list, and gain a deeper appreciation for what they have. It is a soul-searching process, sometimes painful, but rewarding in important ways.

Maintaining a sense of personal worth

Maintaining a sense of personal worth is tied to identity, self-image, and self-esteem. Maintaining as many pre-illness activities as possible and including your child in his or her care can help. Children need to know that they are important members of the family who just happen to have cancer: The illness is not the child's entire identity. Children need dignity.

> I remember one teenage girl who had a crush on her very handsome neurosurgeon. I would always go in early and fix her hair before he arrived. It was so important to her to look her best for him. I felt honored to be someone that she could share all of these feelings with.
> —*Carolyn Walker, a nursing professor and pediatric oncology nurse*

Gentle Reminders for Coping

- Communicate openly.
- Express your emotions constructively.
- Distance yourself from negative possibilities until you're ready to face them.
- Focus on positive aspects.
- Get as much information as you feel you need.
- Seek and maintain support from family and friends.
- Temporarily buffer yourself from overwhelming intrusions, responsibilities, and emotions.
- Live one day at a time.
- Allow yourself to discover personal meaning in the experience.
- Scale back your perspective when making comparisons.
- Take control of what you can, let go of what you can't.
- Reappraise your life in light of altered expectations.
- Maintain your sense of personal worth.

Children's Ways of Coping

Children choose from a menu of coping strategies similar to that of adults. But children are not just miniature adults, and their thoughts and actions reflect the differences. Information management in children can be verbal or nonverbal. A child might ask questions, listen in to adult conversations, or share his knowledge by showing off medical equipment to a visitor or explaining the elements of blood to his classmates. Children use self-protective behaviors and thoughts to regulate their emotions and defend themselves against anxiety, as do adults. However, children often appear more extreme in their reactions.

For example, it is quite common for children to react aggressively to prolonged hospitalization, especially boys. However, this may actually help them to make a better adjustment after being in the hospital, however exasperating it is at the time. Physical exercise and aggressive activities can reduce children's tension. It is also quite common for a child to shut down temporarily and revert back to the comfort habits of their younger years, such as thumb-sucking and hair-twirling.

> Lloyd had a lot of anger, especially when we had to give him his shots. We bought him a child's punching bag and some kid boxing gloves. After his needles, he would go over to the punching bag and punch out his anger and say, "Take that cancer!" Sometimes Rob

would let Lloyd punch him on the arms after he gave him his needle just so that he could feel better.—*Sandy*

Child coping and parent coping efforts overlap and work in tandem, but they are not the same. In the boxes that follow are strategies used by school-aged children who are hospitalized repeatedly, as reported by clinical nurse specialist Jennifer Boyd and nursing professor Mabel Hunsberger (see the Bibliography). Although the children in those authors' study had many different diseases, their actions and emotional efforts are consistent with children with cancer. A few terms for the strategies may be unfamiliar to you, but the examples and the children's words make the points clear. (See charts on pages 67 and 68.)

Boyd and Hunsberger also tell us about the ways children count on adults to help.

Ways Hospital Personnel Can Help

- Talk with and listen to the child.
- Provide information.
- Allow control.
- Be gentle, patient, and positive.
- Be funny, joke around.
- Arrange for consistent caregivers.
- Explain actions.
- Provide emotional support and reassurance.
- Provide competent physical care.
- Provide privacy.
- Respect and value the child as a human being with thoughts and feelings.

Ways Family and Friends Can Help

- Visit frequently.
- Bring gifts.
- Distract the child.
- Provide emotional support and reassurance.
- Talk with and listen to the child.
- Provide information.
- Permit a degree of control and enhance level of independence.
- Provide physical support and personal care.

I decided that I was going to make that room the cheeriest place that you could walk into. I brought posters from home, and cards, and pictures of her with her friends, pictures of the dog, and just plastered everything all over the place. There was a banner that some kids at my school (I'm a teacher) had all signed. I lugged that in. It was a little process, every time we went in, to get all that stuff up. It was a little thing I could do for Melanie. A good friend of mine whose mother had cancer, he said focus on the things you can do for Melanie; positive things that are going to help her. I guess that was one of them.—*Peggy*

Behavior Coping Strategies Used by Children

Strategy	Examples	Children's Words
Distraction	Watch tv or videos Go for a walk Listen to music Deep breathing Doing crafts Playing games Bugging the nurses	"When they're doing it sometimes I just . . . into my pillow or something, scream as loud as I can and it makes me think about how loud I'm screaming and not what they're doing." "Like just try to keep myself busy . . . as much as I can."
Seeking social support	Visiting with friends Having parents there	"I try to phone them (friends), get in touch" "I call my mom, and she comes down and visits with me and brings me stuff." "I was holding my mom's hand."
Avoidance, resistance	Resisting participation Taking a nap	"I was so terrified at this surgery that I wouldn't let them do anything." "I just try to go back to sleep . . . if I can sleep."
Submission, cooperation	Just do it	"Whatever happens I let them do what they have to do to help me get better." "I let them do it and get it over with."
Independent activities	Do things themselves	"I try to get up sometimes." "I usually do it myself."
Emotional expression	Crying, screaming Yelling	"I usually have a good cry before everything because of just all the tension and stuff I hate." "Well, when I get an IV, I'd rather scream and yell during it so I can relieve some of the pain fast." "I was crying because I miss . . . I miss my animals at home a lot."
Verbal expression	Talking about concerns Telling others how they feel	"When it hurts I tell them it hurts. Like I tell them everything, even the slightest, I'll tell them."
Seeking information	Asking questions	"I don't understand, I'll ask the doctor or the surgeon, or whoever it is." "Usually, I look at the needle part. I know when they're gonna poke it so I can be ready."

From "Chronically ill children coping with repeated hospitalizations: Their perceptions and suggested interventions," by J. R. Boyd and M. Hunsberger, 1998, *Journal of Pediatric Nursing* 13(6):330–342. Adapted with permission.

Mental Coping Strategies Used by Children

Strategy	Examples	Children's Words
Distraction	Think about something else	"I thought about other things to not fear the doctors." (During needles thought about) "my kitten."
Self-control		"I just settled myself down."
Avoidance	Not thinking about it	"I just didn't think about it, that's all." "I try not to think about it until they come. That helps a bit sometimes."
Cognitive restructuring, maintaining a positive outlook	Consider the positive aspects such as improved health, know it's in their best interests and will eventually end	"I'm gonna feel better once it's all done over with." "I thought great, cause I've been waiting for it (surgery) for 9 years, or 9 years I've been having seizures, and I want to go to school without seizures now." "I might not want to, but it's all better in the long run."
Confidence in staff	Acknowledge that doctors and nurses are there to make them better	"It makes me feel hap [word not completed] . . . like better cause I know they're going to do everything the best they can."
Endurance	When something is beyond their control, live with a stressor and anticipate its completion.	"I thought OK, let's just get this done and over with." "I just lived with it." "There's nothing important that I do, I just get it over with."
Familiarity, knowledge	Having familiarity with procedures, routines and staff, and prior knowledge of expectations. (*Although to some, memories were distressing.*)	"Well, cause I know what they're gonna be doing and how they're gonna be doing it."

From "Chronically ill children coping with repeated hospitalizations: Their perceptions and suggested interventions," by J. R. Boyd and M. Hunsberger, 1998, *Journal of Pediatric Nursing* 13(6):330–342. Adapted with permission.

Teenagers' Coping Strategies

There is an additional useful set of coping strategies that are helpful to adolescents with cancer.

- Having people (friends, family, and hospital staff) around who understand
- Having parents who are strong (good role models of coping)
- Thinking you can get better and refusing to feel sorry for yourself, and having people around you do the same
- Realizing that appearance is less important than who you are
- Learning new skills
- Taking responsibility for maintaining a conversation with friends.

As a parent, you can help bolster these coping efforts. Allow more leeway than you might usually have done. Normal adolescent activities like hanging posters with positive messages or pictures; listening to music on a personal tape or CD player; writing thoughts, song lyrics, poems, or stories in a private journal; and hanging out may not be active physically, but they are active coping examples.

Encourage your teenager to call or e-mail his or her friends. You can help your teenager's school friends to feel comfortable with visits and be ready to answer their questions and ease their fears. Provide transportation for your teenager's friends, prepare them for what they will see, and encourage them to talk to your son or daughter about the cancer and about other topics.

You can help your teenager to meet new peers, for example, by finding out about Internet chat rooms for teenagers with cancer and passing along that information, without intruding on "private space" by deciding what he or she should do with the information. If there are other adolescents being treated at the same place at the same time, chances are they will gravitate to each other. If your teenager needs a nudge, the social worker might make an introduction or invite your teenager to join a group. Get them together often, to watch a movie or listen to music, and eventually they will get around to sharing their experiences on some level.

Parents can help by being understanding and sensitive to a teenager's concerns (even when you don't think an issue is the most important one to be focusing on now). You can help by being strong enough to face the cancer, the treatments, and their reactions to it. This means not crumbling when the changeable teenager is angry, discouraged, oppositional, babyish, or apathetic. It also means not crumbling when he or she startles you with the fierce power of a hard-to-reach dream. Sensitivity and strength go with the territory of being the parent of an adolescent anyway. As parents, we have to be willing to lead by example, to tolerate negative reactions when we make unpopular but necessary decisions, and to subsume our own desires to support our children's growth and dreams.

Recognizing a Child's Coping for What It Is

Children of any age have innate coping skills—automatic reactions that are part of a child's nature, such as crying; clinging; fighting back; "zoning out"; playing; regressing; or decreasing activity, eating, or talking. We should recognize these reactions for what they are—children's methods of dealing with difficult and painful events and feelings—and encourage our children to express themselves, even if it is not polite or seems like misbehavior.

> Even now, a few years into remission, Cami is physically unsure of herself. Even though she seemed to love it, she kept crying that she wanted to quit gymnastics. She yelled and cried and kept saying her teacher was mean and very, very ugly! We talked it through, and she finally said that she was afraid to do some of the exercises. She is uncomfortable hanging upside down or leaning backwards—anything where she can't see what's coming. She has since switched to karate and is much more confident and happy.—*Robin*

Trust yourself to know the difference between a child who is crying or having a temper tantrum out of tiredness or anxiety and a child who is falling apart. It is draining to shepherd your child through a difficult procedure. When your child is crying or throwing himself on the floor, it is hard to view that as positive. It seems instinctive to do anything to stop your child from crying. We are biologically designed to be uncomfortable at the sound of a child's cry. But crying when you are in pain or afraid is a natural emotional release. Sometimes it simply needs to be lived through.

On the other hand, do not assume that because your child does not cry, he or she is not upset. Psychologist and best-selling novelist Jonathan Kellerman relates the story of 7-year-old Anthony, who had to get frequent injections. He was depressed and withdrawn for days before and after his injections. During the procedure he would sit rigidly, vomit, and suffer in silence, having been taught that he would be a "sissy" if he cried. Working with a therapist, he was able to talk about feeling scared and upset. The therapist explained that other children had the same feelings and that it was okay to have them, to talk about them, and even to cry. Anthony drew angry pictures and practiced letting his feelings out during make-believe injections. Once he was able to protest and cry a little during his procedures, he relaxed, his nausea was greatly reduced, and he bounced back more quickly (see the Bibliography).

Children will surprise you with their natural ways. One little boy found his own way to mark the end of treatment:

> As he was leaving the hospital [after his last chemotherapy], he said bye-bye to everyone: the doctors, the nurses, the janitors, the people in the elevator, the parking people, the people at the information desk, everyone he passed. He said it with a very loud BYE-BYE, a dramatic parade-style wave, and a big smile. It was funny because he had never done that before. I think my 5-year-old is right when he says, "Joey understands a lot more than he can say."—*Jeannette*

Other children's and teenagers' issues and suggestions for coping are found in chapter 10 in the section on special considerations at each age level.

The Family's Coping Strategies

Each family develops its own coping style, with unique rules and specific roles. Family coping is interactive. Members influence, affect, and reflect each other. This can be positive, as when spouses instinctively take turns, emotionally, so that while one is down, the other is up. It can be negative, as the foul mood or irritability of one family member "infects" all the others. The whole family's emotional ups and downs can often be directed by how the sick child is doing. When problems crop up, a healthy family can respond with flexibility, independence, and even humor. They can spot communication problems and generate suggestions for improvement. On the other hand, chronically stressed families can become quite inflexible, and communication often breaks down.

Mark Chesler, a research sociologist and cancer parent, sums up interactive influence in six words: "A hurt child creates a hurting parent." He describes well some of the ways childhood cancer families cope: seeking normalcy, taking one day at a time, finding different ways to cope, relying on others, and becoming partners in health care (see the Bibliography). The strategies are similar to those of individuals but take on greater strength when shared between and among family members.

Parents underestimate the power of their presence. Children are comforted when you are there to protect them, to explain things they do not understand, to be on guard (so they do not have to be), to hold them, and to love them. If you are there, the child does not have to be vigilant and can relax. You, in turn, can relax your vigilance, too, when you are well supported. To handle distress, a family must work together and in complementary ways.

Gentle Reminders for Family Coping

- Be aware of each other's strengths and weaknesses and respectful of each other's coping styles.
- Delegate, share, and take turns.
- Use the "buddy system" to fill in when one member is overtaxed.
- Take breaks; family members each have their own needs and should participate in activities unrelated to cancer.
- All family members need ego and energy boosters so they come back refreshed and ready to tackle the next crisis.
- Keep everybody informed.
- Reassess your goals and expectations often.

Special Avenues for Coping

Storytelling

Since prehistoric times, human beings have always responded to stories, using them as teaching tools and cultural bonds. As storyteller Kathryn Weidener told us, stories are mood lifters; when disease has sapped your joy, stories can bring it back. Storytelling can function as a coping mechanism to both explore and express complicated feelings. It can capture what our children are thinking and feeling, allowing them to grasp the message of the story intuitively and apply it to their own lives.

We offer many suggestions for stories in this section and in the Resources at the end of this book, based on our experiences and the recommendations of others. These suggestions are not meant to be the last word; you will find other stories that are especially meaningful to you and your child.

Picture Book Suggestions

Feelings by Aliki explores emotions.
The Kissing Hand by Audrey Penn and *Owl Babies* by Martin Waddell reassure children afraid to be away from mommy.
Wanda's Roses by Pat Brisson, *The Magic Tree* by T. Obinkaram Echewa, and *The Little Engine that Could* all empower children.
The Worry Stone by Marianna Dengler, *Mirette on the High Wire* by Emily Arnold McCully, *The Adventures of Isabel* by Ogden Nash, *Once When I Was Scared* by Helena Clare Pittman, *Flight* by Robert Burleigh, and *Thundercake* by Patricia Polacco are all about conquering fears.
Applemando's Dreams by Patricia Polacco celebrates the importance of dreams.
If by Sarah Perry shows limitless possibilities.

For storytelling to work as a coping mechanism, the listener must project himself or herself into the story and relate it to his or her life. It should involve a give and take—asking the child (or yourself) what it means to you or how you would feel. Let the child verbalize a reaction.

> Recently, when she was using her medical history to get attention and special treatment, I told her the story of the boy who cried wolf, to teach her not to use that excuse unless she really needed it.—*Nicole*

As nurse specialist Sue Heiney told us,

> Stories help children to see their strengths, by identifying with the main character. In bibliotherapy, parent and child read together, project their own thoughts and feelings into that story, learn that it's normal, learn ways to deal with something, see some humor in the situation. Stories provide us with a language for helping to understand. Classic children's stories tell a normal life story, [which] helps children learn from that story. Stories about a child who has cancer are so close to home, the child can't use his/her imagination and project his/her own issues into story.

She recommends Judith Viorst's *Alexander and the Terrible, Horrible, No Good, Very Bad Day;* Mercer Mayer's Little Critter books; and Judy Blume's stories of real-life issues. For teenagers, she suggests classics such as Daniel Defoe's *Robinson Crusoe,* a story about perseverance, and Isaac Asimov's stories. She observes, "With teens you don't have to worry so much about projection. Their cognitive abilities are such that they can usually express themselves."

Classic fairy tales are full of violence, death, and scary things. They have lasted through the centuries, among other reasons, because they help children address scary things and conquer them. Nursery rhymes, fables, myths, and religious parables are also good sources of material. Older children might respond to fantasy stories by authors such as C. S. Lewis, Lloyd Alexander, Jane Yolen, Madeleine L'Engle, or J. K. Rowling, which give children power and an evil enemy to fight. *Small Steps: The Year I Got Polio* by Peg Kehret, *Peeling the Onion* by Wendy Orr, and *On the Third Ward* by T. Degens are all stories about children in hospitals coming to terms with emotions, limitations, and plans for the future.

Before you choose a book, think about what it is that you or your child needs. At the beginning, you may want nonfiction explanations of illness, treatment, or the hospital experience. Later, you want stories about overcoming fears, being different, maintaining hope, and controlling anger. The best source for other good story suggestions is your local library's children's librarian, but other possibilities include your hospital's family library or a bookstore (regular or on-line), the American Library Association, or Children's Book Council (see the Resources at the end of this book).

For adults and mature teenagers, testimonials by survivors or other parents are often inspiring, but they do not have to be about cancer. One parent recommended C. Everett Koop's book about the accidental death of his son, *Sometimes Mountains Move.* Parents and survivors alike have expressed a connection to stories of holocaust survival, such as Elie Wiesel's *Night* and Viktor Frankl's *Man's Search for Meaning.*

Telling our own stories gives words and meaning to our lives and context to our experiences. Telling the story tames the beast. Hearing the stories of others can provide us with information and different perspectives, normalizing our own fears and feelings. We can decide which parts appeal to us, apply to us, what we might have done differently, and what we need to watch out for. Telling each other our stories bonds us together in a meaningful group—it is our initiation into the "club." We see that we are not alone. We earn the right to participate in the telling of "war stories."

Many personal stories are shared in hospital waiting rooms and support groups. Some people choose to speak at conferences or other public forums to raise public awareness. But not everyone feels comfortable with public disclosure. A more private outlet for telling your story is to write it in a journal or to create poetry or some other art form.

Spirituality

When your child has cancer, you start to ask existential questions about the meaning of life, the purpose of suffering, the existence of God, the nature of God, whether there is life after death, and the effectiveness of prayer. These questions are entwined in the emotions and experiences of a cancer parent. You may question beliefs you have held all your life or delve into issues to which you rarely gave thought. In the words of chaplain Julie R. Swaney, "Being left to the whim of fate is universally terrifying" (see the Bibliography). In the process of discovering your own answers, spirituality can be a powerful source of comfort.

> We are afflicted in every way, but not crushed; perplexed, but not driven to despair; persecuted, but not forsaken; struck down, but not destroyed.
> *I Corinthians 4:7*

Although religion can be part of spirituality, spirituality is not a specific religion. It is not a particular creed or belief or ritual. You do not have to believe in God to be spiritual: Unlike the old axiom that there are no atheists in foxholes, there are atheists in oncology wards. You might believe in science, in ethics, in morals, in yourself, or in "the big picture." Your spirituality is your unique philosophy of life, your view of the universe. Spirituality can offer hope, meaning, direction, acceptance, understanding, and the relinquishing of control (and thus responsibility).

> I'm not sure I believe in God. I don't believe in a figure who sits on high choosing which children get cancer and which ones will die. Illness is part of the human condition, and I have great faith in the advances of science, though they're not perfect. But if someone wants to pray for my child, or dash holy water on him, I say yes. It can't hurt, and it makes the person offering it feel better. It shows that they care, and are thinking about us.—*Joan*

A strong, compassionate faith can boost coping by reducing anxiety, fostering hope, suggesting significance and permanence, imparting forgiveness, giving a sense of being loved and of belonging to something larger than oneself, and either answering questions or removing the necessity of questioning.

> God is that driving force of love within us. When you can't go on anymore, and you have nothing left to give, you reach down deep inside of yourself and you find love. And you pull it out for your child. And you go on. That is God at work. When you're on the floor, and there is nothing left, and suddenly, there is. It's like air coming into the room.—*Lisa*

* * *

> Faith in God got me through, and people praying for us. He's in control. When you're told your child is probably going to die, you totally rely on God.—*Doris*

A person looking through a spiritual kaleidoscope can see exquisite beauty in the patterns of light and color or see unconnected, broken bits of glass that fall apart and change at the slightest turn, distorting the images of the world beyond it. Spirituality can thus become a coping "task"—in that it raises more questions than it answers. This is especially true if it seems as though prayers are unheeded. Faith may not only come into question but can become a focus of anguish and blame, whether directed by oneself or by "well-meaning" others (see chapter 5 for more on this topic).

Rituals, spiritual practices, and prayers are viewed by many people as something they can do to heal in soul, if not in body. When you feel out of control, these demonstrations of hope and faith can feel familiar, normal, and comforting. They can reinforce your place in the "grand scheme."

If you are interested in finding spiritual guidance and you are not sure where to start, ask the hospital staff if there are chaplains available. Often hospitals have access to representatives of many religions from the surrounding communities. Most phone books have listings of local places of worship, but if you do not have a particular affiliation, this may not be helpful. If you do not want to speak to someone directly, try browsing the spirituality section of your book-

> Science and technology revolutionize our lives, but memory, tradition, and myth frame our response.
> Arthur M. Schlesinger, Jr., *New York Times Magazine* (July 27, 1986)

store, library, or Internet book sites. You are likely to find books that span a wide range, from ancient Buddhist practices to New Age approaches. You may also want to look at the philosophy shelf or the self-help shelf.

Remember that you are vulnerable now. This may not be a good time to make any permanent decisions about committing yourself to any new spiritual or religious group, especially one that makes promises of cures, blames you or your past behavior or beliefs for your child's illness, or expects money donations from you.

Children's spirituality

Children, naturally, infuse their view of God with the traits of their own parents.

> If parents are present, open, honest, empathetic, accepting, and loving, then children may likely have an image of God or other spiritual images that reflect these supportive, caring, and accepting characteristics. If caregivers are blaming, judgmental, inconsistent, abusive, manipulative, or narcissistic, children may conceive of God with these traits. If caregivers are passive, overly protective, rigid, or unable to express their emotions in the midst of crisis, then children may develop an image of God who is insulated from their suffering.—*Rev. Dane Sommer* (see the Bibliography)

Children trust what you tell them about God and take every word literally. If you give them conflicting messages, they become confused. If you say God protects His people, or good people, from harm, then surely having cancer means to the child that he or she is very bad. Likewise if cancer is God's will, then God wants the child to be sick as a punishment. Phrases like that are automatic; they are intended to comfort or absolve of responsibility, but as the examples show, they are heard by children very differently. Within the framework of your personal faith, it is most helpful to communicate beliefs that will cherish and sustain your child.

Play

> Children discover grace through play.
> Rev. Dane Sommer, *The ACCH Advocate* (1994)

Walk into any pediatric oncology ward, and you will find bald children playing. They may pause to get medications, to throw up, or to have their vital signs taken, but they keep coming back. This is characteristic of their resilience, their innocence, their perseverance. But it is also something more.

Play is a basic and natural part of childhood. Children learn, grow, and develop through play. It fosters coping and mastery of skills. Play is a vital conduit for expression, creativity, and experimentation. It is a powerful means of stress reduction.

Children express their fears, fantasies, and feelings through play. It is a very effective coping activity, which is why it is common to see a child repeat a theme over and over. For example, relatively small and helpless children often pretend they are superheroes. As children find expression and come to terms with conflicts or worries through play, they mature psychologically. Play allows them to recognize feelings, release tensions, learn new concepts, ease fears, and clarify distortions about illness.

For hospitalized children, play has some additional clear benefits. It provides a much-needed diversion and an outlet for the negative feelings associated with the hospitalization, immobility, and medical procedures. Having this diversion and outlet reduces your child's frustration, anxiety, and feelings of helplessness. Play often gets your child moving around physically, with a chance to release energy, maintain strength, and resume a normal daily activity. It also provides a social opportunity to interact with new children and to stay connected to family members in familiar ways. Best of all, let's not forget that play is fun.

Play can be recreational, therapeutic, or a structured therapy. Even very sick children somehow manage to find the energy for recreational play. Put on your camp director hat or dust off those scouting activity booklets, and have fun whenever your child is feeling up to it. For therapeutic play, or play therapy, a child life specialist, social worker, or psychologist trained in the techniques can work with your child or give you suggestions for games or activities that address a particular issue or help your child develop emotional, social, and cognitive skills. Some suggestions are also found in chapter 10 on child development.

> The child life specialist works with James, one-on-one. She's helped him more than anyone in four years of treatment. Not just distracting him from a procedure, he was so used to them that wasn't the issue. It was more getting him to loosen up and be a normal kid. He walked out of the hospital a full-fledged magician. She tapped into what he likes, what he could do best, and drew that out of him. He put on a magic show for the nurses at the nurses' station before he was released, 3 shows a day.—*Faith*

Medical play involves medical themes or medical equipment in a nonstressful atmosphere. It can be relaxing and fun but also intense and aggressive if children need to act out anger or fear. Medical play can identify fears and misconceptions, reduce anxiety, and encourage expression. It allows the child to reverse roles and be the one in control, the "doer," not the "done-to."

For instance, a child working out fears about procedures might use a doll or a willing grown-up to play the part of the doctor or nurse to act out their angry or sad feelings toward that person. Or, the child may act the part of the one doing a procedure, using a doll to represent themselves or a generic child, sometimes in an exaggerated or aggressive manner.

> My daughter used to line her dolls and stuffed animals up on the floor. Each one got a turn to get their Broviac hooked up to the IV, getting meds, fluids. Each one got its blood

pressure and temperature taken, and each one got a shot. She'd do 9 or 10 of them, every day for months. She had the best doctor kit in the neighborhood.—*Susan*

In medical art, the medical supplies are used to create something—it does not matter what, because the process, more than the product, is therapeutic. Syringes can be paintbrushes, medical implements can sculpt clay, and all sorts of items can create collages.

Rev. Dane Sommer observes that

it is in their play that [children] engage in honest conversation, open negotiation, creative contemplation, and free expression of their emotions . . . [they] find acceptance [can] be themselves . . . [have] no need for pretense or hiding. . . . When they play they are free from adult interventions and expectations, exploring new and splendid territories, free from their worries and concerns" (see the Bibliography).

Humor

Cancer families can and do have a sense of humor. Many families say they laugh at the most bizarre things, and outsiders do not know what to make of them. One Internet listserve group had a lot of fun coming up with a lengthy list of euphemisms for vomiting. The SquirrelTales Web site has humorous stories from parents ("you know you're the parent of a cancer kid when . . ."), as well as malapropisms from children who have trouble with the big words used in treatment. Humor can help you keep a positive outlook and retain a sense of normalcy, as well as release stress and tension.

Humor is an emotional release—good for the body and the soul. It can relax the tension in a somber room, break the ice in an awkward interaction, diffuse an argument, make you feel good, bring people together, and make things seem normal for a few moments.

Sometimes laughter comes at times of great stress or shock, when you do not know how to react or feel. People who laugh at bad news, for example, do not find anything funny about it. Laughter is a tension diffuser. This phenomenon is not unusual but is separate from using humor as a coping strategy.

There are times, of course, when humor is inappropriate. If another parent on the ward has just gotten bad news, you would not go up him or her and tell a joke. Also, put-downs, ethnic jokes, or sexual humor are largely unwelcome at any time. If there is any particularly touchy subject for your child, avoid making jokes about it.

I made jokes about hospital food; I made a joke about steroids: too bad you can't lift some weights now, bulk up, your coach would really be happy. Then I made a joke about getting stuck with needles, and he turned to me and said dad, no more jokes about that. This bothers him.—*Fred*

Staff humor sometimes has a different flavor than that of families. It may seem crass, dehumanizing, or insensitive, but it is part of their human need to distance themselves from never-ending emotional turmoil. Keep that in mind, but do not hesitate to take someone aside and gently let him or her know when something inappropriate was said.

Family humor can bother staff members, too. Leila, a nurse, told us about a father who made sexual jokes or innuendoes when she bathed his son. She knew it was just the father's way of lightening a heavy situation, but it made her uncomfortable.

To bring sunshine into your life, either at home or at the hospital,

- Have a silly word of the day, and make lots of noise whenever anyone uses it.
- Make up weird words for medical terms.
- Put up a bulletin board with cartoons, sayings, pictures, and bumper stickers.
- Play games, and do puppet shows.
- Decorate the room with silly themes, color schemes, streamers, posters, and photos.
- Do imitations.
- Read joke books, satires, comic books, Dr. Seuss, limericks, and Jack Prelutsky.
- Watch comedy shows or videos.
- Sing funny songs, or re-write lyrics to popular tunes.
- Play (nondangerous) tricks on staff.
- Talk in pig latin or rhyme.
- Use clown props such as squeaking hammers, water guns, goofy hats, and masks.

Trish imagines the results of flushing unused medicines down the drain:

> Jane Doe has been arrested and charged with disposal of hazardous materials through her septic system. State environmental officials were quoted as saying, "She was directed to put these poisons into her child. That doesn't mean they're safe enough to go into the GROUND, for heaven's sake. The forest creatures who drink from nearby streams will lose their hair, and the fish are all going to be craving bacon, pepperoni, and Cheetos. We have to make an example of her, or parents will be pouring that hideous PediaSure straight down the drain, and it will be the end of all the local flora and fauna." Parents nearby were heard to mutter, "Jeez, Jane, you didn't have to flush the fluconazole, that stuff costs $7 a pill!"

Wendy responds to the financial stresses:

> Susie and I have been passing the time in the hospital by playing Monopoly. Last night, while playing a hotly contested match, I drew a Community Chest card that read "Pay Doctor's Fee $50." The nurses thought I was nuts when I started laughing out loud. I honestly can't remember the last time I paid a mere $50 doctor's fee! There I was, in the intensive care unit, where the bed alone is probably THOUSANDS a day. The irony was just too much!

Expressive Arts

Some people are not directly verbal. They express their feelings through art or music or dance. Listening to music, playing an instrument, painting, writing poetry, keeping a journal, and play acting are valid and helpful means of emotional release that are used by both children and adults. Many people find solace in these activities.

A teenager might wear a headset and listen to music, shutting out the sights and sounds of the hospital. Infants and children respond to soothing music, and so do parents. There are many organizations that create personalized songs for your child. The music of Celebration Shop, a nonprofit group that writes and sings songs for children in hospitals and camps, holds particular resonance for sick children.

Someone who plays an instrument often uses that as a release, choosing to play pieces that reflect a mood: angry, or sad, or tired, or happy or hopeful.

> My husband plays the piano every day. When our granddaughter was diagnosed with cancer, it hit him really hard. But he finds it hard to verbalize his feelings. He's of the generation in which men don't cry or show emotions. I can tell how he's feeling by the music he plays. And when he's really upset, he can't play at all. That's the worst, because then it all gets bottled up, with no way to let it out.—*Marilyn*

Many survivors and parents create art about their experiences. A poem or a painting can be a tribute by a family member or something left behind for posterity by the one who is sick. *The Jester Who Lost His Jingle* was written by David Saltzman, a young man with Hodgkin's disease who later died. Partial proceeds from the sale of this book by his family are donated for research.

The creation of a painting, a sculpture, or a poem is therapeutic in both the process and the result. The act of creating art is physically and emotionally satisfying. Working with clay, for example, can be an outlet for frustration or anger (pounding) or a rhythmic and centering exercise (kneading, shaping). Having something to show and re-visit privately over the years is a tangible expression of the thoughts and feelings of the creator and a palpable confirmation of the experience.

Child life specialists, social workers, and psychologists should be able to guide these arts in a therapeutic manner. Some hospitals now have music, writing, or art therapists on staff. If yours does not, you can tap into community resources. You might ask your social worker, your local American Cancer Society, or your Candlelighters chapter to arrange for someone to come to the hospital or even arrange for it on a private basis.

> I worked with a 15-year-old bedridden patient. One day he painted an "intuitive painting" and described what his experience was like. He talked about being "shattered" and identified areas in the painting that represented his strengths. In the nine months I worked with him

he never mentioned the word cancer. Art is also very effective in helping a child to integrate with a group and feel "at home" in the hospital. I remember a non–English speaking child who came into the playroom looking traumatized. She just stood there and would hardly speak at all. I went to her and drew some marks on a paper and handed the marker to her. We drew back and forth for a while and finally she did a very lovely and haunting picture of an angel whose head floated slightly above its body. Afterwards she felt safe and comfortable enough to play with the toys and the other kids.—*Janet Ruffin, art therapist*

Hospice counselor Virginia L. Fry has written straightforwardly about how art therapy helps grieving children express their feelings (see the Bibliography). Many of the projects in her book could be adapted for a child with cancer, a sibling, or another family member. Create a memory quilt. Write a poem about one's fears and hopes. Form clay into the shape of a person or thing that scares you, and bash it in. Draw a map of your world big enough to walk on (house, school, store, hospital, or grandma's house) and take imaginary walks or trips. Make worry stones or worry dolls. Make a feelings book: Draw faces that illustrate various emotions, and write what makes you feel each one. Create a "magic" shield from a cardboard pizza plate: Decorate it with symbols that make you feel powerful, safe and protected, using another strip of cardboard on the back to make a handle.

The therapist worked with Alicia to make an album. With the pictures and the writing Alicia [did], it was like taking it off her shoulders and putting it in this album. She chose what she wanted to include; she used pictures of treatment. She would cut people out of her pictures if she didn't want them. She made lists and made us make lists of what we thought of her cancer. It was a tangible thing that she could pick up and put down and organize in a way that felt right to her. She's left it in therapist's office, and she can bring it home if she wants, but she never has.—*Margaret*

One of the most encompassing examples of expressive arts being used in the childhood cancer arena is the ongoing quilt project by the Children's Cancer Awareness Project (see Resources). Begun by a group of parents, it is an enormous creative endeavor that honors and remembers both survivors and victims of childhood cancer. To raise awareness of the struggle, raise funds for research, and make pediatric cancer a health priority, the quilts are displayed, among other places, at the annual march on Washington, DC. Not only is the process of making a square for a child therapeutic for an individual, but those individuals are brought together so that they can support each other and actively participate in fighting cancer on a large scale.

CHAPTER 4

Understanding the Impact on Your Family and Friends

Living together is an art.
—*William Pickens* (1932)

By strengthening and understanding relationships, you can boost your family's ability to build resources and cope more successfully; buffer the strain of hardship; build resilience in your children (both the child with cancer and any brothers and sisters); and make it possible to maintain marriages, partnerships, intergenerational bonds, and cross-cultural alliances that protect and enhance life.

Families take many forms and individuals, their own roles. For every story that fits into a traditional pattern, there is another that does not fit. Out of necessity, we will not be able to cover every possible circumstance but will concentrate on broad strokes and common reactions. The most helpful approach for any family member is to understand multiple perspectives in the family, not just your own.

Mothers

Give me where to stand, and I will move the earth.
Archimedes

Mothers bear the brunt of the responsibility for medical care in most cases, because mothers are usually the primary attachment figure and caregiver or care arranger. Mothers are not saints. A small minority is not able to fulfill the role adequately, but most women fight fiercely for the good of their children. If a woman is a stay-at-home mother, a single parent, or the secondary income for a couple, it is practical that she be the one to take on these duties. It is also much more common for employers to accommodate a mother's child care needs than a father's, regardless of written employment policies.

Even when the mother is the primary breadwinner, she is often the primary caretaker as well. Mothers who maintain their jobs because they carry the primary health insurance or for other reasons often contend with additional pressures when everyone around them questions their priorities, either openly or subtly. When work and care for an ill child cannot be accommodated, some mothers take extended leave or quit their jobs, although they may not do so until they are stretched to their personal limits to manage it all. Careers may be interrupted or lost.

> I have people that say to me, "I don't know how you do it," but most of the mothers I know would do the same. I am a mother. Aren't I supposed to be by my child's side when he is ill? I really don't see what the big deal is.—*Jess*

* * *

> I don't feel strong at all. I'm not a hero, I'm just someone who's trapped. I felt I had no choice. And then, as I walked past the room of a child whose father had left in the middle of treatment, I realized I did have a choice, but the choice to leave was unthinkable to me. —*Maureen*

* * *

> I was at a crossroads. I quit grad school immediately. That door is closed. There was no way to go back to it. I bought a laptop with my student loan and used it to research his illness and contact other parents over the Internet. I'm in a different place now and trying to open a new door.—*Mindy*

* * *

> I was working full-time in sales. My first impulse was, "how can I go back to work"? I can't send him to day care. My employer encouraged me to take family leave. Then they hired someone who worked on flex-time to fill in so I could work part-time; we split our commissions. The schedule never went as planned. We'd go in to the clinic, bags packed, ready to stay for the week, and his counts wouldn't be good enough. I'd start a sale, and she'd finish it and get the commission. It was very stressful.—*Debra*

For women with spouses or live-in partners, being the only one doing all the medical care typically produces resentment and anger. Mothers express the desire for a sharing in these duties, often believing that their husbands or partners do not care about their feelings or are not involved. For them, support means the husband participates in the care of the child.

Brad's care was mine, because Jeff was working, and he had a harder time dealing with it. I got angry when I was always the one who had to tell Brad he had to go to the hospital again. I'd have to pick up the pieces every single time. There were surgeries when I was by myself, because Jeff had work. He said he couldn't cut back, but he was really taking on more work so he didn't have to be there. I wouldn't have left Brad anyway, but it would have been nice to have company. Jeff said, "Well you're already there, why do I have to be?" —*Holly*

* * *

My husband has always been a bit anxious about anything medical. It was distressing to him to take in too much information. Performing dressing changes or giving shots or handling tube feedings wasn't in his realm—it made him really anxious. He's a very loving, capable, helpful person. But he just couldn't do this. Unfortunately, that meant I had to do it all. Resentment started to build up, but I didn't want to express it, because I was aware of his fears. Eventually I let him know how I felt, and we came to a better arrangement.—*Joan*

Researchers Mark Chesler and Carla Perry observe that mothers generally report receiving less support from fathers than fathers report getting from the wives (see the Bibliography). As a result, they found, some mothers end up taking care of their husbands' emotional crises as well as their own and their children's, and resenting the overload. Mothers resent being asked to do one more thing or the implication that they have failed or neglected someone. Yet sometimes, as a measure of control, they do not allow others to step in and participate in the care. They are the main link to doctors and medical information and find it vitally important to learn the medical procedures and be able to perform the required tasks. Mothers often feel guilty for neglecting husbands, healthy children, and household duties. They put pressure on themselves to do it all even if no pressure comes from outside. Many have a very strong identification with the child, and most are intimately involved in the cancer experiences of their children.

I had sympathy pains. I had pains in my back, and I'd limp when he'd have a bone marrow aspiration. I didn't know what was going on. I was taking aspirin and ibuprofen and not getting any relief. This went on for about two weeks. I thought, this is strange. Then I realized that I experienced the pain whenever the thought of a bone marrow went through my mind.—*Val*

Widespread cultural and societal expectations grant permission for women to cry, show emotion, ask for help, be dependent, and act passive. Other people respond to those behaviors reasonably well. By the same token, these norms do not condone women's actions if they seem too pushy, angry, aggressive, or questioning of authority. Aggressive mothers can be quite effective in getting the needed action for their children, but they may temporarily lose emotional support when others react negatively to them. Nevertheless, mothers tell us they make the choice whenever they believe their child's good care depends on it.

Another common thread is that women find it difficult to take relief time. A few mothers talk about getting out with friends, but not many and not often. Mothers with children on treatment rarely take time for themselves, spending what little spare time they have in caring for siblings, husbands, or even helping other families. In general, mothers seem to appreciate the need for a break but need active encouragement to actually take it.

> I had one cousin who came every other week and did my nails. That sounds so vain. But nothing else in my life was normal. I didn't live with my family, shower where I normally showered, or sleep where I normally slept. I had no control over anything in my life. That one thing, it cheered me up, a feminine thing. One hour out of the hospital every other week. It's not so bad to take a break.— *Tina*

Generally, mothers are able to find support. They have good connections at the hospital to medical staff and to other parents. The primarily female staff relates well to mothers and their coping styles. When mothers ask for support, they usually get it—from professionals, other families, and friends. Psychologist Shelley Taylor and her colleagues have coined a new term for the style of coping used by women: "tend and befriend" (see the Bibliography). Under stress, women often do not show the traditional "fight-or-flight" response, the way men do. Instead, they respond to stressful situations through nurturing themselves and their children (the tend part) and forming networks with a larger social group, especially with other women (the befriend part).

Gentle Reminders for Mothers

- Don't try to be Supermom; ask for and accept help.
- Don't be daunted; you can learn the new skills you need. You will stretch and grow, and your child will benefit, as will you. You will become stronger.
- Stop beating yourself up about what you should have known or done, what you ought to be doing better, and matters that are out of your control.
- Take breaks: Let go of guilt long enough to take a walk, take a bubble bath, meet a friend for a cup of coffee, listen to music, or take a nap.
- Don't wait for anger and resentment to boil over; if something is bothering you, say so.
- Share your feelings with family members, and listen to their feelings.

Fathers

Fathers of children with cancer are hurting, too. Yet, because their responses are different from mothers', they may be overlooked or misunderstood. Social worker and psychotherapist Thomas Golden states, "The masculine side of healing is not as accepted a mode of healing as the more traditional verbal and emotional expressions. It tends to be quieter, less visible, less connected with the past and more connected with the future; less connected with passivity and more aligned with action" (see the Bibliography). While his professional focus is on healing from grief, these observations apply quite well to men's general styles of coping.

> Isolation is the worst possible counselor.
> Miguel de Unamuno,
> *Civilization Is Civilism* (1914)

Fathers' coping methods and needs may be at cross-purposes. Traditional cultural or societal expectations dictate that fathers should be strong, brave, and in control; take pain and stress "like a man"; defend and protect the family; be knowledgeable; make rational life or death decisions; and continue their jobs as providers or heads of the household no matter how distraught they are. It might seem normal for men to be angry, active, or aggressive when under duress. In many circles, however, it is not acceptable for them to be vulnerable, sad, or passive or to ask for help. In defining their role, many men are still torn between their emotions and their expected image. The pressure fathers put on themselves to adhere to the ideal makes coping and resolving of issues more difficult for them, and sometimes their families, in the long run.

One feels a bit of a failure. Traditionally, the father is the breadwinner and guards the family and tries to ward off unhappiness. When cancer arrives there is nothing one can do. Our beautiful family has suffered a tremendous blow, and there is nothing that Dad (or anyone else) can do to stop it or improve the outcome.—*Jake*

* * *

I believe a father's responsibility is to take care of his family and wife, to make sure the wife and children get what they need. Their needs come first, your needs are a distant second. During very difficult times, your life must stop, and 100 percent of your effort must be focused on helping them. Of course, you have to maintain your job, but otherwise your personal wants are immaterial. Frankly, I see a lot of men hide behind their job as a way of avoiding family responsibility. It's easier to work than meet the emotional needs of the family. Sometimes you have to be the bad guy with a difficult doctor, you have to make sure your wife gets a break, you have to deal with anything that your wife is having difficulty with. This perspective is not met well by men or women in our culture.—*Ken*

* * *

> It's bad enough dealing with the fact that your child has this horrible disease, but to see your wife in such agony and despair is equally devastating.—*Lou*

To keep functioning and maintain routine roles, too many fathers have to shut down emotionally. They avoid verbal expression of their feelings. Instead, they talk about medical facts or others' reactions. Feeling responsible for protecting the feelings of their wives and children, some hesitate to broach or respond to emotional issues. The wives then see their husbands as uncaring or unfeeling and almost universally expressed a wish for them to show emotions, although some are taken aback when they do. By dint of long social training, men in general are much better at compartmentalizing than women. They set aside the "cancer parent hat" to focus on work or other tasks. To do this, men tend to cut off feelings in a flurry of activity or in a protective wall of silence that gets them through the day.

Not all men fit this picture, but many do. Nurse and bereavement counselor Sherry Johnson found more success by asking men what they are thinking instead of what they are feeling (see the Bibliography). Unfortunately, by not expressing their feelings and needs, these men are cut off from many good sources of support. Stoicism is not strength; it is repression. We should note that under limited circumstances, repression (pushing something so far down that it is out of consciousness) is a helpful strength. It allows both men and women to gain temporary distance from feelings, to avoid being overwhelmed to the point of dysfunction.

> You have to try to keep your wits about you. You're so overwhelmed with emotion. I heard this so many times, well, you're the father. You have to be strong. Yeah, but who do I turn to cry on? Sometimes, I did feel very alone. Because I didn't feel like I could crack in front of anybody. I cried a lot when I was by myself.—*Al*

* * *

> I remember Bill holding Austin on his lap and saying, "Nothing in my life will ever surprise me again." And it was like this big metal gate came crashing down. He didn't want to get close to anybody after that. It was so painful. His child was in kidney failure, on oxygen, yet when people asked how Austin was doing, he'd say fine. He would talk to other people at the hospital and not talk to me or to Austin. It was months before I could say you have to touch this child; he misses you. It took me that long to understand it was his sadness, and I couldn't be there for him, as he couldn't be there for me.—*Rosemary*

* * *

> Like many men, Geoff focused on the aspects he could control—money, medicine. He didn't show much in the way of emotion—he held it all inside. I don't think he gave our daughters much of an opportunity to let things out, either. I think that's one reason they

> both wanted me to be with them—they didn't have to pretend or put on a good show. Geoff often expected Anne to be brave when it was hard for her to do so. She felt safe throwing a fit with me, and sometimes we all need to throw a fit!—*Pam*

Fathers get less outside support than mothers and, as a result, feel uncared for. Rarely does anyone else ask how they are holding up—asking only about the child or the wife. Then again, fathers rarely offer the information themselves. Fathers have very few chances to talk with other fathers of children with cancer. Friends may be of little support, being uncomfortable themselves with breaking down emotional walls. To remedy this situation, both a mother and a grandmother (in separate families) reported having to call up her husband's friend and suggest a phone call or a basketball game as a chance to talk. Single fathers, stepfathers, and noncustodial fathers are at particular risk for having to cope alone. They may have a hard time figuring out what their role should be.

While mothers are jealous of what they perceive as the father having free time or a refuge from medical responsibilities, many fathers report feeling jealous of the time the mother has with the child, in addition to the support and connections she has.

> In times of trouble or pain my son naturally wants his mommy. He doesn't hate daddy, he just wants mommy to be there if he has a choice. As a dad, you feel cut out at times. —*Darius*

* * *

> In our situation, Maureen wasn't working full-time, which was fortunate, because she could devote time to taking care of him. In one way I was grateful, and in another way I was jealous. Jealous that she would have more time with him, when we didn't know how much time we'd have. I was also relieved, in a way, that I could get away and find a refuge at work. I didn't have to face some of the more difficult times. I look back and I wish she didn't have to go through those times and I could have been there more with her.—*Ben*

Too often, staff mistakenly sees fathers as uninvolved, angry, or unfeeling. Even if a father plays a large role in the medical care and hospital time of his child, he may have difficulty establishing a relationship with staff.

> Last time I took the kids to the pediatrician, I couldn't get a word in. She looked past me and spoke directly to my child about which kind of antibiotic would be better for her. When I challenged the pediatrician on this, she said flatly that most fathers don't know anything about their children's medical situations. The nurse who was supposed to teach both me and my wife how to flush lines and change dressings showed the procedure to both of us, let her try it, and left.—*Leon*

Glenda Thompson, a clinical nurse specialist, told us the following story:

> As his 4-year-old son Bobby's disease progressed, Bob withdrew and became increasingly angry with the staff, spending shorter periods of time at the hospital. The night Bobby died, Bob comforted his wife and daughters and asked to be left alone. His tone was very abrupt and angry. Bob wanted to carry his son's body to the morgue. The staff protested, remarking on his recent hostile behavior, and speculated about him damaging the morgue, running way with the body, or harming staff. Bob stated, "I am a policeman and I know what the morgue looks like. No one can stop me from carrying my son to the morgue." Bob wrapped his son in a blanket and carried him in his arms just as he would have carried him in life. He helped me wrap the body in the shroud, kissed his son's head and rolled the pullout into the holding unit. As we walked back to the ward, Bob thanked me for helping him. He stated, "These last days have been rough for everyone. A lot of people do not understand why I wanted to do this. My baby was dying, and I could not do anything to help him or save him. This was the last thing I could do for my son." I realized that Bob was accustomed to being in control of things, being the one that rescues and defends others. Yet he could do nothing to protect or save his own child. The simple act of taking his child on that last walk was his way of caring for his child. I am thankful to have had the opportunity to help this father ease his pain and grief.

There is another telling result that shows the impact of differing parent roles, according to the authors Mark Chesler and Carla Parry (see the Bibliography). Since mothers are usually the link between the family and the medical care system, they are more steeped in the culture of the child's illness. Men get information about their child's illness, treatment, and progress through their wives. This is second-hand information, interpreted and controlled by the wife. Some fathers come to resent the messenger.

> Whenever I had questions, I had to write them down and get my wife to ask the oncologist. I could tell she thought my questions were stupid. She'd tell me what she thought the answer was. I'd have to tell her, just ask him, okay? A lot of times she was right, but I needed to know for sure from the expert.—*Paul*

* * *

> I usually didn't go to the clinic, because I had to work. But I'd call my wife's cell phone, during the meeting with the doctor, to get the scoop on what was happening that day. I could ask whatever questions I needed to, and he and I could understand each other. —*Walter*

Fathers feel responsible for balancing home and work obligations. They feel pressure to pay the bills, maintain health insurance, take siblings to games or music lessons, and mow the lawn. There may be added household or child-rearing responsibilities that their wives temporarily cannot do. Some men chafe at this, just as some women have trouble relinquishing the job. Employers expect fathers to maintain their productivity, although the men are frequently preoccupied or need time off. Careers can be negatively affected in terms of missed opportunities, decrease in income, or delay of promotion. Some fathers regret that they cannot just drop everything and stay with child.

> There's always a balancing act, trying to deal with work. My employer was very accommodating, but I had demands that had to be met. I heard people say they wouldn't stay at the office, they'd be at the hospital. If it were an accident or something short-term, you could drop everything and deal with it. But when you're dealing with something that extends over months or years, you can't just leave everything. I always felt guilty, no matter what I was doing.—*Carlos*

* * *

> Despite everything, I still have to work. When Will is sick and I am not able to spend much time with him, I get very stressed. Yet I have to be professional at work. Some people at work worry over trivial matters, and I want to say, "Hey, none of this matters, your son does not have cancer, lighten up and get a life." However, one has to suppress this emotion and pretend that whatever that person is saying is important and *will be* acted upon. I also have to entertain clients and frankly, I find it difficult to be happy and cheery when my mind is a million miles away.—*Edward*

The high pressure to cope stoically leads some men to escapist behavior. They cannot fight, so they flee. Escape can mean keeping super busy, throwing oneself into work, or doing something physical. More serious and damaging escapes include drinking and drugs or running away and abandoning the family. While it is certainly true that women indulge in these behaviors too, finding escape routes is more common among men. Some escape attempts are adaptive and some are not.

> Before Tyrese was born, we were working on the house. As soon as Tyrese went into the hospital, it was to hell with the house. Now, working on the house is a good outlet for Marcus because it takes his mind off the troubles for a while and gives him a break.—*Dee*

* * *

> My husband's alcoholism just made everything worse. We were alternating working hours: He worked days and I worked nights. I put my foot down and told him he absolutely could not drink when he was caring for our daughter. He needed to have all his faculties, in case there was an emergency. At the very least, he needed to be able to drive. He was able to stop during her treatment. But when it was over, he started in again and just completely went off the deep end. Ultimately, it cost him his job and our marriage.—*Lois*

Fathers who cope effectively say the grown-up response to the stress is to face it and deal with it. The message is "You have handled challenges before, you can handle this one."

Gentle Reminders for Fathers

- Be a full participant in the treatment process.
- Share your feelings with family members, and listen to their feelings.
- Express the impact of illness on your sense of self, your ability to continue to work and provide for the family, and your visions of the future.
- Be willing and able to ask for help, and accept it.
- Explore what you have learned from the experience and how your role in the family has changed for better or worse.
- Share your thoughts, feelings, fears, and hopes with other fathers of children with cancer; don't fight this alone.

Marriage and Partnership

If you're scared, just holler and you'll find it ain't so lonesome out there.
Joe Sugden, *Baseball Is a Funny Game* (1960)

Having a child with a serious illness tests a marriage. The experience of having a child with cancer puts an extra spotlight on the differences between men and women's coping styles. For marriages that already have cracks in the foundation, the cracks may get deeper. A good foundation can bring you through adversity, although it may not be easy at times. Couples that support each other, respect each other, communicate, and compromise are able to cope with the cancer crisis as a team.

When our son was diagnosed, I said to my husband, "If we have to go through this, I am so glad that I have you here to go through it with—I could choose no one better." And it has held true. All I can add is, we have a ton of humor in our marriage. I call us the "clown arounds." Although we have cried together, we have laughed together many, many more times. We have had a few rough moments, but our deep caring for one another has gotten us past them. We are bound together with perhaps fragile threads, but there are so many threads that the ties are strong as steel.—*Anita*

* * *

In the years before Christie's diagnosis it seemed that during troubled times, one of us was more needy and the other could be there for that person. In the days of treatment I desperately needed my best friend. Unfortunately, he needed the same thing from me, and neither of us had the strength to give. We tried very hard to talk—we always presented a united front to the medical people around us and to family and friends. It took a lot of effort. Today we work very hard at caring—I don't understand how he grieves anymore than he understands how I grieve. When he went for a week-long fishing trip, he went with my blessing though I cried for days. I don't understand why he had to go, but I care enough about him that I want him to do whatever he needs to do to make his hurt go away. Those days when I can't be a loving understanding wife I can at least treat him with the common courtesy that I would offer any stranger in pain.—*Lenore*

Differing Coping Styles

Men and women cope differently. Consider the typical scenario, in which the wife wants to share her feelings and the husband needs not to talk. There are conflicting wants and expectations of each other. Each thinks the other is insensitive, and both end up angry, defensive, and distant. If one partner tries to make the other conform to a particular style, there will be a clash.

It's as if you said to your husband, here is a 500-pound weight; if you love me, you will pick this up. And obviously he can't. It's not that he doesn't love you, or doesn't want to. He physically and emotionally can't. Well, that's what you're asking him to do when you ask him to follow your style. I keep thinking that in my head when I'm so frustrated. —*Holly*

* * *

I think in the immediate. What do we need to do right now, to cure Charlotte? I want to know if she can go on a ride at Disney World. My wife worries about what will happen down the road, like will Charlotte be able to have children. I try to comfort my wife. I tell her we'll cross that bridge when we come to it.—*Lenny*

Division of Labor

There has always been a division of labor between been men and women in families. Not because men can only do one kind of work and women another, but because it is more efficient to spread out the work responsibilities. In the cancer world, there are a lot of added responsibilities, and shifts occur in normal roles at home. Work goes most smoothly when all parties are able to share responsibilities fairly and to give each other breaks. One extended family instinctively divided the jobs amongst themselves in a way that made sense for each member's capabilities: practically, geographically, and emotionally. One side of the family took charge of the mother, the sick child, and the medical tasks; the other took charge of the father, the siblings, and the life routines. Together, the two sets of grandparents shared the financial responsibility of hiring household help for the family.

> I stayed by the bedside, all the time. Mitch was my hunter-gatherer. He would go out and get food, go home and get more clothes. He would go to work, go home, feed the cats, take out the garbage, mow the lawn, and come back.—*Debra*

* * *

> I did the shots, even though I hate needles. My wife just couldn't do one more thing to hurt our son. I told her I'll do it, that will be my job.—*Mike*

* * *

> When I was diagnosed at 18, I wanted my mother. She was there everyday, doing all those little things she did when I was little, whatever I needed at the hospital. My dad was a salesman, so his schedule was fluid and he would "drop in" over the course of the day, for short visits. My father's visits created a different experience for me. He reminded me that I hadn't always been sick and wouldn't always be sick. Both my parents made me laugh, but my mother's humor was centered around the hospital and the events there. My father reminded me that there was a world I really wanted to get back to. Both were absolutely essential in my recovery, but had, as I understand it now, different functions. My mom allowed me to be a child in her arms. My dad reminded me that I also wanted to live to grow up. I don't want this to sound like stereotypes that fathers are part of the world, while moms are part of hearth and home. Because I think these are artificial divisions. I think both parents can play either part and do. But I do think it is important that both parts be there. The day-to-day nursing and care-taking which is absolutely essential to getting well, but is inherently regressive, balanced with a reminder/push of the world that lies ahead, a progressive tug so to speak.—*Linda Goettina (Zame), a psychoanalyst and survivor*

Impact on the Relationship

Having little time to be a couple, many parents deeply miss the intimacy, friendship, and support that should be part of marriage. Some parents give up, but most try very hard to hang on.

> How can you love me if you don't understand who I am? That's where my doubt comes from. Part of me feels this isn't working, I want to be out of this marriage. Then, I turn around and say, there's nobody else in this world that knows the pain we went through. He is so much a connection, how can I walk away from this? How can I justify to my son that it's because of this that we're not together anymore?—*Laurel*

When each of you is hurting, you may be unable to support the other. Your partner, lover, friend, or confidant is now less emotionally available.

> You put on the Camp Counselor persona for your kids, you lock it all away from work, and the person you count on the most, your partner, is so tied up in her own version of the same hell that she can't be any more help to you than you can be to her.—*Brian*

* * *

> Our sole focus was on him. It was hard to relate to each other. You're with the child a lot and can't talk freely. The result was some alienation. I felt somewhat distant and somewhat numb. I had no thoughts of ever breaking up or leaving, but she talked on those terms at times. A sense of real love is so much deeper than the surface emotions that can change so quickly. By staying faithful to that love, we were able to get past that temporary difficulty and back to a fully loving, engaged relationship.—*Bert*

* * *

> We were great parents, but lousy spouses. For two years, the only time we were in the same room together was a hospital room. It's very difficult to have any type of relationship. In the first few weeks, the rabbi that had married us came to talk to us. He said, "Remember that you love each other. And this is your child together. Things will happen, you will say horrendous things to each other. You have to know it doesn't count." He was the only person that ever mentioned our marriage.—*Ellen*

Anger is often taken out on each other, because spouses are convenient targets.

> Neither of us ever had much free time to do anything. It became the prized possession. Well, you spent four hours playing golf. When is my time? Well, you went to the supermarket? Excuse me? That doesn't count! That was the biggest issue. You had 45 minutes, and I only had 10. Then you realize, what are we arguing about?—*Laurel*

* * *

> During and after bone marrow transplant we were extremely angry at each other, for no particular reason but that the other person was there to be angry at, and we couldn't *be* angry at our son.—*Madeleine*

Often, there is a tacit agreement to shelve the marriage until later and focus on the children and what most benefits the family as a whole. As long as both parties are comfortable with this arrangement, it can work. You may even find a new appreciation for each other. However, if major issues are festering, the idea can backfire, widening the distance between you. After the crisis of treatment is over, the relationship may deteriorate further. If that happens, it is important to make clear, to each other and to the children, that the break-up was not caused by the cancer or by the child with cancer.

> Spouses need to understand that they are both so scared and hurting that they may not be able to get much from each other because neither has much to give. If there's less pressure, if there's the agreement that this sucks and we're both doing our best and keeping expectations low, it's easier.—*Brian*

* * *

> Our marriage was on the rocks for a long time. Obviously the cancer fight dealt a serious blow, but the flaws in our relationship pre-dated cancer, and I have my doubts if we would have made it anyway. Why is this so important? Because I don't want my son to ever think that he was in any way responsible for his parents' divorce. My point is that our divorce was not caused by the stress of a child with cancer. Our divorce was caused by our inability to deal with each other.—*Melissa*

Some marriages grow stronger, despite and because of the experience.

> I have such deep respect for my wife's talents and gifts. I always did, but they really came out in taking care of our boy with a depth I hadn't completely seen before, and I'm more in awe of her than ever.—*Edmund*

* * *

> Our marriage is better than it was before Alicia's cancer. We spent a lot of time in marriage counseling during and after cancer. The things we learned about ourselves and each other continue to help us work on our relationship. It's probably one of the greatest gifts Alicia's cancer brought us. I also know we appreciate each other and the beauty around us every day in a way that no other experience could have given us.—*Margaret*

Sex

Sex is a delicate and private issue, but it is an important factor in any marriage or adult partnership. Everyone needs personal ways to express affection, love, connection, and intimacy physically. It may bring them closer in difficult times, be an affirmation of life, be an outlet for feelings, relieve stress, or just be a distraction. Sex can be an emotional release, as well as a physical one. Some partners find themselves bursting into tears. Other partners may feel too tired or emotionally drained to have sex or guilty for doing something selfish. Many parents said that it felt like just another chore, one more thing that somebody wanted from them, particularly if they had no time to be together to talk or have a full relationship. Others resented being "serviced," or living like "roommates."

My husband felt neglected. He believes when two people love each other, and they're stressed, they should want to hold each other, and make love. I had no interest in sex at all. It was one more chore, when I already was doing all the care, and was sleep-deprived. I felt he was kicking me when I was down. But, the kids are going to grow up and go away, and my husband is still going to be here. I want to have a good marriage. We're making a conscious effort now to find more time for us. Trying to get the kids down at a certain time, shut the TV off and talk, hold hands, give a backrub. Even just sit next to each other on the couch. It's a start that has made us feel closer.—*Anna*

* * *

On a practical level, our son Gregory sleeps so poorly that we sleep in different bedrooms; one of us "does" Gregory one night and gets little or no sleep. The next night whoever has "done" Gregory the night before goes into the spare room to insure a good night's sleep. In short, we feel knocked out every other day, and the physical separation does not, at the risk of stating the obvious, do our sex life any good.—*Jake*

Gentle Reminders for Partners

- Together with family members, figure out which coping styles and behaviors meet each other's needs and which do not.
- Communicate both ways: Listen as well as talk, and fight "fair" (see chapter 5).
- Compromise must be a two-way street: Meet each other half way.
- Take turns and share duties both at home and at the hospital.
- Support your partner's style of coping and contributing, even though it's different than your own.
- Go together to important events and consultations, such as major surgery. It provides strength and solidarity for yourself and for your child.
- Support rather than undermine each other's relations with children, family, and medical personnel.
- Understand that your child may gravitate to one parent or prefer that parent's support out of habit or because that parent's coping style is complementary to the child's. It doesn't mean that your child doesn't love both parents, only that he or she has very specific needs right now. Continue relationships and offering time with both parents, but be flexible in difficult situations.
- Take advantage of marriage or family counseling if your relationship is floundering.
- Remember that you're on the same team.

Single Parents

Single parents are at greater risk of burnout, because they shoulder all of the burdens themselves. There is no built-in partner to take turns, give you breaks, bring you clean clothes at the hospital, pick up siblings at school, support the family financially, and so on. Quitting work to care for the child may be unthinkable. Practical obligations pull you in one direction, emotional obligations in another. Without someone to share the responsibility of making difficult decisions and living with the results, the task may weigh more heavily on you.

> The best thing about being a single parent facing childhood cancer: all the decisions were mine alone. The worst thing about being a single parent facing childhood cancer: all the decisions were mine alone. I never had to discuss options or compromise on what I felt needed to be done. There was never any question my daughter's treatment and care would be done my way. On the other hand, that left me totally responsible, a burden I felt all the time. If the decisions I made were the wrong ones, there was no one to turn to but me, no one to share that agony with. At times when it was too heavy a load to carry, there was no one there but me. At times when the success was so wonderful I wanted to share the joy, there was no one there but me.—*Yvonne*

It is especially important for you to use and expand your support network to include extended family members, friends, community resources, and support groups. We know one mother who moved 1,000 miles to another state, transferring her child's treatment to another facility, to be near her own mother for support and aid. The aunt of another child stayed regularly in the hospital so that the child's mother could go to her job. This mother, like others in the same situation, frequently called the nurse's station to monitor medical care. In the workplace, colleagues' donated sick leave and vacation time for cancer parents is a boon.

> My 4-year-old daughter and I were staying alone in a Ronald McDonald House. She was not allowed near other people, so she was restricted to her room. I would leave her watching videos while I made quick trips to get food, or videos, or to do laundry. When I explained this to my sister-in-law, she insisted that I call someone to sit with my daughter every time I left the room. I pointed out that there weren't enough volunteers. She insisted adamantly that if a county social services agency found out about this, they would take my child out of my custody. She was totally clueless about the day-to-day realities of single-parenting a special-needs child.—*Rona*

* * *

Hey, I'm a single mom, I work full-time, and I did the chemo thing alone and care for her now alone. And I'm not anything special. I'm just a mom who does what she has to do each day. It ain't easy. There are times when you are doing three things at once, and a line is forming for your attention. Life is now an adventure. When people ask me how I'm doing and I answer "fine," it is a whole new level of a lie.—*Eloise*

* * *

The biggest problem with being a single parent, whether or not your child is sick, is always being "on-duty." The single parent needs to work harder to be prepared for emergencies. I used to keep a packed "hospital bag" in the trunk of my car at all times, so that if a call came from day care that Rae had a fever, I could pick her up and drive to the hospital, prepared to stay. I lost about eight months of work time because I was in the hospital so much. The only reason I stayed employed, drawing an income and covered by health insurance, is because fellow employees at my company donated their leave time. This is a big financial problem: you can't drop back to one income, because you only had one income to begin with. I was very, very fortunate in the generosity of my colleagues.—*Naomi*

Of course, the other tips and coping strategies apply to you, but they go double for you. There are some additional suggestions that are particular to your situation.

Gentle Reminders for Single Parents

- Cultivate partnerships with trusted friends and family, a competent child care provider, home care or visiting nurses, teachers and school nurses, volunteers, and others in the community.
- Educate your helpers about your child's illness, home care duties, procedures, warning signs, and emergency plans. Write these in a notebook, or make up a poster or flyer for handy reference. Make sure they have contact info for you, the doctors, the hospital, siblings, and other helpers.
- Ask your stand-ins to come to the hospital with you, to be familiar with the facility, staff, and treatment protocol and so that staff gets to know them. The child will feel more stable when the stand-in is confident and comfortable. Enlist stand-ins to stay with child at the hospital when you can't be there (several people can share duties).
- Work out guidelines with staff to keep you in the loop when you're not there. Insist that procedures or exams not be done without you, your representative, a social worker, or a child life specialist present; develop a relationship with nurse

Box continues next page

Continued

or supervisor who will call you with updates; request continuity of nursing staff (a familiar face is comforting to a child); ask the social worker, child life specialist, or hospital volunteers to make sure your child gets recreation time (company, time in the play room); and work out menus with the hospital food services provider for projected hospital stay.

- Arrange for flexibility with your employer: Use donated leave time, telecommute, work different hours, cut back on hours, and ask if coworkers or temps can cover some of your hours or take over some of your duties.
- Be reachable: Use a beeper or cell phone, and faithfully charge the batteries.
- Swallow your pride; be willing to accept help, and don't try to be super-parent. Solicit financial assistance (see chapter 2), and have someone live with you such as family or a nanny.
- Join a support group, talk to a therapist, or unload on a friend.
- Give your time only to those things that absolutely require it or are worthy of you.
- Take time for yourself to recharge.
- Use your feet to hold baby or toddler's arms when giving GCSF shots or changing dressings; use a mobile, video, or some other distraction.
- If you have a relationship with a noncustodial parent, do everything possible to improve it and enlist that person's help. Bury the hatchet. Get counseling, use a mediator, and agree to shelve old issues until later. In the unfortunate instance that your ex refuses, cut your losses and get help from someone else.

Siblings

Parents regret that they have little time or energy left to spend on their healthy children, precisely when those children need attention and reassurance. Parents are at a loss as to how to make it better. Time they do spend goes toward meeting basic needs. The most loving caretaker cannot fill parents' shoes. Sibling workshop director Donald Meyer told us, "I'm of the belief that the best thing you can do for young siblings of children with cancer is to educate the parents about sibling issues, so they can head them off at the pass."

> Looking back, maybe we could have done better and given Kate jobs to do so she felt more a part of the process. While we did what was best for Anne, Kate's feelings were just as

> important, and we should have found a way to honor them, too. We didn't do that enough, and I think we're paying the price.—*Pam*

Do not beat yourself up over what you could have done better. As one father astutely observed, "Even if our kids didn't have cancer we'd be sitting here saying I wish I'd done this differently or that differently. We muddle through." The fact is this will be difficult for the siblings, along with everyone else in the family. You cannot recover the losses. The best you can do is to be aware of the sibling's needs, acknowledge them, and foster healthy growth and development in ways that are available and possible, under your particular circumstances. Over time, most siblings are able to incorporate difficult life experiences and make a good adaptation to life.

> Marisa wanted to write a book for siblings when her sister was sick. She wrote some things, but then she moved on, she kind of buried it. Marisa is 18 now. Recently, a lot of feelings started to come out when she wrote about those experiences for her college application essays. She's designing her own degree, combining psychology and child life. She plans to go on to law school after college. Her goal is to be a child advocate. She will be a wonderful advocate for anyone's rights she believes in, she's a fighter.—*Estella*

Children in larger families seem quite often to have an advantage. Multiple siblings serve as a built-in peer support group: someone else who knows exactly what they're going through, more hands to divide up added responsibilities, companionship, buffers from the outside world, less pressure to "be good" or achieve more, fewer comparisons to sick child. This is particularly evident in cases of lasting debilitating effects or in coping with the death of the child with cancer.

Siblings' emotions parallel those of their parents, yet they have a different perspective, due to their age, position in the family, and dearth of resources. It is most helpful to focus on helping the sibling adjust to a highly stressful situation rather than viewing him or her as a "problem child." One mother and sibling advocate shared her belief that cancer is only one aspect of the siblings' lives, and other things will influence the people they become. Although not at any greater risk for mental illness, siblings may have some behavior problems and emotional distress.

Siblings' Reactions and Feelings

Like mothers, fathers, and other family members, siblings have their own emotional reactions to cancer. The following list contains some of their more troublesome issues.

What Bothers Siblings

Worry about sibling's health and ability to cope
Fear of catching cancer
Fantasy that they caused the cancer
Guilt at normal sibling rivalry
Guilt that they're not the sick one
Isolation from family: sibling in the hospital, parents not at home, nobody to talk to
Isolation from peers: fewer social outings, friends don't understand, living at grandma's
Lack of attention; feeling abandoned, rejected, lonely, left out, unimportant
Resentment and jealousy
Acute and chronic stress, posttraumatic symptoms
Long-term worries: health of own children
Sick child gets preferential treatment, rules of discipline change to benefit sick child
Increased responsibilities, chores
Anger at parents, sick child, God, world
Ambivalent feelings toward sibling, parents
Unpredictability of events, lack of control
Embarrassment, shame
Family role shifts
Depression, guilt at negative emotions
Loss of "normal" childhood
Disruption of routines
Confusion, misinformation, lack of information, or limited grasp of information
Anxiety they can't pinpoint or explain

Siblings can experience so many negative emotions without an adult's perspective and ready support. Their world has been thrown into turmoil, but they have no power to do anything about it. The basic emotions of fear, anxiety, anger, jealousy, guilt, sadness, and grief take many forms. Remember, not all of your child's emotions will be cancer-related. They will also have regular, positive emotions. They have good days where they are carefree and able to be delighted with the world and themselves.

- Siblings are *afraid* that they somehow caused the cancer; that they will catch cancer, too; that the sick child will die; that the family is falling apart; and that they will be abandoned.
- Siblings are *anxious* because they do not understand how their sibling got sick, what cancer is, how these horrible treatments can possibly help, the fact that all the adults are acting stressed and worried, and just generally things are not right. Siblings have no control over events, and at any time there might be an emergency. The future is uncertain, and stability is gone: Every day as they go to school, there is no guarantee that mom, dad, or the sick child will be there when they get home. They never know when someone else might pick them up, they might have to stay with relatives or miss an activity, their friends can't come over, or their birthday party might get cancelled.

- Siblings are *angry* at the sick child for getting sick and ruining everything, at parents for not paying attention to them, and at the world because it does not seem good anymore. Everything has changed, and nobody asked them if that was okay.
- Siblings are *jealous* because the sick child gets all the attention and gifts and is excused from chores and does not have to go to school or do homework. Siblings *resent* having to still do chores and homework and take up the slack for the sick child and not even get a present for it.
- Siblings feel *guilty* that they are not the one who got sick, that they're causing more trouble for their parents, that they still yell at their brother or sister for doing something annoying, for thinking bad thoughts about parents or the sick child, and for all the previous negative emotions.
- Siblings *grieve* for their losses and for those of their family—the loss of a normal life and childhood, vacations, and carefree happiness.
- Sibling feel horribly *left out* and left alone. The sick brother or sister is at the hospital or stays home from school. The parents are physically absent or completely absorbed in caring for the sick child. Without being a part of the treatment process, having a job to do, or having any say, the sibling feels like a fifth wheel. Everybody asks about the sick child, but nobody asks the sibling how he or she is doing or notices his or her *A* on a spelling test.

When siblings try to express these negative feelings, they may be met with a dismissal or a guilty pleading request for good behavior and more patience from the parent. Either one can feel bad to the child. In a misguided ranking of worries, adults may downplay the sibling's feelings, saying, "But look at what your brother's going through, that's much worse." In that case, the sibling is likely to stop expressing his feelings, and they fester. Siblings really appreciate parents' genuine reassurances of caring about their plight, too.

A smaller subset of siblings are older, nearly grown. They may have already left the home to work or go to college. These siblings may feel relieved that they are somewhat removed from all the turmoil and have busy lives to distract them. Parents may feel the same relief, in that they can focus more time and energies on the sick child. On the other hand, older siblings may also feel guilty for being "out of the loop," not being home to help, or being so occupied with their own lives that they don't think about the sick child or parents every minute. While they are nearly adults and can handle their emotions with more maturity, they are still siblings, and have many of the same issues as younger children. Parents need to find a balance between overrelying on a older sibling (who needs to live his or her own life and isn't quite ready for the responsibility) and cutting him or her out of the picture (who still wants to be kept informed, continue relationships with the family, and be involved in some capacity).

How Siblings Express Their Needs

Siblings may withdraw; eat and talk less; act out in negative, attention-getting ways; regress to younger age behavior; show increased separation anxiety (such as being afraid to leave mom or dad); develop phobias; have poor self-esteem; or be negative, moody, or irritable. Siblings may have a heightened physical awareness; recurring worries about their own bodies and health; or body-based distress symptoms including bedwetting, headaches, stomachaches, insomnia, vague aches and pains, and changes in their eating and sleeping habits. Their academic performance may slip, or they may get into trouble at school or have trouble concentrating. To protect or comfort their parents, some siblings do not ask for help; they try to act normal or to be "extra good" by suppressing their negative emotions and taking care of others.

> I get the brunt of Mark's resentment. Recently, I spent the whole day with him. We went marketing, did artwork, had lunch out. It was a wonderful day. He said, "This is making up for when you spent all that time in the hospital with Sam. You kept saying we were going to do things together, and now finally we've done something." I do cub scouts, I'm his room parent, I go on class trips, I do the yearbook, he has friends over. But the one day I say John can't come to dinner, he's stamping his feet, shouting it's not fair. Sometimes I get very angry about that. I'm sure parents who don't have sick kids have this. But Mark just throws this extra garbage on me. Take the shovel out and pile it on me. No matter what I do, why even bother, because it's not going to be right. Meanwhile, all his friends want to move into my house, 'cause he's got it so good.—*Barbara*

Without attentive responses, some of these patterns can be long-term. The reverberations may last into adulthood, coloring relationships and well-being. One woman described a grown sibling who continues even now to compete with her for their mother's attention. Another adult sibling worried when his own son had an illness and couldn't rest easy until the doctors tested his child for the leukemia that his brother had years before.

> Jennifer was between 3 and 5 years old during her brother's treatment. Her world view was being shaped. She wanted attention and became a hypochondriac. That stays with her to this day. We've dealt with it through counseling. For her, the world at that time was a terrifying place. They put a Broviac in her brother, and she'd say, "when am I going to get mine? Is my hair going to fall out?"—*Val*

* * *

> Toward the end of Ron's treatment, Andy's personality changed, and he got super attached to me. He didn't want to leave my side. He and Ron have extreme sibling rivalry going on right now, because he never got to enjoy the perks of being the baby of the family. Andy

didn't understand what was wrong with his brother; he just wanted me. He said, "Mommy, come home and take care of me, I'm sick of Grandma."—*Eleanor*

Siblings' perspectives can surprise parents.

Connor wanted to dress his brother up like a skeleton on Halloween so he could ring the doorbell say trick or treat and Brandon could pop his (prosthetic) eye out! He thought that was the coolest thing!—*Tracy*

* * *

As a parent, you view the children in the clinic as invalids. One time, I brought Mike's brother Charlie to the clinic. Charlie matter-of-factly started playing a video game with the kids like nothing was wrong with them. You forget they're just kids.—*Fred*

Parents report changes in siblings' personalities, attitudes, and the relationship they have with the parent. Some are positive changes; others present more difficult challenges.

The hardest thing to watch was what happened to Claudia. It turned her into a not nice person. In the last year or two, she's started coming back around to the likeable kid she was before all this started.—*Henry (grandfather)*

* * *

It forced Michaela to grow up before she had to. A huge chunk of being an innocent teenager was gone. She really stepped up to the plate. She'd get very upset when people would say, "We feel so bad, are you alright"? She'd say, "I'm fine, it's my brother you need to put your energy into." She was so unassuming about donating her bone marrow. Michaela saw it as an accident of genetics that she was the match, not as heroics on her part. This is what you do for somebody you love. She's too together for a 17-year-old.—*Maren*

* * *

Matthew's become extremely adaptable. He gets along with most people. He spent time in a lot of different households, going from grandparents, to aunts, to friends. He dealt with different house rules and watched a lot of siblings interact. He wanted a brother to play with, too. He knows he might have lost his brother. The kids on his camp bus once made fun of Austin for being bald. That really upset Matthew. He never makes fun of anyone. Also, he's close to my parents, because he stayed with them for four months.—*Rosemary*

How You Can Help Your Other Children

Keep the lines of communication open—both ways

Giving age-appropriate information reduces a sibling's anxiety and enhances a feeling of inclusion. It must be an ongoing process of repeating, expanding, and updating the family plans and medical information (even after treatment is over, as the sibling grows and can better understand the details and ramifications). Use a variety of teaching techniques (such as books, videos, workbooks, visual aids, props, and verbal explanations) and a variety of messengers (you, your spouse, medical personnel, and the child life specialist). Educate a sibling's teacher and classmates. Some cancer centers will send staff to a child's school to explain the situation to classmates in easily understood and anxiety-reducing terms. A father told us that hospitals in Milan, Italy, routinely bring the whole family, including the pediatrician, siblings, and extended family, into the diagnostic conference and videotape it. Family members may watch the tape as many times as they wish to help them understand what the doctors said. Children need realistic information in line with their developmental capacities and feel empowered by their ability to explain or answer questions for others.

> Priyanka's teacher allowed her to have five minutes at the end of every Friday to give a "status report" on her brother. She liked the attention and being able to explain everything. The whole class got involved in supporting her.—*Smriti*

Acknowledge siblings' feelings, worries, and needs, and give them plenty of chances to express them. Be wary of minimizing their concerns. Understand that they have different coping styles than adults, and do not expect them to conform to yours. Siblings may not talk about feelings, may hide their distress, may seem uncaring, or may want to stay with friends. Remember that even within the same family, siblings may have different emotional styles. For example, one sibling will want to know everything as a way to reduce anxiety (such as see a scar or understand hospital machinery), whereas the other sibling will want self-protection from graphic realities. Remember also that siblings want to talk about something other than cancer.

Timing is another matter. Siblings may wait until treatment is over before expressing some of their pent-up feelings. They may even wait years to air their grievances. One father noted that his daughter was 22 and teaching at college before she told him of her feelings of being left out and having to be "good" during her sister's illness. When is it safe to let it out? For some, the release feels safer when they're out of the house, on their own, less dependent on parents, and have the distance and perspective they need.

> All the kids had to give a speech on fear in class. My (14-year-old) daughter chose to talk about her fear of her brother dying from cancer. Celeste was surprised that she sounded nervous. Her voice was cracking, and she was shaking a little. I reminded her that when something affects you deeply, it is hard to talk about it without becoming emotional. At the time of his treatment she was in first grade. She never seemed to talk much about the situation except that she missed me. She never seemed to have any problems. So much for my naivete in thinking she came out of this unscathed.—*Delores*

* * *

> Jodi is in a delayed rebellion, which should have hit at 15. I give her more leeway because I know that she knows why she's doing it. She told us, "I had to be so good for so long, and now I don't have to be good anymore." And she's right. If she's an hour late from curfew, she knows we're not happy, but it's her way of taking control.—*Ellen*

Normalize sibling life

Avoid differential or preferential treatment of your children whenever it is feasible. By treating the child with cancer as normally as possible, you are sending a positive, hopeful message to both the sick child and the healthy siblings. If treatment is successful, their relationship with each other will last longer than any other, and it will be more rewarding if they are on equal footing. House rules and chore duties should remain in place. Of course, there will be times when the sick child or the care-giving parent will not be able to perform chores. However, do not just assume or demand that siblings take up all the slack. Enlist their help, stressing that it is a temporary situation and that the family must pull together. State your needs and your appreciation of their assistance. Avoid casting the siblings into a premature parent role as a caretaker of the sick child or other siblings. If there are times when you need them to baby-sit, for example, make sure they get enough time to do something with their friends, too. Take advantage of other adults who offer to help instead.

Because of the focus on the sick child's health, parents may underemphasize sibling's health complaints and symptoms. In that case, the siblings feel unheard and unvalued.

> We thought we were pretty good about making family time. But we were very focused on our son, David, who had leukemia. Our 15-year-old daughter, Bonnie, felt left out. It was almost a year before we found out why she shut herself away. One night, Bonnie said she had a headache. We told her to take some Tylenol. Then David had a leg cramp, and we questioned him at length. Bonnie was very upset. She got physically ill; she vomited. She felt no one cared about her health.—*Don*

A sense of continuity in their lives and relationships helps siblings to cope. Siblings have their own developmental trajectories that need to continue, and they need permission to "go on" with their lives. They need a balance between the focus on cancer and a distraction from it. Teenagers, especially, may need to spend time with friends and continue their usual extracurricular activities such as sports and clubs. Normalize the sibling's relationship with the sick child by ensuring they have time to be together. In addition, give the sibling permission to say flattering and unflattering things about the sick child. Predict absences of the sick child and parents whenever possible. When separations are necessary, leave the sibling with the same caretaker as much as possible, a person he or she is comfortable with and trusts. Parents and other caretakers serve as models for positive coping and a balanced outlook that includes the noncancer parts of life.

Spend as much time as you can with the sibling. More important than the length of time is that it be "individual" time—give the child all of your attention, even if it is only 10 minutes a day. Make the child feel special. Go for a walk or a bike ride, read a story, go out to lunch, play catch, do an art or cooking project together, and ask about his or her day and listen to the answer. Let the child know you need and love him or her, too. Recognize the sibling's own strengths and accomplishments, not just what he or she does for the sick child. Redirect attention to the child tactfully when others focus only on the sick child.

When you cannot be home with siblings, write letters, make audio- or videotapes, talk to them on the telephone daily, or read a favorite bedtime story over the phone or sing a lullaby. Send little notes such as jokes, encouragement, or "I love you" to school in their lunchboxes. Keep a running "conversation" either in a note or with brightly colored magic markers on a poster (roll it up and send it back and forth in a mailing tube). Bring home inexpensive gifts (one mother brought home the mini boxes of cereal from the hospital trays and travel-sized toiletries that were supplied with every in-patient stay), and keep a few little presents on hand to give the sibling when a visitor brings something for the sick child. Ask visitors to remember the sibling if they want to bring gifts. Encourage a friend or relative to "adopt" the sibling and be "Auntie Mame."

Include the sibling in the cancer community

Bringing the sibling with you to the hospital has many advantages. Seeing firsthand what goes on there lets the child see that it is neither a torture chamber nor a vacation spot. At the hospital, they have access to child life specialists and social workers as well as siblings of other patients. Like the sick child, young siblings may need opportunities to explore experiences through medical play. Encourage contact with other siblings to serve as a support network and peer group that can understand their situation. Other siblings can commiserate and share coping ideas.

To keep them involved in the process and give them something to do, let siblings look at blood tests in the lab or watch medications being made up in the pharmacy. If the sibling is young, consider bringing another adult along to the hospital, too. That adult is there to be a buffer, to pay attention to them, and to stay with them when you take the sick child in for a procedure. Older children or teenagers can keep a hospitalized sibling occupied, take him to the playroom, run errands for a child or parent (such as getting a video or food) who is stuck in the room, distract the child during simple procedures (such as blood draws, dressing changes, or mouth care), and generally provide a normalizing atmosphere.

> At our hospital, they allowed siblings to have sleepovers. Colin (age 5) was excited. He had missed me and resented the fact that I was often away from him. We were planning to have fun. As it turned out, it was a very bad night for Ross. Colin had to help me get towels

when Ross was throwing up and call the nurses. The next morning Colin said, "You know what I learned, that it's really not fun when you're this sick." The night of fun I had envisioned wouldn't have been as helpful.—*Mary Jo*

* * *

We brought our other children to the hospital under limited circumstances. They often came to the clinic because that's where the child life therapist was, in the playroom. We didn't try to hide anything, but we tried to protect them from the scary things. The biggest challenge was providing a sense of stability for them. You know how it is, you wake up in the middle of the night with a fevered child whose blood counts are down, you go to the emergency room and end up in the hospital for two weeks.—*Maureen*

Allow siblings to participate in the care of the sick child. Give them a nonthreatening job to do, so they feel important and included. One 5-year-old held her baby sister's hands during central line dressing changes, flushed the nasogastric tube, and built obstacle courses in the living room for physical therapy. A teenager might work with the child life specialist to learn some basic therapeutic play techniques (subtly uncovering her own issues at the same time). Siblings might make a tape for the sick child, telling him what is going on at home, reading stories, telling jokes, or singing songs. Siblings can make decorations for the hospital room or child's room at home, bring school assignments home, or assume care of a pet. Have the sibling make a photo album or a scrap book—the siblings might like to do these projects together. Older children can be included in planning sessions.

Take advantage of sibling programs such as workshops and summer camps. One particularly good program that is held regularly is Sibshops, a program begun by Donald Meyer of the Sibling Support Project at Children's Hospital and Regional Medical Center in Seattle, WA, for siblings of children with developmental disabilities. Sibshops offers ongoing peer support programs across the country for school-age children. They have been adapted for siblings of children with chronic illness, including cancer. The Sibshops model addresses siblings' needs well. The children play games and share insights with each other in a fun atmosphere that is "therapeutic, but not therapy" (see the Resources at the end of this book for contact information).

Pediatric oncology program nurse Cathy Chavez described another useful program: an annual fall sibling retreat.

In one special activity on the last day, parents or grandparents write the siblings a letter. The letters are secret until the group hikes to a special place, where the children receive the letters and read them privately. It is a moving experience. The children treasure their letters, long after the event.

Positive Possibilities for Siblings

Out of difficult experiences, it is still possible for siblings to find positive personal meaning. Examples of creative growth or benefits are

- Knowledge and education, which instills pride and self-confidence in knowing about the illness
- Maturity and responsibility
- Compassion, empathy, and awareness of people's problems
- Adjustment to differences in people and social competence
- Perspective on priorities and a positive outlook
- Appreciation for the "little things"
- Appreciation and empathy for parents
- Tolerance, insight, flexibility, and resilience
- Vocational choices such as child life, advocacy, nursing, medicine, and social work
- Coping skills and problem-solving abilities
- Loyalty—"No one else can beat up my brother"
- Self-discovery and knowing what they want
- Stronger relationship with sibling and family closeness
- Enhanced self-esteem
- Spirituality
- Knowing the value of friendship (people who did not abandon them in time of need)
- Temporary perks, such as the Make-a-Wish Foundation, celebrity visitors, extra gifts, and being first in line at Disney theme parks.

My daughter Karen jokes that she's broken because of what happened to her brother. I explain to her that there's a lot of beautiful light that comes through those cracks.—*Holly*

Extended Family and Friends

The quality of your relationships with people beyond your immediate family during a crisis depends a lot on the quality of the relationship you had before your child got sick. When the relationships are good, people rally and come forward readily. Strained relationships or differences in beliefs (such as medical, religious, or parenting styles) can cause rifts. Old wounds can be reopened. The sick child's grandparents, aunts, uncles, cousins, and so on are all affected.

The greatest thing in family life is to take a hint when a hint is intended—and not to take a hint when a hint isn't intended.
Robert Frost, The Figure a Poem Makes, *Collected Poems* (1939)

If your family lives far away or is emotionally unavailable, you need to seek support elsewhere. Not having family nearby can be a source of added stress and emotional distress. Not having any other relatives nearby, one child's parents made the decision to move, so that her Navy father could be on shore duty and participate in her care. Although it was difficult for the child to adjust to a new hospital and staff, in the long run it was better for her and everyone else if her father could be with the family. Another parent describes her family's lack of support and one way she reached out to get what her family needed:

> Our family and friends did practically nothing for us. Selfish and self-absorbed people do not change when your child gets diagnosed with cancer. At a holiday family get-together, we sat for 4 hours and no one asked us how we were doing or if we needed anything. My mother-in-law says, "This is your life now—stop complaining about it!" Make-a-Wish Foundation built Max a tree house; our neighbors called it "the contraption" and complained that they have to explain what it is to their guests. One of my "friends" e-mailed me a joke about a funeral! My father stopped by the hospital while Max was having a toxic reaction to chemo, and after 5 minutes left me in the hall crying to join the rest of the family at a restaurant for dinner. No one came back to the hospital or even called us to see if Max was ok. What a major let down—and an unforgivable act. One night, I couldn't sleep because I was so angry that no one was acknowledging my beautiful little boy for all he had been through and how brave he was. I wrote a letter to the mayor of our town and asked her to recognize him. Three days after his final chemotherapy treatment, she presented Max with a proclamation for his courage and declared August 18th as his day. I can't tell you how grateful I was to her and how much it meant to all of us.—*Gail*

Impact on Family Members

Grandparents and great-grandparents of the child with cancer struggle with what seems an unnatural progression of the circle of life. One great-grandmother told us, "It should be me. I'm old. I've lived my life. It shouldn't be the baby." Dee summed up her own mother's anguish: "She has feelings and worries about her grandchild who is sick, and feelings and worries for me, too. It's almost like it's double for her." Marilyn, speaking to her adult daughter, put it this way: "You were my baby, and you were hurting. I'd put my arm around you, and smell your hair, and it would take me back to your childhood." Grandparents may feel powerless, in that they are not in charge of the sick child's care, have no authority to make medical decisions, and cannot protect either their own child or the grandchild. Some grandparents may feel the need to "parent" their child is so strong that they try to direct the care of either the sick child or the healthy siblings. This invariably results in a clash of wills. Most grandparents, as well as other family members, take comfort in doing whatever jobs they can to help.

> The greatest impact was at the beginning in the turmoil of emotions: anger, fear, sadness, a feeling of devastation. I questioned, why, why, why? There was a feeling of disbelief that this could happen to people I love and to such an innocent child. I felt helpless, not being able to shield and protect my loved ones. These are feelings and sensations one can never forget and sometimes too easily recall by just hearing a song. No matter where I am, when I hear music from Lion King, which came out at that time, it brings me right back to that spot. Later on, I realized how fortunate we were to have each other to lean on.—*Alexandra, grandmother*

* * *

> As a grandparent my first thoughts were a sense of horror and fear of the future, but especially helplessness. The most frustrating feeling was that I was powerless to do anything to make it all better, to make it all go away and to not be able to protect my granddaughter and my son and his wife from the consequences of this terrible disease. In the past my wife and I were always able to come up with a solution to make things better for our children, but in this case it was a medical decision that only my son and his wife could ultimately make. There was nothing we could do but provide comfort and assistance to my son and daughter-in-law during their time of need. My only solace was that I firmly believed from the onset, that with prayers and confidence in the medical decisions that my son and his wife made, that at some future time my granddaughter would be totally free from the disease.—*Lenny, Sr., grandfather*

* * *

> Grandparents have the magic touch. I can get Janie to do the necessary things her mom can't. I don't get involved in the usual power and control issues between mother and child. Who cares, as long as it gets done.—*Cecilia, grandmother*

Other extended family members have their own reactions. They can be quite distraught, particularly if they have a close relationship to the parent or child. Other children in the family, as well as the sick child's friends, are upset by separation from the child, changes in the child's appearance, the emotional upheaval in the adults around them, and their own fearful fantasies about cancer. Like siblings of the child with cancer, they benefit from information, normalization, and inclusion. Some parents keep family and friends updated with newsletters, Web sites, phone chains, or ever-changing recorded answering machine messages.

Parents' own siblings and friends are jolted with the realization that they, too, might be vulnerable, thinking it could happen to me and my child. Helpless, unsure of what to do,

> Beware of allowing a tactless word, a rebuttal, a rejection to obliterate the whole sky.
> Anais Nin, *The Diary of Anais Nin* (1944)

they either jump in to help or pull back. They tend to feel better and be of more help if they are kept fully informed and given suggestions. One child's aunt and uncle coordinated and recruited blood donors from their own circle of friends.

Misconceptions and misunderstandings can cause problems if not corrected. For example, family members may promote old-fashioned, superstitious, or misguided ideas that do not mesh with modern medicine. Usually, this is the family member's idea of protection, an expression of their anxiety and worry and attempt to help.

> There is a never-ending impact. My niece is always in my prayers. I've never accepted the possibility that she will die at a young age. It just won't happen. I always pray, too, that my children won't get sick, and then I feel guilty.— *Vicki, aunt*

* * *

> My aunt is one of those amazing people. She zoomed in, took care of the house, took care of the kids, took care of us. She was my rock and my support. Didn't faze her a bit. Big ugly goopy scar on his eye, she just dives right in, does dressings. Constant e-mails, constant calls. We didn't have that from anybody else.— *Trish*

* * *

> I was talking to my brother, who is certainly no expert. When I told him what my son's diet was, he said, "That is so much fat. Don't you worry about his heart?" But the doctors told me to put him on a high fat diet because he was so underweight.— *Debra*

Ambivalence About Visitors

Patients and parents frequently feel ambivalent about visitors coming to the hospital and, at times, to the home. You want support and company and certainly do not want to be alone. But you and your child also need rest and privacy. You may not have the energy to put on a happy face for visitors who seem to expect it or at least are relieved when that is what they see. You may feel overwhelmed, embarrassed, or like a poor "host." On the other hand, families who do not receive any visits can become resentful and feel abandoned. The most helpful solution is to have rules and cues: Conduct visits in a lounge or playroom; set time limits on visits, arrange for your nurse to come in at certain time and shoo visitors out, or have a "secret signal" the child can give the parent that means, "I'm done." The better the communication to extended family and friends the more likely you will be able to arrange a visiting schedule that is comfortable for everyone.

Blended Families

Stepparents, step-grandparents, and stepsiblings are in limbo. They may not know their place or their role. If they are not in the inner circle, they often feel left out. They may feel guilty for not feeling as bad as they would if it were a sick blood relative. There may be more resentment at the disruption of their life's plan. The shorter the time period of the relationship, the more exaggerated this response may be. The nature of the relationship between ex-spouses can either help or hinder the family's experience, both practically and emotionally. Custody agreements and financial arrangements may need to be altered. Blended families may also have more hands available to help ease the care taking of healthy siblings and household duties.

> When Rae was alive, Jerry told people, "I love her as if she were my own." It was his mantra. Months after her death he finally admitted that losing a step-child you've only known for a year or so is not the same as losing your own child. He said that if the child he raised became seriously ill, he would go to pieces; that he is not as strong as me. I felt lied to; though a broader reality would be that he wished he could have loved her as if she were his own.—*Naomi*

* * *

> My wife has a medical background and is our daughter's natural parent. There were many ways for her to help. I am a step-parent. I felt left on the sidelines, helpless. What could I do that was useful? What I could do was to make good moments, because we never knew how many good moments there would be. It made it nice for me to be Grandpa.—*James, grandfather*

* * *

> When treatment started, my older boys went to live with their father during the week and came here on the weekends. While their dad is very supportive of my situation, he's *not* unhappy about having his boys full-time. The person it hit the hardest was me. It's really hard to "let go," even if they are going somewhere where they are loved. Now that treatment is over, the boys have expressed a desire to continue going to school there. They are with me every weekend, so we do get quality time together. Knowing that makes it easier for me to put selfish desires aside and respect their thought-out choices. I didn't take it as a personal rejection, and my ex and I were very careful to set up the choice in such a way that the boys did not feel like they were choosing one parent over another. I honestly believe that it was the support and input of extended family that helped the boys adjust. It would have been a completely different story had they been in the same house with me full-time and able to see the stress and worry. As it was, they could have a "normal" life at their dad's and not have to think about and deal with what their brother was going through 24/7.—*Diane*

Help Them Help You

Family and friends are deeply affected. Fears and misconceptions about cancer may alienate them from you. They may feel grateful that their children are healthy and feel guilty for those feelings. They may attempt to buffer themselves or their own children from distress and potential grief by staying away. Often, they are at a loss regarding what to say or do to help you. Give them something to do, and most likely they will do it. Helping makes them feel useful and less despairing. People often say, "If there's anything I can do, please call me." Make a list of tasks that need to be done and be prepared to suggest something. Do not wait for them to call you.

Keep in mind that everyone has a different capacity to help and may actually say "no" to a task they do not feel able to do. Whether they can offer time, money, or simply moral support, a little bit from each goes a long way toward easing your life and is not a burden on them. It may not come from the ones you expect. Sadly, nearly every cancer parent can tell you they lost at least one person, who just could not cope. Cancer parents will also tell you that those they kept or gained were that much more precious. At least three cancer support organizations were started by friends of cancer parents.

> We had a group of friends, with all our kids the same age. They really rallied to help us. They took turns baby-sitting our older daughter at the drop of a hat, when the younger one was sick. One of them was a nurse, and she helped me get used to the nasogastric tube. —*Heidi*

* * *

> My husband's parents were there for financial help, as they have tended to be over the years. They are not capable of being there for you physically or emotionally. It's not their thing. In retrospect, it's been a very interesting year. My father-in-law was diagnosed with prostate cancer. I spent a lot of time in the hospital with him. He started to ask questions about Luke's treatment. I'd say, when they gave this stuff to Luke it really seemed to help when we did blah dah dah. It was eye-opening for him to realize intimately what this kid had been through.—*Liz*

* * *

> One friend who is really a strong support for me is a counselor, so she's a good listener and helps me focus. Once, I was having a tough time at the hospital, and my husband had just gone home and was sleep-deprived. I couldn't call him and say, "I'm a mess." I called her. She said, "I'm getting in the car, and I'm coming down." I only needed it one time, but I know that if I get in that spot again, I have somebody who's going to jump in this mess with me.—*Josephine*

* * *

> People don't know what to do. I found that if people were upset, they were kind of lost. If I gave them something to do, even something small, from then on when they saw me they didn't have a look of dread, they had a smile. They weren't thinking, "Oh my God," they were thinking, "Yeah, I did something nice for her."—*Maureen*

Give this list to anyone in your support network.

Help List For Family and Friends

You can help. Do not be surprised if your offers of assistance are initially rebuffed. There are some things that the parents of a child with cancer want and need to do for themselves, but there are many other things they will welcome from you. Offering something specific is better than saying, "If there's anything I can do. . . ." Do not wait for them to call you. Call them. If none of the following suggestions work, ask what else you can do.

- *Respect the family's privacy, confidentiality, and needs.* Do things their way. Honor their boundaries. Abide by their wishes. Do not undertake holiday shopping, major house repairs, or a public fundraiser without consulting the family.
- *Listen.* Be a sounding board without giving advice, trying to fix the problem, or belittling the feelings being expressed. Let them talk out their feelings or decisions with you without judgment. Platitudes (such as it's God's will; don't worry he'll be fine; well, at least you have another child; or you can still have more children) are not meaningful and are often upsetting to the family. But do not be afraid to talk about the cancer. You will not remind them of it; it is already on their minds. On the other hand, they do want to talk of other things besides the cancer.
- *Learn the basics about the illness.* If you feel comfortable with the idea, try to learn something about the child's illness and treatment. You do not have to read medical literature, but listen when the parents tell you what is going on. It will help you to understand better what the child and the family are going through. Also, it will make it easier for them to talk to you.
- *Visit the hospital.* Keep visits short. Be sensitive to the child and parent's receptivity. Do not take it personally if they are having a bad day and the visit needs to be rescheduled. Provide transportation for family members, friends, and especially for the child's friends to visit as well. Because children and teenagers cannot drive, they have fewer opportunities to visit.
- *Run errands.* Do food shopping, get the car inspected, wait for a repairman, pick up dry cleaning, shop, or take a pet to the vet.
- *Provide food.* Single portions and disposable containers are both helpful. Find out what the sick child can and will eat and bring extras of those. Have take-out food delivered on clinic days (the child will probably be nauseated from chemotherapy, but everyone else needs to eat).

Box continues next page

Continued

- *Do chores.* Take care of laundry, housework, yard work, snow shoveling, and pet care. If you are unable to do these services yourself, you might screen and hire workers or arrange for volunteers to do any of these tasks.
- *Baby-sit.* The main need is usually care for the well siblings, but if you are able to care for the sick child also, do so.
- *Be a fairy godmother to the siblings.* Spend time with them, do something fun (such as going to the movies or the zoo), write them notes or cards. If you bring a gift for the sick child, bring one for the sibling, too.
- *Be a chauffeur.* Offer to drive to and from the hospital on clinic days, drive school children to soccer practice or ballet class, or be on call for emergencies.
- *Give parents a break.* Spend one day a week with the family at home or the hospital, letting the parents take a nap or go out alone. If possible, stay overnight at the hospital so the parents can spend a night at home.
- *Accompany the family on medical visits.* Be a runner for lunch, be an extra pair of hands, keep siblings occupied, or just keep them company. Be prepared to stay all day and bring some cash.
- *Give blood or platelets.* Even if you are not the needed blood type or the family has been excluded for medical reasons, give anyway. You might help someone they know at the hospital. Offer to keep track of blood donations—who gave when and how much. Recruit donors and call to remind people when they are allowed to give again. Find out the necessary information from the hospital's blood bank.
- *Do an Internet search.* Assemble articles, information, and a list of Web sites on whatever subject the family needs, from medical topics to education to hobbies.
- *Coordinate fundraisers.* Consult with the family first, to get permission and instructions. Community groups such as the Elks or Kiwanis clubs, school or scouting organizations, philanthropic organizations, religious groups, and interest clubs are all sources that may be tapped. See the Resources at the end of this book for additional help.
- *Stock an overnight bag.* Fill it with sample-sized toiletries such as shampoo, soap, toothpaste and a toothbrush, laundry detergent, deodorant, razors, magazines or books, snacks, and a water bottle.
- *Be the press secretary.* Update the rest of the family with calls or notes. But be sure to get the information straight first. Offer to start or maintain a family newsletter or Web site.
- *Give the gifts that matter.* Send cards, balloons, videos, art supplies, toys, fun hats or scarves, movie or electronic game rental certificates, a portable CD or tape player and tapes or CDs, books and magazines, or stuffed animals to the sick child. For the adults, give phone cards, gift certificates for groceries, frozen dinners, relaxation tapes, paperback novels, notebooks, extra bed linens (for the child's bed), a beeper, a laundry bag and marker, or casual clothes for hospital wear that can be slept in. A certificate for a ther-

Box continues next page

Continued

apeutic massage would do a parent a world of good. Provide thank you cards; Fill them out with something generic, stamp (but don't seal) all the envelopes, and write in the return address. You could offer to keep a list and fill out all the cards and address and send them yourself. If you are able to make a larger gesture, you might give an open account at a video rental store, a gasoline credit card, air travel, an electronic game, a cellular phone and service, or a stay at your vacation home.

- *Give cash.* There are expenses not covered by insurance, such as parking, meals, gasoline, telephone bills, nutritional supplements, experimental treatments, and so forth. Even an envelope stashed in the car with a few dollars for tolls and parking is thoughtful.

The Cancer Community

It is very comforting to know that you are not alone. Families in the cancer community can gain so much, trading resources, medical knowledge and tricks of the trade, emotionally supporting each other, and banding together in activism. The cancer community can almost become a "club"—not one in which you sought membership, but one where you can find people who understand firsthand what you are going through. One mother confessed that she found it easier to talk about life and death issues with cancer friends than to make small talk with "normal" people.

Not all of these encounters will be positive. Cancer strikes people from varying backgrounds, each with his or her own issues and coping styles and belief systems, which may not jibe with yours. You will not like or get along with all cancer families. In one example, Reuben noted that on a hospital ward with limited resources, parents can get proprietary about rocking chairs or pull-out beds. Also, some people participate in an almost morbid one-upsmanship—but the "I'm worse off than you" game is unwinnable. If you do clash with another family, take a step back and remember that their pain and distress colors what they say and do, and you are both pretty sensitive and vulnerable.

Not everyone chooses to align themselves with this community. Some parents do not want to associate themselves or their children with what they see as a negative image and thus make no lasting relationships with the community. However, most do benefit in some way from relationships and interactions with other families.

Great and lasting friendships are formed by both parents and children with other parents and children and also with staff. Friendships formed in adversity are very powerful.

Lean on Me

Sometimes in our lives,
We all have pain,
We all have sorrow.
But, if we are wise,
We know that there's
Always tomorrow.
Lean on me
When you're not strong.
I'll be your friend
I'll help you carry on.
For, it won't be long,
Till I'm gonna need
Somebody to lean on.
Please, swallow your pride,
If I have faith
You need to borrow.
For no one can fill
Those of your needs
That you won't let show.
You just call on me brother,
When you need a hand,
We all need somebody to lean on.
I just might have a problem
That you'll understand.
We all need somebody to lean on.
(chorus)
If there is a load
You have to bear
That you can't carry.
I'm right up the road,
I'll share your load,
If you'll just call me.
Call me.
—Bill Withers (1972)
Reprinted with permission.

Molly informed me that she was packing her bags and running away to live at the hospital. She said, "The nurses and doctors love me, and I love them. I can order food whenever I'm hungry and watch Cartoon Network. You and Dad can always come and visit me, and even sleep over. I will miss you." With that, and a quick peck on the cheek, she left my room and started packing. I guess we're lucky that she's comfy there, but when I was a kid, I always wanted to run away with the carnival!—*Bess*

* * *

I did make many friendships at the hospital, mostly on the annual amputee ski trip. I became very friendly with a great person, John. He passed away two years ago, and I miss him dearly. I keep in close touch with his mother, and I feel that is how I keep a part of John. —*Monica, long-term survivor*

Cancer parents pull together to help each other and other children in meaningful ways.

There was a toddler repeatedly abandoned by her family on the hospital unit. The nurses were struggling to feed and care for her while juggling a large patient load. She'd toddle after any adult, calling them "mama" and "daddy." It was putting all the other families over the emotional brink. Some of us would get our own kids to sleep in the evening, then sit in the lounge and listen to her. Several of us took to going into her room to rock her and play with her or bring her into the lounge with us. Finally, my husband called the state child services division. From then on, the toddler got much more attention from the "support staff," and her young mother was called in and taught at least the basics of her child's care. — *Trish*

Along with the support of these relationships, there are added emotional highs and lows. What happens to other children affects us greatly. We celebrate when children we know are doing well, and we are heartbroken when other children hit bumps in the road, relapse, or die. Many parents have noted feeling discouraged because they see only sick children, and not the survivors, at the hospital. When they do meet survivors or hear their stories, their hope is boosted.

One day, we went in to check counts, and there was a teenager there who was 17, on an annual visit. I could have kissed this boy. You may be hearing about 5 people having problems, but they've treated 280. The rest are doing well at home or at college. You don't hear about them. If nothing else, they should get them all together and take a picture and put it up on the wall beside all the memorial plaques.—*Maggie*

The death of a child on the ward is devastating to other parents. Comparable diagnosis or treatment regimen or a close relationship with the grieving family can compound the reaction. Feelings of sadness, grief, and anger at cancer and the unfairness of it all surfaces. Fears for your own child may intensify, increasing anxiety about the effectiveness of your child's treatment and heightening your vigilance. Survivor guilt is a strong reaction. Acknowledge your feelings, get reassurance about your own situation from your child's doctor, talk to other families, or seek grief counseling.

These intense feelings and a subconscious need to defend yourself from the emotional assault may cause you to pull back. You, who were so angry at the insensitivity of others' words to you, find yourself not knowing what to say or do. Parents suggest, "I'm so sorry," a hug, sharing a good cry, writing a note or letter including some remembrance of the child, or sending flowers or making donations in the child's name.

There was a little boy who had the same diagnosis as my daughter. Going to his funeral was the hardest thing. So many emotions were running through me. My heart broke for my friend. What struck me most is when she said, "You never saw him when he was well. You only knew him when he was sick." I wished I could have shared that part of her child's life, too. I sobbed for the entire three-hour drive home.—*Heidi*

* * *

One day, at the hospital, I ran into the mother of a child who went through treatment at the same time as my daughter. Her daughter had relapsed, was on life support, and the

> doctor had just told the family they should turn off the machines. I sat and talked with her, put my arms around her, and cried with her. She told me how her daughter had been well for a time, but then got sicker and sicker. She had gotten my end-of-the-year letter, and it made her mad because our life was continuing so normally, while she was in the pits again. She meant to call me, but didn't know how to break the news, and didn't want to bring me down. Here I was, going blithely along with my life while she suffered. I felt so horribly guilty—that I hadn't contacted her in all that time, that I sent the stupid holiday letter, that my child was doing well, that I couldn't do anything to ease her pain. I felt like I had no right to comfort her, that I had no right to be happy. Cancer stinks.—*Nora*

Your child reacts to the death of another child with grief and anger as well. Your child abruptly confronts his own mortality, even at a very young age, asking you difficult questions and needing honest answers. Your child may become more fearful, anxious, or depressed; have nightmares; fight procedures; or withdraw. Encourage your child to express these emotions verbally, in writing, or through expressive arts. This may be difficult for you to participate in, because of your own strong emotions. Do consider enlisting the help of a therapist. Relationships and sights witnessed profoundly affect sick children.

> Molly's major problem during all of the commotion in inserting lines and sedating for the "A" line was when a nurse hooked up some oxygen. This freaked Molly out, and she kept trying to tell them that she "wasn't dying like Didi," and she didn't need any extra air. I think that she was reminded of one of her last images of her beloved friend, all hooked up and with that "thingy" in her nose. I politely requested that they remove the oxygen and just keep it on standby, as it was obviously doing more harm than good. They did. Chalk up one for mama bear.—*Bess*

Helping other families is gratifying, yet it can be an emotional drain. Easing someone else's emotional burden adds to your own, as painful memories mingle with new stories.

> I've been talking with two friends who are dealing with cancer right now. I don't want to be in that world again, but I feel a responsibility to help because of what my daughter went through.—*Josephine*

* * *

> I love being able to help other people, to give them hope. But it can be very tiring, worrying for them and their children and knowing just how they feel. It always brings up old feelings about Adam. I do feel this is a way of healing ourselves though. When a child dies it is horrible. When I cry for their child, I am crying for all the suffering Adam went through and for myself. I know some of those tears are for the pain that I felt watching him suffer. I did not have time to cry while he was ill. He needed me to be strong.—*Maxie*

The Rest of the World

Parents often say the rest of the world has no clue what they are going through. However, it is not your responsibility to educate the world. It is important to choose well the time, place, and person with whom you will share your private life experiences. The decision to share your story or not is a decision made more than once. In fact, you may make that decision more than once a day. You may handle it differently a month, a year, or a decade from now. Talking about an ordeal can be therapeutic, empowering, cathartic, or normalizing.

> I really enjoy sharing my experiences with people. I would much rather people ask me what is on their minds rather than stare and gawk at me wondering if it was a shark, escalator, or even a birth defect that left me with one leg. I can say honestly I am not going to walk up to a complete stranger and just start babbling on and on about what happened, but I do not mind people asking me questions. I'll tell you what you want to know.—*Monica, long-term survivor*

Conversely, putting the experience into words can seem all wrong, a degradation of intensely private information. Although he was not talking about cancer, the actor Edward Norton spoke in an interview in *Parade* Magazine (see Rosen in the Bibliography) about reticence: "There's a Hemingway story about soldiers coming back from World War I and telling people about their experiences, then feeling really cheap afterward. That's how I feel whenever I've given over my own complicated human experiences to the gristmill of anecdote. So I guard against it."

You may bristle at remarks from strangers or even friends, especially those who complain about trivial matters or criticize your actions and decisions. Cancer parents, particularly if they have had minimal support, sometimes get a chip on their shoulders, assuming that no one will understand or appreciate their difficulties. You cannot tell by looking at a person what he or she has been through in life. And they cannot tell by looking at you either. Give them the benefit of the doubt and be gentle when you can.

> We were in a shopping mall and a boy said, "Do you know you're bald?" And Mia said, "Do you know you're rude?" I would have chastised her under normal circumstances, but I was like, "Go, girl, go," that day.—*Natalie*
>
> * * *
>
> I was at a swim club and noticed a pale, thin little girl with a pretty hat. Then I noticed the pin in her shirt, and I knew immediately that she had a Broviac. She was "one of us."

I approached her mother, and she started to dish me off, until I told her that my daughter was a cancer kid, too, it just wasn't apparent because she'd been done with treatment for a while.—*Alice*

Cancer affects all of the people in your child's life. Knowing how they are affected, how your relationships influence each other and can help you to cope, will help you to deal more effectively with the stresses of your child's illness.

CHAPTER 5

Handling Emotions and Communicating Well

The pessimist complains about the wind.
The optimist expects it to change.
The realist adjusts the sails.
—*William Arthur Ward* (1989)

Your quality of life is improved greatly when you are able to handle emotions and interact with other people successfully. In this chapter, we show you how to work with uncomfortable feelings and recognize the development of childhood emotions. We present examples of the major steps for good communication and give you guidelines for standing up for yourself and for settling conflicts with others. Bolstering these areas can help you to strengthen your sense of yourself and your relationships while on cancer's emotional roller coaster. The ride is not smooth, but the point is to stay on track and not go off the rails.

These four skills will help to ease and support your day-to-day functioning in relationships:

- Handling emotions effectively
- Communicating cooperatively
- Asserting yourself responsibly
- Resolving conflict amicably.

Handling Emotions Effectively

The primary focus of this first section is adults, although parts are applicable also to children. Specific childhood emotional development is discussed later.

Fear, anger, guilt, jealousy, shame, grief, and a global sense of being overwhelmed have a powerful impact. This is true whether you are the one suffering or you are the one bearing the brunt of another person's emotions. Feelings rarely come one at a time. They tend to pile up and to get jumbled together. Nevertheless, they can be handled effectively and with kindness to yourself and others.

Strong negative emotions can cause great disruption in a relationship. We all have first-hand experience of them but have different ways of responding to the upset. For example, if a man thinks that it is cowardly to reveal that he is frightened, he may disguise his fear and show only anger through sarcasm, yelling, or blaming others. In response, if his wife is frightened of anger in others, she may become anxious, withdrawn, appeasing, or vague. The result is a mess—misunderstanding, poor communication, and continued anxiety and conflict. The situation can be remedied by a focus on either handling the angry feeling better in the first place or by changing the pattern once the problem is identified.

Action Steps for Handling Emotions

Acknowledge the emotion for what it is.
Don't deny or run from the feeling. Instead, recognize it as a signal of distress. Identify the emotion. Are you feeling guilty but trying to push it away? Are you worried that if you are sad today, you are failing your family? Are you angry but smiling through clenched teeth?

Clarify the trigger for the emotion.
Look for the source of the troubling feeling. Do you act irritable and short-tempered when tired? Do you feel guilty if you can't make things perfect for your child? Do you feel anxious in the face of the unknown? These are a few of the triggers for negative emotions.

Develop alternatives for handling the emotion.
Go into problem-solving mode. Do something to improve the situation. Alternatives may include soothing (such as reassurance, a hug, or music); self-talk messages or teaching such messages to children; activation of quick coping strategies (such as counting to 10, deep breathing, or finding a distraction), setting limits (on behavior, time, resources, or tasks), removing yourself from the scene until you can regroup, and asking for help.

Emotional upset tends to ricochet in a family, just as a ball thrown hard against a wall will bounce around the room. Out-of-control emotions bounce from one family member to another. Many families have one person who is known to be the emotional ball-catcher. When too many emotional balls are in the air, however, one ball-catcher per family is not enough.

When their own emotions overtake them, some people withdraw. You might find that some of your friends disappear in the face of cancer or that a particular family member retreats. Siblings might withdraw when parents are preoccupied or absent a lot. When a child is extremely or terminally ill, his or her own parents may start to withdraw in anticipatory grief. Usually this withdrawal is a temporary coping mechanism that enables distance from harsh realities. But the child withdrawn from feels lonely, abandoned, and afraid. There are effective action steps to handle painful emotions instead of withdrawing.

This is easy to say, but hard to do. It takes practice to handle emotions maturely. If many adults find it difficult, imagine how that difficulty is magnified for our children. Children learn from the models we demonstrate every day—whether they are good models or not.

When in crisis and under strain, emotions can feel very threatening. Out-of-control emotions threaten the teamwork needed to deal with cancer, as well as with family and work life. Suppressing them is not the answer. But turning down the heat, diffusing the heat, and sharing the heat works. It is more effective to work with emotions than to try to work against them.

Uncomfortable Feelings

You most likely have many common feelings stirred by living with cancer that are negative and distressing. Identifying them will help you to accept them and work with them better. Moderation is the key, as with so many things in life. Feelings, including strong negative feelings, are normal. Problems generally arise only if the feelings both persist over time and are extreme. At one extreme is a blocked absence of expression and awareness of emotions; at the other extreme is an intense and out-of-control reactivity that is disruptive to daily life.

Fear and anxiety

Let us create a mental picture: Fear is a state that occurs when you stand at the very edge of a high mountain ledge in imminent danger of falling off the cliff; anxiety occurs when you stand at the bottom of the mountain and imagine what it would be like to be up there on the edge of the cliff. Living with cancer is a long journey, sometimes you are on the cliff edge, sometimes you are contemplating the cliff.

The strongest initial response of most parents is fear for the child's life. Later come fears of the unknown, of making decisions, of a child being in pain or being mutilated, of not being able to perform medical care for the child, and of a family falling apart, and also worries about long-term physical and emotional implications, financial problems, and job stresses. Fear and anxiety rise and fall with the ups and downs of treatment and follow-up care. Sometimes they are specific, like waiting for test results; sometimes they are nameless.

It is said that our anxiety does not empty tomorrow of its sorrows, but only empties today of its strength.
Charles H. Spurgeon, *Gems From Spurgeon* (1859)

As a parent, you are experienced with the struggle to control your fears and anxieties to function for your child. For your child too, the fears spurt and the anxiety comes and goes, even when it is expressed differently. Without expression, fear and anxiety can wear both adults and children down.

I watched the red Daunamycin flow through the IV tube in the hospital into my son's beautiful and pure body for the first time. Once it entered his veins, would he literally feel sick instantly and start throwing up? How sudden would it be? I finally asked one of the nurse practitioners, and she said it was more of a gradual thing, within a few hours and days. That made me feel a little better. Not knowing what to expect is the hardest to bear at first. Once he went through a complete cycle of chemo, and we got to know what to expect from each of the nine different drugs, it got a little easier. The fear of the unknown was taken away to some extent.—*Gabriela*

* * *

My fear? I have no idea what the future holds. I have plans and dreams for Will. I want to teach him to play ball and to drive and to go out for a beer with him. I have no idea if he will be around to do these things.—*Edward*

* * *

When Casey was a toddler, she was afraid of monsters in the closet or under the bed. She had trouble going to sleep at night, so I borrowed an idea from a friend. I took an empty spray bottle and told her it was "monster spray." Any time she was afraid, she should "spray" this magic stuff. It would ward off any monster and keep her safe. Periodically, I would "refill" it. She seemed to believe in its "power."—*Susan*

Fear and anxiety can be managed. Chapter 3 contains techniques that can diminish them. See especially the sections on parent, child, and family coping strategies.

When my son was first diagnosed, I thought my life would be over if he died. After a few weeks I realized that I was a person before he was born and would go on if he left. It doesn't make sense that I was so tied to my son that my thread would end if his did. I thought of my own mother. Would her life end if mine did? No, she is one entire, complete, complex person and would go on living a life. I tuck thoughts of loss in a drawer, hoping I never have to open it. But my time with him I spend better than I would have if this had not happened. I listen to him more carefully, touch him more often, I stop whatever I am doing to be with him.—*Jenny*

Anger

Perhaps the most common reaction after the first shock is anger. You might be angry at the cancer, the loss of childhood and family normalcy, the rigors of the treatment regimen, the lack of control, the bearer of bad news, and the financial burdens, and often you are angry at God, the medical team, and other family members for not making the nightmare go away. Many survivors and parents are angry at debilitating effects and the continued need for interventions, which seem to add insult to injury when a child has "suffered enough." Anger can become an automatic response directed at anyone or anything experienced as threatening.

> I was frustrated and frightened at my daughter's inability to eat and angry that nobody was doing anything except uselessly sending her food trays. I admit to hurling one particular tray of food all the way to the end of the wing. Boy it felt good! Another time, the night staff repeatedly woke my daughter up calling nurses over the intercom. I stormed the nurses' station, reminding them, loudly, that they carried beepers for a reason. I threw in a few choice profanities at the top of my lungs. The next day an inflatable punching bag appeared in our room. Yes, I beat the you-know-what out of it and left it deflated in the hall.—*Julie*

Because anger is often viewed as socially unacceptable, some people learn to hide and disguise it. They take out their anger in harmful, indirect ways. Suppressed anger may take the form of "the silent treatment," being negative or sarcastic, overreacting to trivial things, picking fights to justify an angry reaction, or projection (accusing someone else of being angry, instead of recognizing you are the angry one). Unchecked anger damages relationships; therefore, it needs to be kept in-bounds. Some people turn anger in on themselves. But that puts you at risk for depression. For your own and your family's sake, it is more helpful to recognize your anger and that of others, to keep control of yourself, and handle it appropriately.

Depending on the situation, there are times to diffuse anger by talking yourself or others down, by solving a problem, by assertive behavior, by soothing, or by safe ventilation. Once anger is identified accurately, you can choose the best strategy for channeling it. Psychotherapist Thomas Golden tells the story of a father who bought a cheap set of china, took it to a dump, and proceeded to smash every piece to smithereens (see the Bibliography).

Parents report great relief in venting, tending to choose as targets people who do or say stupid, thoughtless things. A parent gives an example:

> I was using a handicapped placard for parking. I pulled in to pick up some groceries, and some yahoo in a pick-up pulled up and said, "You look fine to me." As I was pulling my son out of his seat I said, "It's for him." The Einstein then said, "Well you're carrying him." The next thing I knew I was at the other end of the parking lot. I'd pulled my son's hat off to show his bald head. I was running after this guy's taillights shouting some not so nice

> things about his soul. I'm not very proud of that moment, but I will say this: I think sometimes when we are very, very pent-up, people come into our lives who serve a very specific purpose of letting us get it all out.—*Melissa*

Guilt

Parents commonly feel guilty for any ways in which they are unable to protect their children. In the cancer world, there are many variations on this theme. You may feel responsible that your child became ill at all or guilty for not recognizing symptoms sooner. You may feel guilty if you cannot follow all of the treatment instructions perfectly, control the outcome, prevent the pain, get to your other child's school play, concentrate on your job, be strong for your spouse, go to all medical appointments, or stop the nagging of your in-laws to change doctors because they found a better one on the recommendation of the local deli owner.

> They tried another medication, and we were waiting to see the results if he went back in remission. I had an important meeting that day, so my wife told me to go ahead to the meeting. But now I regret that I wasn't there when the bad news came.—*Ben*

* * *

> I spent yesterday at the hospital having many scans done to rule out thyroid cancer. It's very strange, as I know I should be extremely thankful that I don't have cancer, but I can't help but feel guilty over the fact that my son has it and I don't. How am I supposed to feel good about that?—*Jill*

Other family members or even perfect strangers may try to put blame on you through statements or questions that appear to question your parenting abilities, your genes, or your treatment choices. Parents we spoke with lashed out in anger at these suggestions but often felt guilty themselves about the exact same issues. Comments that make you angriest are ones that touch a nerve.

Although it is rarely discussed openly, many survivors and their families feel guilty for surviving or for surviving well. The unfairness of it all is troubling—no child should get cancer, or suffer, or die. Why have my child and I been spared? Gratitude for what feels like a gift breeds guilt when comparisons are inevitably made to equally deserving patients and their families. Survival seems so arbitrary and tenuous—therefore, everyone is vulnerable. This feeling colors relationships with families whose children died. You might be less likely to keep in contact, afraid that the family whose child died will be angry or jealous and reject you (however, this is not a common reaction from bereaved parents). Sometimes survivor guilt keeps people from expressing concerns (about effects, for example) that, in their minds, pale in comparison. Older patients may wonder if there was some purpose to their survival and feel they must make their lives "worth it." Survivor guilt can lead to some positive soul-searching, but if taken to the extreme, it can rob you of some of the joy of survival.

> When I talk to other parents whose kids went through transplant, or who have major lasting effects, or died, I feel guilty. As difficult as treatment was, I sometimes feel like we got off easy. He does have some effects, but they're so minor compared to some of the things I've seen, how can I complain?—*Joan*

* * *

> I do have a little guilt. I used to have more before graft-versus-host disease, but after that I know that Adam suffered almost like a POW, so the guilt is small.—*Maxie*

* * *

> At first when my friend John died I was very upset. I did not understand why he had to suffer through all of that, move on with his life, and just when he was beginning to start living again, it came back. Why did he die and I didn't? It is unfair to John that I am still alive. I was afraid to talk to his mother because I thought she would be mad or angry that I was alive and her son was not. I have grown to accept that that is just the way things work.—*Monica, long-term survivor*

Whatever it is that you feel guilty about, it is important to recognize that you are not omnipotent or perfect. You cannot control the universe or even yourself in every moment. Decide on the priorities for your family, yourself, and your child. Tackle your responsibilities. Learn from your mistakes, but don't beat yourself up over them. Then throw out the guilt. It does not serve you, and it does not help to make things better.

Jealousy and resentment

What cancer parent or child has not wished they were spared? Probably you will feel jealous, from time to time, of others who are healthier and less burdened; this is another norm in cancer families. Simply viewing a television program or movie or taking a walk through the park, mall, or grocery store can be upsetting, because it seems as if all the world is happy and carefree, and you are not.

> Going food shopping was surprisingly difficult. I wandered around the supermarket, dazed. It all seemed so trivial. I wanted to scream out, "My little boy has cancer, and I don't care what food I buy." I would look at all of the other Mommies with children and be so envious of their "normal" life. I was usually in tears by the time I left.—*Sandy*

Remember that the wounds seem obvious to you, because they are so painful. However, others can't tell what you are going through, and you have no inkling of the traumatic experiences they may have endured in their lives. Some parents take a more positive viewpoint and consider the average person fortunate for being ignorant about childhood cancer. Feeling jealous does not mean that you wish cancer on another family, only that you wish that you, too, were so "ignorant."

Parents, children, and siblings can all feel resentful of the illness; the painful and intrusive nature of treatment; the loss of normal life and activities; the extra duties, chores, and financial burdens; the changes in plans; the added worries; and the extra time, money, and attention that is lavished on the sick child. Feelings of resentment often breed feelings of guilt, because we feel selfish for having these thoughts. For this reason, resentment is often unspoken and festers under the surface.

> I sometimes resent like hell the fact that my son has leukemia. There are things that I would like to do, and I can't do them because we have a hospital appointment. I might receive a phone call inviting me out with some friends, but I invariably turn these down because I know my wife has had Will all day, and I feel that I should be at home.—*Edward*

* * *

> In the beginning, I hated my husband, because he was more patient than I am. He calmed my son better than I did. He never lost his cool. He was there for me and the children. St. Rick, that's what I called him. One day, about two weeks into the whole thing, he had something bad happen to him. I saw him slump to the floor, and put his head in his hands. For a split second, I was glad. It was a relief to see him suffering like I was. I never told him these feelings, but he knew it.—*Isabelle*

* * *

> I was envious that out of all my friends and family, I had never smoked or drank alcohol, and here was my only child with cancer, and they all had multiple healthy children. That was appalling to me at first and seemed so unfair.—*Marlena*

Conversely, you will feel relieved when your child is not the one with the bad news this week or this visit. Parents tend to keep quiet about making the comparison to other cancer families. Jealousy is not discussed very much, but it is a typical feeling in the basket of emotions.

Shame

Shame is related to what we are, whereas guilt is related to our behavior. You might feel guilty for doing or not doing something, but shame is related to your sense of self. Shame is closely tied to embarrassment and humiliation. Most of us have a story to tell about the most embarrassing moment in our lives.

Shame is a powerful controller of actions and emotions. For example, more people than you might have guessed avoid medical examinations because they feel shame about their exposed bodies. They are embarrassed to show any imperfection, vulnerability, awkwardness, discomfort, or humiliation for their nakedness in the presence of a fully dressed staff. Cancer treatment involves intrusive examinations, with multiple strangers looking at you, touching you, talking about you, and asking you questions about your body. Children are taught from a very young age that their bodies are private, so the new messages they are getting confuse them and make them uncomfortable. Is this a good touch or a bad touch? This is particularly troubling for a child if a tumor location involves the private parts or if treatment affects their sexuality or reproductive capabilities. Sensitive medical staff make sure that patients are not exposed physically or psychologically in any unnecessary ways—your child should always be examined in a private room or have a curtain pulled around for privacy.

An adult may feel ashamed of negative feelings, of an inability to cope or help with care, or of poor behavior in a difficult situation. People who are very markedly sensitive to criticism often develop shame-based anger. They tend to hear criticism even when it is not present, and the constant expectation of criticism makes them feel bad about themselves. To rid themselves of shame and a sense of unworthiness, they criticize others and develop an angry, blaming, shaming pattern against others.

Cancer assaults the body and may assault the self-esteem of both the child and the entire family. Be on the look out for shame. You do not want it to control your emotions or your freedom to act in positive ways. It is important to reassure your child that there is nothing to be ashamed of—not the illness itself, physical appearance, or fears or reactions to treatment experiences. One of the best antidotes for shame is laughter. When we can laugh at a situation that embarrasses us, we take away the power of shame. It is our way of expressing acceptance of our vulnerabilities as normal, not shameful.

Grief

Sadness, sorrow, and grief are all related to loss. It is universally hard to come to terms with significant losses, and it takes time. A natural period of grieving occurs in the presence of cancer. We grieve for the loss of innocence, for lost dreams and time, and for changes in relationships and plans. Although many people outside the cancer community misunderstand our grief or think that it means the prognosis is bad, this is not true. Every family member needs the time and emotional room to grieve for whatever levels of loss they are suffering, from diagnosis all the way to death, should it occur. They need the opportunity to express the sad feelings in their own way, sometimes to others and sometimes privately.

> I mourn the loss of her babyhood, for her, but mostly for me. Seeing other babies learning to talk and walk saddens me, because at that point in her life when she should have been doing those things she was lying in a hospital bed simply surviving. She eventually caught

> up, but it took a long time and a lot of help—her baby book doesn't follow the same path as her sister's. In the long run, it doesn't really matter, but I really missed that exciting and wonderful phase.—*Marta*

Grief and sadness may look a lot like depression—unhappiness, loss of appetite, and tossing and turning and worrying rather than sleeping at night. Grief is normal and to be expected. However, if your sorrow is ignored, denied, suppressed, or cut off in some other way, there is no natural outlet for it to run its course. Allow yourself and your family members the chance to talk about the losses and stresses. Make sure you have someone to talk to and lean on. Every family member needs to have emotional support. Grief takes its own course, although depression sometimes prolongs it. You do not need to know how to diagnose depression. If you are concerned that you or another family member is depressed, ask for additional help. See chapter 2 for suggestions on finding psychological help. See chapter 8 for more information on depression screening. Also see chapter 12 for more discussion of grieving for a death.

Fantasies and superstitions

You might call fantasies and superstitions beliefs rather than feelings, but they are intimately tied in with emotions. Parents confess to "silly" superstitions. During treatment, parents hesitate to tell good news or progress for fear of "tempting fate" and inviting something bad to happen. Alice voiced fears of staying in a particular hospital room, because she knew of two patients who had died there. Superstitions can linger after treatment ends. For example, Maxie refuses to go to her son's checkups alone, since the only time she did she got news of her son's relapse. The decision to save or throw away leftover equipment and supplies after treatment ends often is related to superstition. Parents continue to temper reports of their child's long-term progress or success with caveats.

Fantasies can seem very strange, almost disturbing. Nora told of her fantasies about going to a very ill child's funeral, not because she thought or wished the child would die, but as an expression of her connection to that family. Fathers and mothers both fantasize about running away with the sick child. Siblings fantasize about the child dying or of being the sick one themselves, getting all the attention and gifts. Parents sometimes pre-plan a child's funeral or imagine what they would do if their child died, then feel horribly guilty for even thinking about it. Fantasies are not always a manifestation of wish fulfillment; they also can be a form of emotional rehearsal, or an attempt to inoculate yourself against a dreaded scenario through repeated imaginings. They can be a way to imagine something positive, too, although it is embedded in a negative picture. As long as fantasies and superstitions are not disrupting your ability to function normally, do not be troubled by your natural inclinations.

> Sometimes I see myself being brave as the parent of a relapsed child. I think in an odd way I'd like the attention it brought me. In my logical mind I don't think this way, but sometimes such thoughts flit at the fringes of my consciousness. I probably had such fantasies before diagnosis, too. But the reality of cancer is very different than any fantasy. There is nothing glamorous about being a cancer parent. It's just very sad and hard.—*Jenny*
>
> * * *
>
> I had a fleeting fantasy from time to time of driving the car off the road into a ditch or something, just so I could go into the hospital for a few days and get a break. Except with my luck, it would be fatal. I didn't want pain. I didn't want to die. I just wanted to rest. I think the main reason I didn't do it is because there was no one else who knew how to take care of my child.—*Alice*

Spiritual or existential distress

For many people in times of crisis, faith is a great comfort and an effective coping mechanism. For others, faith not only comes into question, but also may become a focus of anguish and blame.

Expectations of a loving, omnipotent protector may, in some instances, lead to great disappointment and to the question so many parents struggle with: Why does God allow children to suffer? Parents are terribly disturbed by the suffering and death witnessed. For some, including children, the answer seems to be that illness must be a punishment, leading to guilt and self-isolation. Others see suffering as part of the human condition, a sign of God's presence, or martyrdom—something to be endured. Numerous parents expressed a connection to the suffering of biblical figures such as Job or the Virgin Mary.

> Everything fundamental about unjust suffering was already said thousands of years go in the Book of Job, and still those who are afflicted have to live it for themselves.—*Naomi*
>
> * * *
>
> When Danny relapsed, I was rocking him, saying, "I know you don't understand the pain." It made me think of Jesus on the cross. I can't wait to speak to the Virgin Mary. Like Mary, we watch our child suffer and don't have much of a say about the outcome.—*Kathy*

In response to this distress, people may solidify their beliefs, change religions, or come to a new philosophical or theological understanding. For example, an atheist whose child died may embrace the idea of an afterlife, because the thought of seeing the child again is comforting. For some who come to embrace faith, the possibility of nothingness is unthinkable, lonely, sad, and frightening.

> I used to think religion was a crutch, but now I'm limping!—*Alice*
>
> * * *
>
> I finally got the nerve up to convert to a religion different from the one I grew up with. For years, I had been afraid to convert for fear my parents would be hurt. During our son's illness, the most meaningful acts of kindness came from strangers who acted out of pure compassion. I finally made the decision to change. I feel I have finally come home.—*Gail*

Others find no theological answer good enough. Out of anger, or a feeling that it offers no comfort or support, they reject religious faith.

> I was never very spiritual, and I'm still not. But I don't think I ever can be now. I can't comprehend a God who would allow a child to suffer so, who would allow some to die in pain.—*Mike*
>
> * * *
>
> I was abandoned by my church when I fell on my knees in prayer! Instead of embracing me, "my church" came into my home when my daughter was critically ill, removed all her clothing and toys, and told me that I needed to get my head out of the clouds and face reality that "God" knows best and that my child was going to die. She didn't! These people who were supposedly "so linked" to God and so knowing of his ways were very, very wrong but in the process took away all my hope and almost destroyed me at a time when I needed to be incredibly strong.—*Paula*

Other people find their faith takes a few bumps and remains intact, but altered. They cannot answer existential questions, so they may stop asking them.

> My child experienced a bona fide miracle. The doctors said that no one had ever survived multiple organ failures post-transplant. Days went by and she did not die. Instead, she slowly got better, left intensive care, and was discharged. Unfortunately, about six weeks later, she relapsed and died. This left me bitter. I cannot understand why the Lord would grant a miracle, only to snatch it away. I cannot say there is no God, because I witnessed a miracle. I do say that the ways of the Lord are too mysterious for us to understand, so I don't even try.—*Naomi*
>
> * * *
>
> I had to abandon the exaggerated sense of individualism that I had—the sense of me, and that God can heal my child. God deals with us as a people. This experience completely disabused any naïve notion of God as Santa Claus. God is with us in this insanity—coaching, encouraging, but God isn't going to fix things, magically.—*Val*
>
> * * *

I had a number of well-intentioned friends who told me that the answer was to keep praying and not give up. But I came to a point where I said, "God, there is nothing more I could ask, than I would give my life for this, for my son to be well, I wish I could take his pain. Now I'm putting this, myself in your hands." That's not giving up, that's giving over. Not by badgering God, but by trusting God to be present and then to be quiet.—*Maureen*

* * *

God's got a lot of explaining to do when we get up there. He can't pass this off as the greater good. I'd like to think that God does the best he can. When our son was in the hospital, I like to think that God wasn't off in Hawaii lying on a beach, but was there with us.—*Ben*

When those around you voice beliefs different from your own, your distress can be compounded. Pressed on you, their platitudes or directives to pray or participate in other rituals, even expressing the belief that prayer saved another, can provoke your strong, angry, and hurt feelings. Please remember this before you offer your own views to another cancer parent. Religion is such an explosive issue in the "normal" world, why wouldn't it be in the world of pediatric oncology? The biggest arguments seem to arise in the gaping chasm between what philosophers have long termed faith and reason. Human beings have struggled with that debate as long as they have existed, and we are certainly not going to resolve it here. Listen and speak with respect for another's belief. You are not going to convert them any more than they will convert you.

Gentle Reminders for Resolving Spiritual Distress

- Minimize the patient's pain and distress.
- Give caregivers breaks from the "trenches."
- Encourage the exploration of questions and feelings.
- Talk with clergy, the family, and counselors.
- Boost coping skills (see chapter 3, the section on spirituality as coping mechanism).

Positive Emotions

Positive emotions have a place on the cancer journey, as well. There is pride in the new skills acquired, in the proven ability to handle crisis and stress, in pulling together as a family, and in maintenance of a positive attitude. There is also gratitude for help you have received, for a new lease on life, or for new perspectives and priorities. There is joy in achieving remission, in survivorship and manageability of effects, and in friendships forged.

What is confusing for cancer families is that positive emotions can be uncomfortable, too, because they may be tempered by guilt, fears, and limitations.

Children's Emotions

Children experience the same set of emotions as adults, but not in the same way. They react differently, have different triggers, and show their emotions in different ways than do adults. Children's minds are imaginative but immature, so their emotions may seem out-of-sync with our own, but they are perfectly real to the child.

Children's emotions develop as they grow and mature. *Basic emotions* are present and are expressed from infancy onward: happiness, anger, sadness, and fear. Babies are also capable of showing interest, surprise, and disgust, as most parents observe.

Self-conscious emotions begin to develop later, in toddlerhood: shame, embarrassment, guilt, envy, and pride. Each of these feelings is related to a sense of self, either a blow or a boost. By age 3, a child's self-conscious feelings are linked clearly to self-evaluation: They know when they've done something to be proud of or have been caught with "a hand in the cookie jar." During the school-age years, these emotions are linked to achievement-related behaviors (such as grades, learning to swim, and music recital performances) and moral behaviors (such as stealing vs. participating in a scout troop's efforts to clean up litter in a park). Children take their cues about what is prideful and what is shameful from the grown-ups in their world. Whatever the family's cultural norm, children most often feel pride for intentional achievements and shame for unintentional lapses or violations of the guidelines.

For children facing cancer, the most pervading emotion is fear. A child's biggest fears are primal: separation from parents, pain, and death. A child being treated for cancer may also fear bodily mutilation or rejection from peers and society. As with adults, sometimes their fears or anxiety seem generalized—not about anything specific—although in working with a counselor you can usually find the root of it and then address it. Your child's fears may seem unwarranted. Perhaps your son is afraid of getting x-rays, or your daughter is terrified of thunderstorms. Fear can also manifest itself in stranger anxiety or in a tentativeness about anything new or different, especially in babies and young children. As we've said elsewhere, unpredictability and the unknown both make children's fears much worse. Addressing fears directly, allowing them to be expressed without judgment, belittling, or fluffing them off, will help to alleviate them. Accurate, but not overwhelming, information is comforting. A nurse talks about her experience:

> In my opinion, patients' biggest concerns at diagnosis are that they are dying and nobody is telling them. Think about it. All of a sudden all these relatives show up, mom and dad are crying all the time, everyone is sooooo nice to them, the word cancer keeps coming up,

they never mention death, it must be true! When I have sensed a lot of fear in a child, I will often visit with them for a while and then gently say, "You know, you're not dying right now. You are very sick and we want to make you better, but you are NOT dying. Did you hear that? You are not dying. If we think you are dying, we are going to tell you, ok"? Often, I can feel the entire room breathe a sigh of relief. It's important to put a name to your fears. —*Cathy Chavez, pediatric oncology nurse*

Anger, jealousy, and resentment tend to get all wrapped up in one another. Children are generally pretty good at expressing these emotions, although not always verbally. They are angry and resentful at the same things we are: the unfairness of it all, the intrusion, the pain, and the loss of normal childhood. Ask any cancer kid and he or she will give you a laundry list: missing birthday parties, not being able to go swimming or to school ("well, that part might be okay, but I miss my friends"), having no hair and feeling "yucky" all the time, and everything the doctors and nurses do hurts. Siblings have their own reasons to be angry, jealous, and resentful (see chapter 4). In an infant or toddler, anger is shown typically through crying, body tension, and twisting away from the source of the anger. Older children may cry or shout; have temper tantrums; strike out physically or verbally; refuse to share; whine; act sullen; act tough or mean to other children; and experiment with swearing, insulting, and back talk.

Steven's been sick a lot lately. He's had a bacterial infection that is recurring, that has required lots of blood draws, finger sticks, and IM [intramuscular] shots of antibiotics. He's a few years off treatment and had been doing really well at his checkups, not needing EMLA and not being upset when his name was called for the lab. Now we're back to square one. He's afraid, but he's also getting resentful. It's so pitiful to hear him cry, "Why me, why is it always me?"—*Joy*

Children, like adults, feel guilty at times. They see their families' distress and may believe that they are the cause of that pain. Even fairly young children can be hard on themselves. An adolescent might feel guilty that he is taking up the parent's time and energy when that parent is needed at home or feel guilty that he is annoyed because the parent is there all the time when the parent is trying to help. Young children and siblings often feel guilty that they somehow caused the cancer. Siblings feel guilty for thinking bad things about the sick child or the parent. Guilt is one of the negative emotions children may hesitate to express. They may cry, withdraw, lie, or act out angrily. They may seek to protect the family from their feelings, be embarrassed or ashamed, or feel that they will get in trouble or cause more pain and anguish. It is important to make it clear to the child what is out of his control, what is not his fault, that you are not angry with the child because you have to take care of him or for anything he did or didn't do.

Sadness, for children, usually comes and goes. Our children, like us, grieve for their myriad losses. Isolation, separation from parents, siblings, and friends; loneliness; disappointment; and spiritual distress can contribute.

Acknowledge the losses, for they are great. Even the smallest thing to you may seem considerable to your child. A child who cries is not wallowing but is voicing his or her sadness. Your natural instincts for soothing will kick in: hold and hug her; pat her hand or rub her back; say, "I know, you're right, it's awful"; let her cry it out; give her a tissue and wipe her tears; encourage her to find and focus on something positive; and use a little humor.

Some astute children realize that although their parents are there to help, what's happening is happening to them, to their own bodies, and not to their parents, grandparents, siblings, or the doctor. They can not hide under the bed or run away from cancer. This knowledge, with its hints of mortality, is sad and frightening. Most adults don't learn this until much later in life and even then have trouble coming to terms with it. It is helpful for children to talk to other cancer kids, so they do not feel like they are the only ones in this position.

Emotional reactions to specific triggers and suggestions for coping with them are discussed wherever appropriate throughout the book.

How children manage their emotions

As they grow, children develop strategies to adjust the intensity of experience to a comfortable level, to manage their emotions. Babies rely on their families for stimulation and soothing, although they learn quite early to turn away from the negative and to start sucking to seek the positive. From about age 2, toddlers talk about and actively try to control feelings.

Preschoolers have vivid imaginations, which make them especially prone to magnifying fears. They need help to calm them in the face of such scary events as imagined monsters, the dark, or stormy weather. They are very observant about how adults handle stress and feelings, learning quickly to make use of what they see. Parents can help by suggesting ways to handle their fears. Both parenting and temperament have a strong impact on the development of a child's strategies for handling emotions.

A father describes how he both allowed and helped his son to manage his strong feelings:

> I remember the radiation visits. I'd carry Luke into the hospital (that was my real role, wasn't it, to carry Luke everywhere he wanted to go but couldn't go on his own) and hold him on the way up in the elevators. We'd get off, and I'd carry him about half-way down the hallway. Then, he'd insist on being put down. He'd practically bound in, showing off to his friends, the radiation techs, and docs. After the treatments, it was the same thing in reverse, him walking out under his own steam, but never making it quite all the way to the elevators before collapsing in my arms again. Funny, I'm crying just thinking about how brave he was and how hard he worked to please them all.—*Mike*

By age 10, most children have developed their own set of ways to manage emotions. For events with outcomes at least partly under their control (such as a test or a dispute with a friend), children opt for problem-solving and social support. For events beyond their control (such as a distressing medical procedure), children tend to distract themselves or reframe the situation mentally. Because of their cognitive gains and the growing ability to reason and to delay their impulses, school-age children can use internal means to handle feelings.

A mother describes how her daughter took control of a repeated, uncomfortable procedure to control her anxiety:

> Melanie decided on a definite pattern, telling us firmly who should get the shot ready and who should give the shot. There was great comfort in routine.—*Peggy*

Adolescents can generate a diverse set of emotional coping strategies. They are better able to be flexible in adjusting to the demands placed on them than younger children.

How children learn to show their emotions

Children learn to express their own feelings by learning to recognize and understand the feelings of others. They do this through sensing an emotion in others, through relying on another to give them cues in an uncertain situation, and through empathy—the ability to both grasp another person's perspective and to feel *with* him or her. Children expand their understanding of others as they progress through childhood: Their brains grow and learn, their language develops, they observe the family environment, they discuss feelings, and they engage in make-believe play with brothers and sisters. In school, they learn other cues in a larger social network of relationships and experiences. They learn that people may have more than one emotion at a time.

Children are very tuned in to parents' signals and will react to what they perceive, although it may not always be accurate.

> I made it a point to get myself up every day and put on my make-up, to normalize myself, the day, and to present my "best" self. The one time I did not do it, we'd gotten some bad news. My daughter noticed and immediately said, "What's wrong?"—*Aggie*

The show of emotions is governed by rules in any society. As a part of their development, children learn to make the distinction between what they feel inside and what they show on the outside. They learn when, where, and how they may express emotions. Society teaches children to communicate positive feelings and inhibit the display of negative ones.

By age 7 or 8, there is general conformity to the rules and a conscious awareness and understanding of the rules. Earlier than that, children may comply, but they do not fully understand the value of the rules as a cultural standard. Needless to say, the rules may vary quite widely from cultural group to cultural group.

A child who is hesitant or has trouble communicating feelings may need some encouragement. One way to elicit a reticent (or pre-verbal) child's feelings is to make a visual aid. The simplest would be a paper plate "puppet" with a tongue depressor for a handle, with a happy face on one side and a sad face on the other. Or, make a wheel (out of cardboard, a paper plate, or other heavy paper), flash cards (punch holes and put them on a key ring), or a booklet with pictures of faces and typical statements that might describe the child's feelings. You might choose I want my Mom/Dad/Grandma, I'm scared/angry/sad/embarrassed/jealous/proud, I miss my friends, I want to go home, Thank you, That feels good/better, That hurts, I like you, Yuck, I hate shots, Do not disturb, I can't do it, and I want to try. Let your child choose and illustrate the statements, then use the aid to indicate his or her feelings in a particular situation. Another way to elicit a child's feelings is to teach the child how to say the words for happy, sad, scared, lonely, and hurting in sign language. It may be easier for the child to express his or her feelings in a nonverbal manner.

Communicating Cooperatively

Effective communication involves both talking and listening. It requires both sending and receiving meaningful messages. If either of the two parts is missing, miscommunication happens. Miscommunication causes misunderstandings, upset feelings, arguments, delays in action, escalation of problems, unresolved issues, gaps in information, and unwanted absences or intrusions. Miscommunication makes a mess, but communication generally creates cooperation. Communications skills teacher Dennis Rivers has a useful Web site and book on cooperative communication skills and related readings (see the Bibliography).

Major Steps for Good Communication

Give a whole message

Whole messages are direct and clear. They establish a framework for the listener to hear your intent and your message. Express the intent of your message as clearly and completely as possible. For example, ask for what you want as the outcome:

> I would like your help to brainstorm options for tutoring programs for Johnny. John and I are trying to collect ideas from as many sources as we can before we make a choice for Johnny.

Give the listener a way to understand your experience and intention. For example, give "I" messages about your observations, feelings, understandings (which includes your knowledge, interpretations, and evaluations), and hopes:

> I am worried because Mary is not eating [combines feelings and observation]. Fortunately, you alerted us that she might have periodic trouble related to the chemo effects, but the problem seems to be lasting longer than we thought it would [conveys understanding and observation]. I hope you will talk with her and examine her to see if something might help her [expresses hope and the intent of the communication].

Avoid inflammatory messages. Accusatory "you" messages are opposite from "I" messages and can be damaging. Try not to say "you always do this" or "you never do that," because it stops open communication. Instead the listener will get angry, defensive, or offensive or maybe all three.

The introduction of "always" and "never" statements into a dialogue drags in exaggeration and old grievances. Instead of a clear whole message, it becomes a muddy one with multiple messages. It is hard to avoid accusatory messages when you are hurt and angry. Sometimes the best you can do is catch yourself and apologize. It is not necessary to abase yourself with overapologizing, but it is not helpful to withhold apologies when they are warranted. This is true whether you are speaking to a doctor, a spouse, or your child.

Be a good listener

First of all, put yourself even with the person's physical level. Standing over someone who is trying to say something difficult will only intimidate him or her further. Privacy may be helpful or necessary. Watch for nonverbal cues (such as looking down or away, wringing hands, jittery hands or feet, not looking you in the eye, or pacing) that may indicate that the person is uncomfortable, upset, angry, anxious, or holding something back.

Become an active listener. This starts with trying to understand the experience of the other person, which means the intent of the communication and his or her "I" messages that reflect the experience. Of course, people often do not communicate clearly, so it helps to have some tools to get past the blocks. If you are willing to listen actively and to acknowledge the other person's experience but do not understand the message, try the following steps to clear up the confusion or conflict:

- Ask for clarification.

> I understand you will be late. Are you saying you want me to save dinner for you, or you will eat before you get home?

- Paraphrase or summarize the message you are hearing.

Let me see if I understand. You are faced with a tough choice here and you want me to be a sounding board, but you don't want me to give advice. You want to sort out your own feelings.

- Give feedback.

You seem to be saying two things at once, that you want to do this by yourself and that you need my help. I am willing to let you do it or help a bit, if that makes it easier.

- Communicate openness and empathy.

I know this has been a tough time for you. You didn't get much sleep last night, so you are tired and cranky today. I can see why you would be irritated with me for pushing you to do your homework. We'll find a better way.

Smooth the way with questions

Use open-ended questions, those that give the listener free rein about how to respond rather than just with "yes" or "no" answers. These types of questions open up and move a dialogue along, because many responses are possible. They are creative and invite the responder to be creative, too.

What did you think of the new physical therapy routine?
How can we add to the plan we began to discuss yesterday?

Beware of giving criticism disguised as a question. Such veiled barbs are not really questions. Instead, convert the barb into a real question or request with an improved message. For the following question samples the background situation is a difficult moment between a father and his teenage son. Originally the father was trying to find out whether his son had put the recycling bin out at the curb for the weekly collection. The son replied that he was busy and his brother should do it anyway. The father's response was barely concealed and annoyed criticism:

Did you really think you could get away with that?

A more clear and direct message with a request would be

The recycling is your job in this family. If you want to discuss changing the assignment of chores, we can do that on the weekend. In the meantime, will you please take out the recycling bin, as we agreed? [Clarification of understanding, openness to renegotiate at a specific time, making a clear request]

Look for the positive

Give praise, encouragement, and thanks. Everyone likes to be valued and appreciated. It warms relationships when you express the positive. Children (and adults) have many experiences of being "caught" for "bad" behavior. All of us respond better in an atmosphere with more room in it for being "caught" at being "good." It can be hard to offer this or to find the positive in an atmosphere filled with distressing emotions. Nevertheless, it is usually possible to find a positive place to make a beginning.

> Turn your face to the sun, and the shadows fall behind you.
> Maori proverb

Conspiracy of Silence

One major barrier to open communication is the conspiracy of silence that surrounds certain issues. Every family has unwritten rules about what can be said openly and what cannot. Some family members or friends refuse to discuss cancer, the possibility of death, the realities of long-term effects, their feelings, and their fears. Even hospital staff has subjects they avoid. This refusal can stem from a misguided attempt to protect you or themselves from painful feelings, from awkwardness or discomfort because they do not know what to say, from a superstitious fear that talking about negative things might bring them about, or even from their own inability to cope with the situation.

The unwritten rules trickle down to even the youngest family members. Children quickly discern which subjects should not be talked about—either to protect their parents from additional pain or out of fear that their expressions will be met with anger or rejection. It is especially important that a child's emotional expressions be encouraged and not suppressed to keep the child from feeling isolated.

> This inability to share emotions and questions can distance children from the people who nurture and provide support . . . children live, and tragically, sometimes die, with the awesome burden of comforting those who should be their source of comfort.—*Rev. Dane Sommer (see the Bibliography)*

Asserting Yourself Responsibly

Responsible assertion involves standing up for personal rights—yours or your child's—in an appropriate way. Like cooperative communication principles, responsible assertion is a direct and clear form of communication. It is respectful of your own or your child's needs and rights and of the rights and needs of others. The aim of responsible assertion is mutuality, which allows for fair play and often leaves room for compromise to resolve conflicts.

> Yes, I want to help you with your homework, and we can take the time after dinner to do it. But right now I need to finish getting this meal on the table. I can't do both things at once, and I hope you can be patient. What do you say?

The only time compromise is not suitable is when important issues of basic integrity are at stake.

> I understand this order seems right to you, but the dose is different than what Dr. Smith told me. I don't mean to be disrespectful, but I must insist that you check on this drug dosage. I cannot allow you to inject this into my daughter's IV until we are both certain it is correct.

The examples above set clear limits and give a whole message without attacking the listener. Contrast this with nonassertion and with aggressiveness. Nonassertion violates your rights; aggression violates the rights of others. Nonassertion erases your own or your child's needs. Typically, the goal for nonassertive behavior is to avoid conflict and to give in to others. This can take the form of silence, expressing yourself in such an apologetic tentative way that you are not effective, or allowing others to dictate to you. It conveys a lack of self-respect and inferiority. If you become a doormat, do not be surprised when people walk all over you.

> Oh, okay, I guess I can take the time to go to the dry cleaners, too. Maybe it was selfish of me to say I am busy this morning.

Aggression trespasses on other people's needs. It is disrespectful, because it is focused on winning, often at the expense of others. It does not foster mutuality. Typically the goal is to dominate the relationship or to prop up one's own sense of self by humiliating the other person.

> You're really selfish to think of asking me to go to the dry cleaners for you. I already do much more than my share of chores in this marriage. What's the matter with you?

Resolving Conflict Amiably

Conflict is a natural part of life in all kinds of relationships. It is to be expected at home, at work, in the medical system, and in the community. The question is not whether a conflict will arise but how to negotiate and navigate conflict to a comfortable solution. The first step is to spot when a conflict is being set in motion or has already happened.

> My husband handled some things differently than I would have. For instance, while I was in the hospital with Luke, Mike told our other son that Luke had cancer, then sent him off to school. His teacher said Tommy came to school, poured this information out, and sat there and cried. I wanted to be there to talk to Tommy together and comfort him. It took me two years to forgive Mike for that. It still upsets me. It was a poor judgment call.—*Liz*

Conflict stems from differences. It can be triggered by different values or goals or a simple act of thoughtlessness. It can be a product of poor communication, in which differences are unrecognized, fuzzy, or exaggerated. Personalizing an issue, which is often the result of differing life scripts, can stimulate it. Regardless of the source, conflict needs to be recognized and addressed. The problem needs to be solved jointly. The goal is to resolve the conflict effectively and to preserve an amicable relationship.

> We had a couple of roommate conflicts. There were times I didn't feel comfortable leaving Anne alone in the room. I didn't feel that she was safe. One time, the father of a child we were rooming with was using foul language. I went to the social worker, and she spoke with him. Another time, I couldn't sleep because Anne's roommate had the TV on all night. The nurse said that the child couldn't sleep without it. I felt that since she was the patient, her needs took the front seat. But that was a challenge. Now, if it had kept Anne from sleeping, I would have insisted on turning it off.—*Pam*

* * *

> While we were in the hospital, a close family member asked if she could do a little housecleaning for me. The next day, I was informed by my partner that the woman called everyone she knew to discuss her opinions of my lifestyle, using the illness of my son to justify her comments. In her opinion, I should "grow up and be a responsible parent for the sake of the kids." I certainly didn't need her implying that I was responsible for the illness or unable to care for him. I was fuming mad. She wrote me a letter, apologizing. I realize everyone deals with things in their own way, and she is someone I have to deal with over the years, so I do have to come to some sort of understanding with her. Although I might be able to forgive, I don't think I'll ever forget how salt was rubbed into an open wound.—*Kim*

In his work *The Eight Essential Steps to Conflict Resolution* (see the Bibliography), professor Dudley Weeks outlines the following important action steps. We give our own examples to illustrate his steps:

- *Create an effective atmosphere.* Pick a comfortable time and private place for discussions. At the hospital you might choose a private lounge or small conference room; at home, wait until the children are asleep, or hire a baby-sitter and sit in your parked car if you have nowhere else to go that is private. In conversations that you think may get out of hand, offer to follow basic ground rules, and ask the other person to do the same: no yelling, name-calling, belittling, or airing old grievances.

- *Clarify perceptions.* State your own understanding of the issue, and ask the other person for his or hers. In addition, you might also state what you think some of the obstacles are and your optimism that a mutually satisfying solution can be found.
- *Focus on individual and shared needs.* Both are important. For example, many conflicts are about simple things like requests for more flexible work schedules, accommodations in treatment arrangements, and taking responsibility for noticing what needs to be done around the house. Compromises are usually more acceptable when both parties see that individual needs fit in with shared goals.
- *Build positive shared power.* Explore how much more effective you can be if you act as a team to accomplish a goal. Also, create ways for shared decision-making rather than one party being in control and one being bossed.
- *Look to the future; learn from the past.* There is an old sports saying, "Don't stay with a losing game." In other words, if the way you are operating is not helping you to reach your goal, then assess the picture and start trying some new things that will give you a better chance as you go forward.
- *Generate options.* Be creative and come up with new possibilities. Don't become bogged down by limiting yourself to one choice versus none or having to choose only between competing alternatives. If the two of you cannot think of new options, ask a third person to contribute.
- *Develop "doables."* Select something you both agree can be done. The idea may be only a first step, but it sets the stage for later doables.
- *Make mutual benefit agreements.* The resolution has to work for both parties. It might involve a compromise, combining some of what each of you wanted. It might involve a trade (I'll give you this and you'll give me that, and we will both get something important). It might be a pact to do something positive or to stop doing something negative.

It is not always easy to resolve a conflict or arrive at ideal solutions. When a conflict drags on, the most helpful path may be to seek a neutral third party to mediate. For limited disputes, you may choose a trusted and fair friend or relative, one who can be objective and is respected by both parties. In very contentious situations or when the problem is chronic, a psychotherapist (such as a marriage counselor, social worker, or psychologist) is likely to be of greater assistance with personal relationship conflicts.

Our Encouragement

Relationships are supported by the four aspects discussed: handling emotions well, good communication, responsible assertiveness, and effective conflict resolution. With those as a solid foundation, your family's problem-solving capacity is improved greatly.

We would like to add a note of encouragement for times of extraordinary strain. It is a sign of strength and not weakness to recognize when your resources are severely depleted or challenged. Under those circumstances, it is a healthy choice to widen your support network. Seek professional problem-solving guidance. Mental health professionals, such as psychologists, social workers, and marriage and family counselors, can be useful to you by seeing your situation with a neutral, fresh perspective. For example, a miscommunication is readily resolved when the problem is identified and a joint solution is reached. An out-of-control emotional situation can be brought back into control in a way that works well for the family as a whole.

CHAPTER 6

Reducing Stress

You can't always get what you want, but if you try sometimes,
you just might find, you get what you need.
—Mick Jagger and Keith Richards

The hardest thing had to be waiting for results. It was the uncertainty. If it seemed like it was taking too long for the top numbers to come back, I would worry. If it seemed like the nurse was avoiding us or she didn't look me in the eye, I would panic. And of course, for my husband, sitting in his office, waiting, waiting, waiting. Sometimes I would forget to call him. He would call me, asking why haven't you called me. Oh, I forgot. If you don't hear from me, everything's fine. He said no, I don't know everything's fine. He was picking his fingernails off and chewing his cuticles. And pulling out bunches of hair from his moustache. He finally had to shave his moustache, because he would sit there and pick at it.—*Carly*

Life is full of stresses—from the physical world around us, from society, from our bodies, and from our minds. The normal stresses of life do not go away when you have a child with cancer, they get compounded. Newer, bigger stresses increase the weight bearing down on you. While you cannot escape the realities of cancer treatment, you can shape your responses. You can make yourself feel better. If you are able to relax and be calmer, you will be much better equipped to handle the next crisis.

Dealing With Symptoms of Stress

The body responds to stress automatically with a series of biochemical reactions. For example, stress hormones are produced that affect bodily function. If the stress is temporary, the response is turned off, and the body quickly returns to normal. When the stress is chronic, such as when you are dealing with cancer treatment and effects, the response continues, and the results are noticeable. Here are the common symptoms:

Symptoms of Stress

Headache, migraine, backache
Muscle tension, neck-aches
Fatigue, weakness
Stomach upset, ulcers, indigestion
Constipation, diarrhea
Acne, rashes, hair falling out
Teeth grinding, picking at self
Pain intensified
Irritability, short temper
Hypertension
Stuttering, stumbling over words
Easily distracted, oblivious to environment
Feeling lost, confused, incompetent
Cold hands and feet
Suppression of menstruation
Loss of sex drive, impotency
Existing ailments get worse: asthma, diabetes, arthritis
Susceptibility to cold or flu
Contributor to depression
Tics, tremors
Sleep disturbances, insomnia
Weight gain or loss
Muddled thinking
Indecisiveness
Can't mobilize self

Parents find it most difficult to take time for themselves and report that they wish they had done so more often. Try to overcome your reluctance by realizing that you are doing your child a favor. You cannot take care of your child if you are falling apart. You may not be taking a week's vacation to Tahiti, but an hour or two can do wonders. Several stress-reducing techniques do not require you to be away from your child. Relaxation exercises are portable; you can do them at the bedside or even in a waiting room. Keep in mind that children, too, get stressed. They can reap the benefits of relaxation and tension release as well.

> One thing Mitch and I will argue about. He always encourages me to get on the phone, call my friends, and go out. And I don't do it. I think I feel guilty. Why do I deserve to go out and have a good time when my child is home sick? But you need to recharge your batteries. I didn't do it enough.—*Debra*

Start by examining your own stresses and reactions. How stressed were you before your child was diagnosed? How stressed are you now? Make a list of the things that really get to you. Note how often they occur, such as daily or weekly. Think about how you usually react to these pressures. Choose one or two at a time to change. What can you avoid? Which job can you give someone else? Start with the little things. If it is something over which you have no control (such as waiting for blood test results), what you can address is how you react.

Suggestions for Immediate Stress Reduction

Do something physical

Physical activity is a terrific tension release and has the added benefit of keeping you healthy, alert, and energized. Exercise each day, at the hospital or at home.

- Take a brisk 20-minute walk.
- Take the stairs and not the elevator.
- Rip up phone books.
- Punch a punching bag, a pillow, or the bed.
- Do jumping jacks, stretches, or run in place.
- Do shoulder and neck rolls or "windmills."
- Use a treadmill, ride a stationary bike, or swim.
- Knead dough or clay.
- Get out in your garden and yank weeds.
- Practice aerobics, tae-bo, karate, or dance.
- Play racquetball, volleyball, or tennis; jog.
- Go for a bike ride, jump rope, or rollerblade

Relax

Practice yoga, tai chi, or meditation. Use breathing, visualization, and imagery techniques (see the exercises discussed later). Get a massage; your hospital may have a massage therapist available to you or your child. You and a partner can offer each other massages. Use lotion or oil to make it more soothing; put a drop of vanilla in mineral oil for a bit of aromatherapy.

Get away, physically

Go on "escape-ades." Go for a walk after hours with your child in a stroller or wheelchair at the hospital. Explore a little. Take a bubble bath or long hot shower. Rest or nap for half an hour. Go for a drive or a walk in the park. Hire a baby-sitter and go to dinner or the movies. Don't be afraid to go alone. Running errands doesn't count as a getaway.

Get away, mentally

Read an adventure novel or a mystery, something that is not about cancer. Do a crossword puzzle. Take a mental vacation. Listen to music. Daydream.

Release emotions
Cry in the shower, in the car, or at night in bed. Talk out your feelings with a good listener (your spouse, a friend, a counselor, the clergy, or even your pet). Talk to other cancer parents. Keep a journal. Draw, paint, or write poetry. Scream at the world (out of earshot of the kids, of course).

Do something fun
Whenever your child feels up to it, do something fun with him or her.

- Have a picnic indoors or out.
- Continue your hobbies: crafts, needlework, model building, and collecting.
- Search scouting handbooks for projects.
- Do makeovers or paint nails.
- Make "fortune-tellers" (with positive predictions) and paper footballs.
- Use craft supplies to make "swaps" (miniature doodads to pin onto hats and extras to swap with other kids).
- Hang posters on the ceiling.
- Learn something new from library books, such as origami, sign language, magic tricks, or handwriting analysis.
- Play musical instruments or have a parade.
- Have a checkers tournament; play cards.
- Put together jigsaw puzzles; use a flexible "board" to roll up and carry the puzzle.
- Get a lava lamp, bubble tube, fiberoptic source, or electrical impulse display.

Suggestions for Long-Term Stress Reduction

Take care of your body
Eat right and regularly. Avoid junk food from the vending machines when you can. Eat healthy food, with less fat, sugar, and sodium, and eat smaller portions more often. Get some sleep; the regularity of it is almost more important than the amount.

Organize your life and be prepared for emergencies

- Organize medical supplies in a bureau or closet, out of sight but accessible, all in one place, so you know when you are running low on something. Use a makeup caddy or tackle box for small supplies. Stackable, plastic pull-out drawers work well for larger supplies. Label them for easy access.

- Maintain complete medical and insurance records. Put all of the paperwork into a three-ring binder. Use an executive organizer, journal, calendar, or spiral notebook to log medications, blood counts, hospitalizations, reactions, surgeries, feedings, transportation and lodging costs, emotions, feelings, and events.
- Carry paperwork (such as treatment information, appointment slips, insurance cards and necessary forms, authorizations, referrals, and your child's latest health reports) with you at all times (use a folding file, briefcase, or plastic storage container in your car's trunk).
- Carry a list of phone numbers of your child's school, your spouse's and other family members' work, the insurance company, doctors, the pharmacy, the hospital, baby-sitters, friends, and neighbors.
- Use the calendar or a poster on the refrigerator to chart school and activity schedules so that family or friends taking care of your kids at home know what they need each day (such as library books, a ride to soccer practice, clean dance clothes, or help with homework).
- Put kids' names in their clothes so the person doing laundry knows whose is whose.
- Post phone numbers of the pediatrician, hospital, oncologist, baby-sitters, and cell phones, and list medications. Also list who is available in emergencies on which days, at which times, and for which tasks so you don't have to worry about them or waste time making phone calls.
- Manage your time properly; do not overbook appointments.
- Expect delays: Bring books, coloring supplies, travel-sized games, string for cat's cradle, electronic games, dolls, craft work, crossword puzzles, homework, journal, snacks (save them for after the procedure if your child is not supposed to have anything beforehand), paper and pens (for hangman, tic-tac-toe, and dots), and cash for food.
- Bring someone with you to the clinic (to listen, drive, get food, keep siblings company, mind the children so you can confer with doctors alone, and help digest what has happened afterward).
- Do as much as you can before you go to bed (such as make lunches, pack backpacks, make up formula, set out clothes, pack hospital bag, and take a bath or shower).
- Prepare for procedures so that you and your child know what to expect (see chapter 8).
- Do what you can for your child ahead of time at home (such as hydrating with fluids or getting a urine sample).

- Check your insurance, and get referrals in advance.
- Keep your car in good shape, with full tank of gas. If your car is unreliable, arrange a long-term, temporary trade with a family member; get help to finance repairs; or trade yours in and lease a newer model.
- Keep extra clothes, towels, plastic bags, wipes, and an emesis basin (a "throw-up bucket") in the car.
- Pack an emergency overnight bag for your child and yourself, and keep it at work, in your trunk, or at day care so you don't have to make an extra trip home to pick it up.
- Have physicians call prescriptions in so you do not have to wait for them to be filled. Take advantage of the delivery service. Call ahead for refills, or have standing orders for ongoing prescriptions. Have a back-up pharmacy in case the first one has trouble getting an item. Pharmacists can also offer palliative complements such as acidophilus (which may help avoid gastrointestinal distress and bladder or yeast infections). Just be careful not to use anything that might interfere with treatment (ask your doctor first).

Set realistic goals

Brainstorm. Develop action plans to get over hurdles. Evaluate progress periodically, and set new goals.

Delegate

Keep a list of tasks, and let other people do them. Does it really matter if these are done your way? Let them go; when this is all over, you can get back to doing them yourself.

Prioritize

Keep routines as normal as possible, but let go of anything unnecessary or stressful. So, don't clean the house, buy classroom cupcakes instead of baking them, and sell off this season's tickets. You do not have to coach basketball, run the PTA, or go after a high-powered promotion. Do those next year.

Stay on an even keel

Take one day at a time; do one thing at a time. Focus on good things that happen, however small. Do not jump to conclusions or take everything personally. Be forgiving. Is it worth expending your energy on getting angry over something that couldn't be helped or predicted? Count to 50 before you react. Be flexible.

Keep a sense of humor

Do not be afraid to laugh. Read joke books. Watch cartoons, TV comedy shows, and old movies (especially the Marx Brothers, the Three Stooges, Jerry Lewis, Laurel & Hardy, and Abbott & Costello).

> A young doctor came in to our hospital room and asked my friend and me if there were any problems. I raised my hand and said, deadpan, "Yeah, rhabdomyosarcoma." Laura raised hers and said, "Leukemia." We started laughing, and the guy just stood there. The nurse practitioner came in saying, "Don't mind these two."—*Alice*

* * *

> Even when I didn't feel like it, I made sure to do something impulsive, crazy, or stupid whenever possible. Late one evening in the cafeteria, there was nobody behind me. Not sure which entree to pick, and the lady behind the counter is getting impatient. I say, "Hang on. . . wait. . ." and do this thing with my fingers pointing different directions on top of my head while sort of nodding a little. "All right. The secret alien transmissions tell me to get the VEGETABLE LASAGNA!" Sure, it was totally stupid. But the cafeteria folks were at the end of a long day, and they thought it was funny. And from then on, I had to do the "transmission" thing every Monday and Thursday. They'd ask, "So, what is the Mother Ship telling you to eat today?" So for 10 minutes once or twice a day, I was out of Cancer Land and into Fun Land. That was enough to clear my head and stop the panicky thoughts for a while.—*Leon*

Consult a professional

Social workers, marriage counselors, psychologists, psychiatrists, child life specialists, biofeedback experts, and massage therapists are all able to help you relieve your stress.

Stress Inducers to Avoid

Minimize or avoid the following items, which can cause or aggravate stress.

- Alcohol
- Caffeine
- Drugs, such as diet pills, controlled substances, or overreliance on sleeping pills
- Anyone who makes you feel anxious, guilty, pessimistic, or overwhelmed.

> I would recommend that you stay away from anybody that makes you feel bad. That's a really big thing. There was one woman who would be screaming in the hall, "They're killing my daughter," and she wouldn't go along with what the doctors wanted her to do. It was really bad, and I just stayed away from that person.—*Judith*

Stress-Reducing Exercises

The same mechanism that turns on a "fight-or-flight" alarm can turn it off. The relaxation response (a term originated by Herbert Benson in 1975, see the Bibliography) can be actively initiated using simple techniques that can be done by anyone, anywhere, at anytime. They do not cost anything or require any materials. These are widely available techniques that you might find used in yoga, in relaxation and stress workbooks or Web sites, and from various sorts of therapists.

While a quiet, private place to lie down might bring optimum effect, you can do the exercises in an ER, if you have to. The exercises here are examples of typical relaxation, imagery, and breathing. You can adapt them to your needs, have someone else read them to you, or make an audiotape of yourself reading them.

Focused Breathing/Deep Breathing

Breathing is an involuntary activity. Most of us don't think about how we do it. When we are stressed, our breathing is shallower, irregular, or rapid. We may even hold our breath without realizing it. This kind of breathing is part of the body's response to stress but also keeps the cycle going.

Lie down, if you can, with your knees bent and feet flat on the floor or a bed. You could also do this sitting in a chair. Put one hand on your chest and one on your abdomen. Become aware of your breathing. Do your chest and shoulders rise the most? That's shallow breathing. To become more relaxed, try abdominal or diaphragm breathing.

Breathe in slowly through your nose. Keep inhaling, even when you think you cannot take in any more air. Feel your abdomen rise. Feel the air fill your lower, middle, and upper lungs. Breathe out slowly through your pursed mouth, making a soft whooshing sound. Keep exhaling, even when you think you have no more air to expel. Press with your palm on your abdomen if you wish. Continue for several minutes. A purifying breath is a deep breath that you take in through the nose, hold briefly, and release through the mouth in short, forceful puffs.

Next, try one of the exercises in the box. The first one is our own. The second is adapted from *Breast Cancer: A Psychological Treatment Manual,* edited by Sandra Haber, PhD, a collaboration of 10 psychologists, including the coauthor of this book, Carol Goodheart (Copyright 1995. Adapted with permission of Springer Publishing Company, Inc., New York; see the Bibliography).

Focused Breathing/Deep Breathing Exercises

Inhale slowly and deeply through your nose. Exhale through your mouth, making a quiet, whooshing noise as you blow out. Take long, deep breaths that raise and lower your abdomen. Focus on the sound and sensation of your breathing. Imagine with each breath, you take in relaxation. Relax your face, your jaw. Imagine with each exhale, you are breathing out tension. Breathe in relaxation to the rest of your body, one part at a time. Do this for at least 5–10 minutes. If you like, you can count your breaths or sigh with each breath.

* * *

Breathe comfortably and easily. Imagine your breath as a warmth, a comforting presence that enters your body and brings peace. Feel the warmth and peace spread throughout your body as you breathe. Calming all your body. Become aware of any part of your body that feels tense. Bring your breath to that muscle or area, and become aware of how much more relaxed it becomes as your breath touches it.

Relaxation

In the following box is a progressive relaxation exercise also adapted with permission from Dr. Haber's book. At first, you may want to have a partner read this to you as you try it. If you have a therapist, he or she can make a personalized relaxation tape for you.

Progressive Relaxation Exercise

Lie down in a comfortable place. Breathe easily and regularly. Focus on your breathing. As you inhale, feel your breath bring peace and calm to every part of your body. Do this for a few minutes.

At your next inhalation, point your toes and stretch the bottoms of your feet. Hold your breath, and as you do so, hold your feet in the outstretched position. Then gently exhale and relax your feet. Breathe comfortably for a few minutes.

At your next inhalation, tighten your leg muscles and stretch your legs. Hold this position as you hold your breath, then gently exhale and relax your legs. Breathe comfortably for a few minutes.

Feel your legs becoming warm, heavy, and relaxed.

When you next inhale, tighten the muscles of your buttocks; hold this tightness as you hold your breath. Gently exhale, and relax your buttocks. Breathe comfortably for a few minutes, then inhale and tighten your stomach muscles; hold this tightness as you hold your breath. Gently exhale and relax.

Box continues next page

Continued

Feel your whole lower half of your body becoming heavy, warm, and relaxed.

Inhale, and make your hands into two fists and pull your arms straight down, as if you were pulling them out of their sockets. Hold your breath and hold your hands and arms in this tight position, then gently exhale and relax your arms and hands. Breathe comfortably for a few minutes, then inhale and pull your head down and touch your chest with your chin. Hold this position as you hold your breath, for as long as you can. Breathe comfortably for a few minutes, then exhale and relax your head and chest muscles. Now your whole body is feeling warm, heavy, and relaxed.

Breathe comfortably for a few minutes, and when you next inhale, raise your shoulders up to your ears and hold them there as you hold your breath, for as long as you can. Then exhale and relax your head and neck.

Breathe comfortably for a few minutes, then inhale and scrunch your face up and tighten all of your facial muscles. Become aware of how much tension you are carrying on your face and tighten all of those areas. Hold this position as you hold your breath, for as long as you can, and as you exhale relax your face muscles, and feel all of the tightness dissolve.

Now breathe comfortably for awhile. If there is any part of your body that still feels tense, visualize your breath as a ray of soft warmth that can be directed to that tight place to relax it and heal it. Stay in this position as long as you wish.

Think of a code word for the way you feel when you are relaxed so that you can return to this position any time you need to. Practice saying your code word and feeling your whole body relaxed, warm and heavy as it is now.

Other forms of relaxation, using a combination of breathing, relaxation and imagery, are also helpful. This centering exercise is also adapted with permission from Dr. Haber's book.

Centering Exercise

Stand with your feet about 10 inches apart, knees bent in skiers' snowplow position. Keeping your knees bent, allow your body to fall forward until your head is hanging down as close as possible to your feet. Breathe deeply. Using your fingertips to maintain your balance, and keeping knees bent, slowly raise your heels off the ground. Experience the vibrations that go through your legs and into your body as you do this. Stay this way for as long as you can, then slowly return your heels to the ground, keeping knees bent. Slowly raise your upper body to an upright position and then raise your arms above your head. Explore the space around you and become aware of the space you own in the world. As you do this, stay in touch with your own inner center, and say out loud if possible, "I'm alive!" or "I'm okay."

The next exercise in the box is adapted from an excellent resource, *The Relaxation and Stress Reduction Workbook,* by Martha Davis, Elizabeth Robbins Eshelman, and Matthew McKay (adapted with permission of New Harbinger Publications, Oakland, CA; see the Bibliography).

Eye Relaxation

Put your palms gently over your eyes. Block out the light. Use a mental image to see the color black. Continue for a few minutes, focusing on black. Lower your hands and slowly open your eyes.

Meditation

The Relaxation and Stress Reduction Workbook also explains meditation and gives examples of exercises, one of which is adapted here. Meditation facilitates relaxation by focusing your attention on one thing at time. What you choose to focus on is not important. It can be a word, syllable, a name, or a group of words (mantra), or you can gaze at fixed object. Thoughts and emotions pop into your head, are acknowledged, and released. Do not try to make sense of them. Just let them be.

Meditation Exercise

Close your eyes and focus on the place where your body touches the cushion or chair, or itself. Pay attention to the places of contact. Focus on the way your body takes up space. Take several deep breaths and be aware of your breathing. Notice where your breath rests in your body; try taking it from one area to the other: into your upper chest, your stomach, your belly. Feel your abdomen expand and contract.

Mantra meditation: choose a word or syllable, even a nonsense sound, or the word "one." Chant silently to yourself. Say it over and over within your mind. When your thought strays, note it, then bring attention back. Notice sensations, then return. Let it find its own rhythm. Try chanting aloud. Let the sound of your voice fill you as you relax. Notice whether the sensations are different than in silent chanting. Try to stay aware of each repetition of each syllable.

Breath counting meditation: follow the ins and outs of your gentle breathing. Close your eyes or fix them on a spot on floor about four feet in front of you. Take deep but not forced breaths. Focus your attention on each part of the breath: inhale, turn, exhale, pause, turn, inhale, and so on. Pay attention to the pauses. Notice bodily sensations. As you exhale, say one. Count each exhale until you get to four. Start over at one. If you lose count, start at one again.

Gazing meditation: gaze at an object (a flower, a stone, a statue). Notice everything about it. Use a soft focus. Trace its edges with your eyes. Experience its qualities.

Imagery/Visualization

Visualization is the process of creating visual images in your mind and focusing on them to improve the quality of life. Imagery is very personal. A man, a woman, a teenager, and a 7-year-old will choose very different images. Any visualization exercise can be adapted. Let the person think of the most safe spot, where he or she feels the best, such as the seashore, the mountains, or a cozy room.

You close your eyes, empty your mind, and sketch a scene of that special place, with all the sights, sounds, and smells. Perhaps you take a path, a staircase, or a hot-air balloon to get there. Imagine what you would feel and do there. Let harsh images fade into more relaxing ones (colors soften, lights dim, focus softens, loud or upsetting things "morph" into more pleasing ones). Imagine a goal for yourself, and see yourself doing it.

The following visualization exercise was adapted with permission from Dr. Haber.

Visualization Exercise

Close your eyes and breathe comfortably. Take yourself to a wonderfully peaceful place: the sun is shining, the sounds of the wind chimes play in the background and songbirds fill the air with joyous songs. The sun shines down upon your body and brings with it the sense of hope. As the sun touches your body it creates the beginning of a new you. See and feel the sunbeams touching your body, and visualize a new you slowly and gracefully emerging from yourself, bathed in the warm caresses of the sun. The new you is you at your best: strong, calm, whole, beautiful in body and spirit. You feel competent and powerful. You are peaceful and relaxed.

Keep this image of the new you before your eyes. Watch as you move about in the sunlight, moving gracefully in the breeze, doing anything you need or want to do. Enjoy this you. Keep this image as you do this visualization and take the image with you after you finish, so that you an always see it and recharge your sense of hope in yourself and your life.

Anger Expression

Expressing anger in a safe, protected environment can be an exhilarating experience. Try the following exercises, which are adapted with permission from Dr. Haber's work (with the exception of guided combact, which is an idea gleaned from a Sibshop experience):

- Stand or sit in front of a couch or bed. Hit the bed with your fists and forearms or a tennis racket.
- Stamp your feet, kick a bean bag chair, or lie down and kick your feet on the

bed while shouting "NO, NO, NO, WHY, WHY, WHY, I hate ____, I won't ____, I want ____!"

- Stand with your feet about 10 inches apart, knees slightly bent. Make two fists. Bend your elbows so your arms with clenched fists are in front of your chest. Extend the lower jaw. Breathe deeply. Say, "off my back" (forcefully), pulling your arms behind you very strongly until your elbows pass behind the rib cage. Repeat several times. Get louder and louder with each one.
- Try guided combat: Bop each other with foam bats, yelling out what you are mad at. "I'm mad that ____." Follow strict rules, such as no hitting above the shoulders. Stop immediately if anyone calls for a time-out. However, this is not a good exercise for children with low platelets.
- Go for a run or a fast walk.

If you try to add all of these stress reduction techniques to your "to do" list, you will only stress yourself out even further. Pick and choose according to your needs and circumstances. Choose the kinds of activities and exercises that you naturally gravitate toward or would enjoy doing.

CHAPTER 7

Alleviating Trauma

It is hard to fight an enemy who has outposts in your head.
—*Sally Kempton,* "Cutting Loose," Esquire (July 1970)

Treatment is finished. We just go back to the clinic every three months for checkups. He's back at school and getting back into all his activities. But I feel worse now than I did when he was on treatment. I was too busy then to worry. Now I have plenty of time to think about it, and I'm scared. I have trouble getting to sleep because I'm replaying things in my mind. My family keeps telling me I should be happy. I am, but all these "what ifs" keep going through my head.—*Nadia*

Is cancer experienced as a trauma? The word *trauma* conjures up images that most of us would rather not think about, like war or violence. Yet the culture of cancer is couched in the language and imagery of war: fighting, battling, winning, losing, heroism, tragedy, courage, victim, veteran. These words pay homage to the difficulty, the effort expended to get through the ordeal, as well as the dire possibilities and the "patriotic" optimism for "our side" to win.

In this chapter we show you the adult trauma picture, followed by the child's, so you can recognize the signs of distress that are important to pay attention to. Then we consider recovery, the practical steps to take when traumatic stress occurs. Lasting impressions and healing complete the chapter. If you find it hard to read about trauma specifics right now, skip to the section on lasting impressions. However, if your child is on treatment now and you skip over the trauma recovery part, make sure to return to the section on practical help for children.

What Is Trauma?

Both you and your child need a way to get through those parts of cancer's emotional aftermath known as "traumatic stress reactions." Traumatic stress fuels anxiety. You, we, and everyone else react to severe stress by trying to protect ourselves and recover from this anxiety, naturally.

Trauma occurs when a person suffers a terribly distressing event, his or her ability to cope becomes temporarily overwhelmed, and he or she doesn't simply bounce back. If this happens to you or your child, you might find yourself re-experiencing the bad event again and again in your mind and having bad dreams. You cannot just "let it go" or not think about it, as people may be advising you to do. You might become hypersensitive—super alert—to sensed danger triggered by sights, sounds, or touch. You might avoid more and more situations that make you anxious. You might feel shut down or numb. But remember, help is available. Do not fear that you will always feel this way.

The experience of childhood cancer is emotionally distressing for you, your child, and your family. Trauma reactions may be set off by the aggressive medical treatments, the side effects that are hard to endure, and the many physical and emotional demands. Children undergoing active cancer treatments are assaulted by physical intrusion—surgeries, amputations, chemotherapy, radiation therapy, bone marrow aspirations, feeding tubes, and transplants. It is not surprising that the children may look like acute trauma victims for a time. As a parent, you suffer assaults from watching your child undergo these experiences.

> Going to the hospital was always extremely stressful. I worried about what Lloyd would see there. There were very sick and some very scary looking children there. There were a few times when [we] had to deal with roommates who were yelling, crying out in pain, or throwing up all the time. You just wanted to scream and run out of there, but you couldn't. I came home from the pediatric cancer ward feeling like I had just been let out of a chamber of horrors.—*Sandy*

Acute stress hits you during this active illness phase. Chronic stress replaces it over time. You are in pain if the disease is progressive rather than controllable. You are anxious when the treatment ends successfully but fears of recurrence begin to set in. You have strain and worry about handling any continuing disabilities or limitations. Lengthy and difficult treatment, ongoing maintenance, steroid medication, degree of bodily injury, and continuing needs for advocacy because of late effects are all factors that can make you more vulnerable to trauma.

When the outside distressing events are finally past, the internal distressing thoughts take over. If your upset reactions are ignored and go unresolved, adjustment to your child's disease and any long-term physical effects is hampered. Also, relationships suffer, emotional growth and development are stunted, physical health may be compromised, and your self-esteem takes a beating.

Our modern, technologically focused medical treatment approaches encourage practical coping, but too often the important need to deal with feelings emerges only after cancer families show signs of burnout or overload. The costs are high when emotional issues are ignored or delayed.

> If I sit and think about the day he was diagnosed, or see pictures from before he was diagnosed, I cry. I cry worrying. Falling asleep is [a] problem. I just went to my doctor the other day and unloaded on him. I told him I compulsively worry, and I'm tired of worrying and I'm tired of being down. My doctor said, "I'm blown away. When your son was on treatment, you were a laugh a minute." But some people are that way, that's how they get through it. He was surprised. [Now] I've started to get the help I probably needed earlier. —*Maggie*

The end of treatment does not end the impact of the experience. Describing that impact as trauma validates the awfulness of the experience and normalizes the feelings you carry with you long afterwards. Having a child with cancer *is* traumatic.

Posttraumatic Stress Reactions

Many children with cancer and their parents have some posttraumatic stress symptoms. Almost no one has all of them. Trauma reactions occur commonly, but full-blown disorders or permanence are rare.

Adults' Trauma Picture

"Electrifying" events, such as diagnosis, relapse, bad side effects, a conflict with your medical team or in your family, and especially any situation in which your child was in pain or his or her life was threatened are common roots of posttraumatic responses. Sometimes you cannot point to a specific occurrence, but the total cancer package and fears of relapse are enough to cause posttraumatic stress symptoms. The adult trauma picture can apply to parents, other adult family members, and survivors and siblings who are now grown.

> We had one really bad experience, when my daughter was not medicated sufficiently. It was just after major surgery, during her brachytherapy [a form of radiation], so it was an extremely stressful time. We thought we'd had everything worked out with the pain team, for

> plans A, B, and C. Then the team went home, and we were stuck with the oncology fellow [doctor receiving training in a specialty], who sat in a routine meeting with his group, while we ran back and forth getting increasingly frantic as the baby was suffering. He was not responsive, and we weren't capable of being rational at that point. We did get through it, but it wasn't resolved very directly. Now, when I tell that story, I still get angry. My heart pounds and my face is red and I have to fight not to cry. It passes quickly, but I'm surprised how strong those feelings still are.—*Nicole*

A posttraumatic stress reaction can be triggered by foods, smells, an off-handed comment, an article or television program, vicarious experiences (such as having some other crisis in the family or hearing a story about a newly diagnosed family), or during periods of stress or fatigue. Anything that reminds you of either a specific event or the whole period of time can trigger a response.

> I nearly fainted the day Olivia asked about the "throw-up bucket." She had a common virus. As we headed for the door to go see the pediatrician, she asked if we needed to take the throw-up bucket. During her entire treatment, we kept a bucket in the truck for emergencies. Once her treatments ended, we naturally removed the bucket. But that simple question sent me back. I started to sweat, my knees got weak, I had to hold onto the furniture for support. Suddenly we weren't headed to the pediatrician for a common bug, we were headed to the hospital for a high fever or a treatment. It took every ounce of strength I had to calmly say, "No, we don't need the bucket today."—*Patty*

* * *

> I was standing at the washing machine, getting ready to start a load of towels, when I popped open the new bottle of Surf. The smell of it almost instantaneously transported me to the laundry room at the Ronald McDonald House. Before I knew it, all the fear and pain came rushing back. There I was, 2:30 am in the laundry room, unable to sleep, washing clothes, and inside I was gripped with fear that the test she was scheduled for the next day would reveal something horrible. I was physically in my laundry room, but mentally, I was back there. After a few minutes, I was able to "snap out of it," but I was unable to sleep well for some time after that.—*Wendy*

* * *

> It's important to me to help other parents through what we've been through, but it can take a toll on you. I trained to be a parent support counselor. One of my friends, whose child was treated at the same time, joined, too. In a training exercise, we sat back-to-back and pretended she was a mom calling me for support. She made up a story, and said that things weren't going well, and I started to cry. It wasn't even real. Sometimes I'll hear a story from newly diagnosed parents, and it catapults me right back into the storm. The desire to help them is strong, but reliving the experience is draining. Sometimes I have trouble getting to sleep, for thinking about them.—*Susan*

Symptoms of physical illness, especially those that were present at diagnosis, are one of the most powerful triggers for flashbacks or the "panic mode" described by parents.

> After five years, I'm much better. I can face some things with the total calm and competence that I used to. Then there are times when I'm not so good. Vomiting will do it to me every single time. I just want to cry, and my insides cringe. Vomiting and the knot in her tummy were the only symptoms Becky had. The common denominator for most things that send me close to the edge is the unknown factor. If I don't know what is causing her symptoms/problems/pain/fever, I feel my nerves twitch, and the word cancer pops right into my head. She has a fever for no apparent reason. She gets a bug and I don't catch it, too. If something is happening that I can't point a finger to a culprit, the culprit then becomes cancer in my mind.—*Louanne*
>
> * * *
>
> You know, you bury it pretty deep. You think you're over it, and wham! My son is six years in remission—he's healthy, no worries, right? But a few months ago, he had this weird bacterial infection. For eight days, he had a high fever, couldn't eat anything, just lay there on the couch. He lost 15–20% of his body weight. The pediatrician took a lot of blood and ran a lot of tests, but couldn't find an answer. He ended up getting four shots of heavy-duty antibiotics, which took care of it. But I was a wreck. I couldn't sleep, I couldn't concentrate at work, I had a constant headache. I just kept thinking it was a relapse. What made it worse was I was right in the middle of switching jobs. Here I was, filling out forms and reading about insurance to make sure that, "if something happened," we would be covered, and the whole time I'm thinking that something already happened. I actually thought about staying in a job I hated and giving up a good career move because I was so worried. Boy, am I glad I didn't do that!—*Russ*

Many parents experience increased nervousness for several days before follow-up visits. They feel tired, cranky and irritable, and often it takes them awhile to realize that it is because they dread the hospital visit. The stress of knowing that your child will be upset is enough. If you add fears of relapse, a long day or drive, and having to be "on" for your child, the result is PMS syndrome: "preparing for medical stuff."

> My husband would say why are you worrying so, you'll make yourself crazy. John would worry the night of, but I would worry for 4 weeks. If you put a pin in him, he would explode, that's how the tension would go. By the time I got there that day I was pretty much prepared for whatever would happen because I worked on it for 4 weeks, where he was ready to strangle the docs. Another dad told me that too. "I'm up all night in cold sweats."—*Faith*

The fears can be displaced. Instead of worrying about cancer, you worry about a freak accident or chemicals in the water or school shootings. Obviously, those things merit appropriate concern, but the focus on them is more vigilant than it would have been had you not already been through one traumatic experience. Parents can feel a strong pull to be overprotective of all their children in reaction to these feelings.

> I can vividly imagine being in a car accident with the kids. I'd be screaming at the EMTs you don't understand, you can't let her die, she survived cancer! One weekend, my in-laws came to take the kids, so we could have some time together. I know they're perfectly capable, and take very good care of my children. But as I buckled the seat belt, I had a moment of doubt that I'd ever see them again.—*Nicole*

* * *

> My fears for my children manifest in strange ways. I think about school bus accidents, intruders, fires, stuff like that. What frightens me is things over which I have no control. I have to let my kids go out and have a life. I don't keep them shut up in the house. We follow the "safety rules" (don't talk to strangers, buckle up, don't play with matches), and when I get squidgy, I take a few deep breaths, reassure myself, and keep going.—*Marta*

Dreams are vivid showcases for both memories and fears. Parents often dream alternate outcomes for distressing events, including that the child died.

> It was a dream that our whole family was on a ship. The ship began to crash into the dock. Our family got separated. I don't know why. As everyone was scrambling to get off the ship, Stan and I gathered the kids. Eric was no where to be found, so Stan went looking for him. I took the other kids and got off the ship and went to the car and waited in the parking lot. Stan eventually got off the ship but couldn't ever find Eric. I woke with the vision of him being crushed in the crowd screaming for me. I've always wondered if this nightmare was about unresolved fear of losing Eric.—*Sue*

* * *

> The nightmare happened after we found out that my other son would need surgery for a hernia. The same surgeon who operated on Justin was doing Tyler's hernia repair. The nightmare was that both boys were in surgery at the same time. The operating rooms were made out of glass, and I could see in. Dr. S. was running back and forth between the two. My husband was at work and I was alone [in real life we both were there]. When the surgeries were over, Dr. S. came out to the waiting room and said that he was able to get all of Justin's tumor [something that didn't actually happen in the real surgery] but that Tyler's hernia was cancer [a big fear I had at the time] and that there wasn't anything that could be done for Tyler. At that point I ran screaming from the hospital and woke up. —*Emma*

* * *

> I've had a few dreams lately but instead of being about Andy, they are about his dad [who also had Wilm's tumor as a child]. I have dreams that Larry, Andy's dad, develops another form of cancer, like leukemia. I think Larry and Andy are interchangeable in my dreams. It's hard to know which one I'm really worried about. Probably both.—*Diane*

As these stories show, the trauma symptom picture for adults can take many forms. You may relive distressing events, be chronically anxious or overprotective of your children, or feel guilty about what you did or did not do during a traumatic event. You may have panic attacks, sleep disturbances, a heightened awareness of physical symptoms or ailments, frequent thoughts about relapse, an inability to plan for the future or make decisions because of fears of relapse, residual anger over traumatic events, depression, or apathy.

To avoid distressing emotions, you may avoid any situation or person that triggers memories or cut yourself off from having any emotions at all.

> "Coasting" is the way I've often described it. I zone out. I forget things unless they are written down or right in front of me. I get the job done—take kids to activities, work, plan a birthday party, whatever. But I don't feel as fully engaged as I could be. Part of it is brain overload, but also I think it's biding my time, waiting for something to happen. There's a story by Herman Melville called Bartleby the Scrivener in which the main character coasted through life, waiting for the something big and wonderful to happen to him and not engaging in anything. Of course, it never happened.—*Helene*

You may suffer from bodily reactions to the traumatic stress, including headaches, stomach upset, ulcers, susceptibility to colds and flu, fatigue, insomnia, muscle tension, neck and back pain, or difficulties with concentration and memory. Do not be daunted by symptoms; recovery is discussed after the following sections on children and interactions between parent and child.

Children's Trauma Picture

Among children's symptoms there are important differences related to age and developmental level. Remember, siblings can exhibit these reactions as well as can children who are sick. The basic pattern of reactions for children older than 3 is similar to those of adults, although they are expressed according the child's level:

- The experience of an event as distressing that anyone would consider distressing
- The re-experiencing of the event repeatedly in various ways
- Response symptoms of numbing (feeling blank or shut down); avoiding scary

experiences or people; and increased arousal, or super sensitivity, to sights, sounds, and touch.

In the following box are typical symptoms of posttraumatic stress in children. Any of these symptoms can come and go over time or can be triggered by an experience, a return visit to the clinic, or another reminder.

Posttraumatic Stress Symptoms in Children

Emotional and Behavioral Symptoms

Nightmares, night terrors
Repeated play expressing the trauma
Severe separation anxiety, fears of being left alone—even just if you're in another room
Acting out or withdrawing from strange or new people or situations
Heightened fears, overreacting to triggers
Reliving an event
Marked change in activity level
Feeling like a victim
Frequent outbursts of uncontrollable temper
Isolating self, apathy
Yo-yoing self-esteem
Difficulty making decisions
Hopelessness about the future, refusal to make plans or participate in favorite activities
Continual nervousness, irritability
Distraction
Heightened awareness of body, symptoms
Difficulty in school

Physical Symptoms

Headache
Muscle tension
Heart palpitations, racing
Sweating
Nausea, nervous stomach, change in appetite
Loss of concentration
Swings in energy level, high energy one minute, low energy the next
Unusual fatigue or insomnia, disruptions in sleep

Remembrance and association are strong for children. Many cancer veterans report that, for instance, the smell of rubbing alcohol nauseates them. One mother told us of her daughter's refusal to ever again drink apple juice, because she associates its smell with an occasion of vomiting.

> He still to this day will not eat peanut butter and jelly sandwiches, or potato chips, because that's what he ate during treatment. So now, it's more in his head, but he really doesn't want to have it. The other day, he tried a potato chip and he goes, "Oh, this is really good, mmm I can't believe it I really like it." But then he said, "You know, I really don't think I want to eat those again."—*Judith*

Children may not always understand or be able to verbalize their strong traumatic response feelings.

> She can't remember being bald, throwing up all the time. She can't remember her central line. She doesn't remember the most frightening days for her immediately following her surgery. Recently, though, we took the Daisy scouts on an outing to the rescue squad center in our small town. The paramedics showed the girls their offices and the ambulances. They practiced simple procedures on the girls. Olivia was very excited when this trip began. But once the paramedics opened the back of that ambulance and started going over all the equipment, Olivia became more and more silent. We weren't very far into the presentation when she looked at me with huge eyes and said she wanted to go home "NOW!" I tried to calm her down and asked her if she remembered some of the items. I got an emphatic, "NO! I want to go home."—*Patty*

* * *

> My older daughter, not the one who was sick, has her own fears. She is absolutely terrified of needles! She won't do any of the breathing or distraction. That's her sister's realm, and she wants nothing of it. I remember once while her sister was on treatment, she had a urinary tract infection, and the doctor said they'd do a culture for me while we were there. She flatly refused to give a urine sample. She got very agitated. Maybe she thought they'd find she had cancer, too.—*Alice*

Teenagers may understand intellectually why they are having a reaction, but the emotional impact continues anyway.

> There's one thing that bothers me. I can't ride a bike. I tried to get on a bike when I was on vacation in Ireland, and I suddenly couldn't breathe. The same thing happens when I have a stress test [to monitor heart effects of treatment]. They put me on a bike, and I stop breathing. Right before I was diagnosed, I was on a 4-mile bike trip. I got dizzy and had to walk home. Then I was diagnosed with ALL [leukemia].—*Gloria, long-term survivor*

Infants and toddlers react to traumatic stress but without the words to tell us about it. They show their fright and overload in other ways. For example, a baby may startle easily, cling, become less responsive and rarely smile or coo, be irritable and hard to settle down, and show great fear of strangers. As soon as the older baby becomes mobile, he or she will try to get away from specific situations. Toddlers do the same things, but as they learn language they may also overuse or underuse any words associated with the trauma.

> My daughter was treated from the age of 8 months to 18 months, which should have been a period of enormous leaps in growth and development. Instead, she retreated into a small

> world that included just the two of us. She clung to me like a little monkey, afraid to let me put her down. She was afraid of other people, even other children at the place where she got physical therapy. It took about a year and a half after treatment ended before she began to rejoin the world, to start growing and developing again, learn to crawl and walk and talk. For a long time, she was terrified of doctor's offices, even when she wasn't the patient. The sight of an exam table with that crinkly paper would set her off. Gradually, her tendency to panic subsided. Now that she's a little older, it's more subtle. She'll get that look in her eye, and I know she's scared but trying to keep a lid on it.—*Irene*

Interactive Reactions

You and your child strongly influence each other's reactions to an upsetting event. Your way of presenting the event and ability to handle your own anxiety influence your child's appraisal and handling of the event. Equally important, your child's response to the event, such as pain or fear, has a big impact on your response to the event, in the moment and perhaps long afterward. Anxiety can spiral out of control when you and your child feed on each other's frantic escalation. Conversely, a calm focus, soothing, and a quick return to normalcy feed each other's sense of getting through a tough time together and intact.

> When my son was first diagnosed, I saw a mom who was reacting pretty badly. Her kid was having a spinal tap, or something, and she was screaming and crying, "You're hurting my baby" and "I'm sorry baby." The nurses had to take her into another room, and her kid was screaming louder than she was. I didn't know what was going on, and I was scared about what they might do to my son. But I could see that she was only making it worse for her child, and I vowed not to ever do that. No matter how bad it got, I would hold him and be there for him and save my freaking out for later.—*Angela*

A group of researchers (Margaret Stuber, Dimitri Christakis, Beth Houskamp, and Anne Kazak; see the Bibliography) reported the following results, based on families' responses to a posttraumatic stress disorder reaction index. Their findings may help you to recognize your own family's reactions as normal and motivate you to take positive steps to remedy your situation as needed. It is not just the child who has gone through an ordeal; the parents have, too.

- Most survivors of childhood cancer are doing well psychologically two years after the end of treatment.
- A significant percentage of the children (12.5%) report symptoms of posttraumatic stress (examples are bad dreams, fearful thoughts about cancer, and nervousness).

- ♦ A high percentage of the mothers (39.7%) and the fathers (33.3%) suffered from posttraumatic symptoms (examples are anxiety about relapse, upset feelings when thinking about cancer, and re-experiencing disturbing scenes).

By this and other measures, most children go on to function well. This is heartening. Yet we must find increasingly better ways to help the children who are still struggling long after the cancer. And we must directly address the unsettling number of parents in our cancer community who continue to struggle. The continual drain of anxiety is a key factor in this struggle. Family by family, the sooner we recognize and reduce anxiety, the more we can ease the toll taken by traumatic stress.

Despite the fact that posttraumatic stress symptoms are quite common in parents of childhood cancer survivors, it does not mean that all or even most parents have a diagnosable posttraumatic stress disorder. It does mean that help would make life better. Often, the best help for the child is to help the parent. If cancer is a "family disease," then resolving the effects of trauma is a family process, involving all members who are affected.

> My husband has flashbacks sometimes, to painful moments in Lloyd's treatments. I don't, because I think I let out all of my emotions shortly after each event happened. I let myself feel the pain as it was happening, and so the farther we get from the chemo treatments experience, the less and less I seem to think about it.—*Sandy*

* * *

> I think it's very important that we not see parents as having the full PTSD syndrome. They may have symptoms of it, but that's not the same thing. I've found that children's coping is highly correlated with that of the parents. That's why the psychologists are more likely to intervene directly with the parents. Another bonus is that the mother is a central figure for the family; if she gets the help she needs, the other children (and probably her husband) benefit as well.—*Donna Copeland, PhD*

Recovery From Trauma

For every cancer family there are terrible moments and trying events. The family in the following story found that they could not prevent a problem, but they worked hard to contain the damage it was causing.

> Our baby, Charlotte, developed a severe burn reaction [from one of the chemotherapy drugs] that covered her entire diaper area. She was in a lot of pain. We used burn treatments and wiped her with sterile pads, and the doctor gave her a protective cream before subsequent rounds. That was okay for awhile, but once the radiation started, it got worse. She would

> just wriggle her bottom, and cry, and make this horrible gasping sound. We were frantic. My Mom and I must have asked everyone in that hospital for ideas. Finally, a radiation unit nurse mentioned Domeboro solution, which she said had been used on elderly radiation patients with some success. Within minutes of the first soak in this solution, her relief was visible. Her tense little body relaxed. The relief was only temporary, but we could see it was working. After that, we used this treatment routinely, along with her antibiotics and antifungal medicine. Even now, my Mom says she still thinks of the awful feeling of helplessness and how important it was to keep trying to find relief for Charlotte. Charlotte's skin is still sensitive, and once in a blue moon, she'll make that gasping sound. Even her sister remembers that sound and how it showed how much pain Charlotte was in.—*Marta*

When the issue is comfort and not cure, there is always another avenue to try, always room for improvement, always some way to manage the anxiety of painful events.

Practical Help for Children

To be effective, help must be tailored to your child's abilities. Of course, the best medicine for trauma is prevention whenever possible.

One father was able to relax his baby daughter and get her to sleep by crooking his index finger and gently stroking from between her eyes down the bridge of her nose. Most parents respond in automatic and natural ways to a distressed infant, by physical soothing, rocking, crooning, stroking, and letting the child suck on a pacifier or fingers.

> I nursed Justin for a very long time, much longer than I had expected, but I'm glad I did. It worked for both of us. I think the nursing played a major role in how well Justin did. Nursing him helped me too, emotionally. I felt it was something I could do for him, giving him comfort and security. It was solace for both of us during a time of trauma and turmoil. —*Emma*

Older children also benefit from physical soothing such as hugs, holding, back or foot rubs, or stroking an arm. These commonsense responses help regulate your child's physiological reactions and move the experience from a distressing one to a reassuring one.

> I would agree that the treatment experiences affect even young children, but at least some of it is in a positive way. For instance, if a toddler were in pain or frightened, and her parents were right there to comfort her, that's what she will have learned—that even though one might be distressed, there are people there to soothe and support.—*Donna Copeland, PhD*

Allow children to react to the trauma and to talk about it. Talk to them about what scares them and what they can do to make themselves feel better. If you are attuned, you communicate to your child that those reactions are manageable. Toddlers can respond to talk about the event even before they themselves can put their experience into words. One idea is to write a story (use a spiral notebook, blank book, or staple or tie plain or construction paper together): call it your child's story and write about what has happened; what might have scared him or her; or what might have made him or her mad, or sad, or comforted. Draw pictures or put in pictures from magazines. Read it to the child, let him or her add pictures or words, and talk about feelings as you read it. Toys and doll play can serve the same purpose.

Older children usually respond well to talking about troubling experiences and turn actively to trusted adults for help when distressed. At first, a child may not be able to talk readily about the upset, due to the anxiety that surges. But with each conversation or other expression, no matter how brief, the child has the chance to become less anxious, bit by bit. The repeated process of talking and expressing works like an inoculation, with small doses of emotional "vaccine" used to help build up tolerance and work against big "infections" of trauma. This repeating and revisiting process, in small, tolerable doses, leads to emotional mastery.

Children are capable of showing anger at any age, from infancy on up. Their anger may be expressed as a total body experience: tension and crying, yelling, throwing things, threatening to run away or retaliate, or saying, "I hate you." Anger is a natural response to the experience of being provoked, and medical procedures can be highly provocative. Encourage the child to punch a pillow or punching bag, bash some clay, bang pots, play drums or other musical instruments loudly, throw bean bags at a target, run around the yard, or scribble a picture of something that makes him or her angry and then tear it into a million pieces.

As a parent, you develop your own ways to help your child, based on common sense, experience, and intuition.

> Nicky slept with us because we felt he needed the security. He displayed some of the signs of a temporary condition called ICU Psychosis. It happens to people who have a bad experience. He would wake up screaming and push us away when we tried to hold him. After a few seconds he would realize it was us. This went on for about two or three weeks. After he started sleeping normally we tried to get him to sleep in his crib a few nights using techniques that worked in the past, but he just wasn't secure enough. So we decided to let him sleep with us for a while longer and try to get him in a bed later. We figured he needed the comfort and security after what he'd been through. He just recently started napping in a "big boy" bed in the afternoon.—*Neil*

Gentle Reminders of Children's Needs to Recover From Trauma

- Soothing—stroking, rocking, holding, calming, or a supportive attitude
- Time to recover from a hurtful or frightening procedure—try not to schedule procedures close together, if possible
- Opportunities for distraction and another focus besides illness and treatment—friends, social events, or developmental activities
- Outlets for aggressive responses and large motor activities—pounding, kicking, or swooping play
- Encouragement and praise for all attempts to manage and cope, not just for successes—success may come only in fits and starts
- Help to master the trauma, with opportunities to repeatedly express the trauma, the memories, and the meanings, in tolerable emotional doses and in a safe setting—through talk, stories, drawing, toys, dolls, or plays
- Structured play and play materials to recreate and communicate the trauma—available in many hospitals and clinics and in private settings for use by therapists and parents
- Empathy and an "emotional container" to integrate the strong feelings aroused by the trauma—when the listener is able to tolerate and hold the strong emotions, the child's emotions can be safely expressed
- Time to make "sense" of what happened to them, to understand their own experience in their own way.

Sometimes parents are so traumatized by an event themselves that they freeze up during it, or they are so overwhelmed by their own emotions that they cannot respond to the child. In that case, the greatest gift a parent can give the child may be to get the help needed to move from being overwhelmed and paralyzed to being responsive. In that way, you can help yourself and your child to recover.

Some children benefit from assistance beyond what even very responsive parents can provide. Under those circumstances, it may be helpful if parents participate in a child's therapeutic sessions with a psychologist, social worker, or other specialist. Parents stand to gain

- Greater understanding of your child's internal world related to the trauma experience
- Appreciation and collaboration with the helping process being offered to your child
- Models for communication about feelings that can be used at home also
- Support for your own reactions and responses.

When you are involved too, you will learn how to be more supportive and less frightened during those times when your child is remembering and grappling with feelings associated with the traumatic illness.

Steps for Adults

The first step is to recognize and understand the symptoms. It is easier to cope when you understand what is happening to you. Afterward, you need many of the same practical helping aids that children do, but in grown-up forms: soothing, time to recover, safe outlets for feelings, and help to master the trauma through talking about the memories and their personal meanings. A stance of silence, isolation, and trying to keep a "stiff upper lip" makes it harder to recover. Coming to terms with the experiences and reconnecting with your own internal world, your life story, and your path to the future are central to recovery. As you do that, you will feel less anxious, angry, and despairing.

Along the way, you may use any of the stress management and coping strategies presented throughout this book. However, the most important element is the opportunity to return again and again to the memories, as often as you need, until the trauma is worked through and your anxiety subsides. It takes time and happens only gradually. Start a personal journal. Take a fast walk around the neighborhood when you feel like you are jumping out of your skin and need room to breathe and think. Talk to other parents, join a support group, or consult with a trained professional counselor familiar with trauma and cancer; maybe do all three. But expand your network and talk to someone. Choose someone who is trustworthy and truly able to listen to you, one who will not hurry or judge you. When you are getting the help you need, symptoms will lessen; episodes of distress will not last as long or feel as if they are taking you apart.

> In the depth of winter, I finally learned that within me there lay an invincible summer.
> Albert Camus, *L'Ete,* (1954)

Lasting Impressions

A common thread for cancer parents is that "it is always with you" to some degree. Even while getting on with life, even as days go by without thinking about it, the specter of cancer remains for a long time. Some of the altered perspectives of cancer parents are startlingly similar to those of bereaved parents.

Loss of Normal, Being Different

Being normal is something that children and adults in the cancer world think about a lot. While on treatment, it is important for most children that they be treated like the person they were before they got sick. When a child or a parent is feeling discouraged, they often express the desire to just "be normal"—wishing that it would all just go away and that they could have their lives back.

From the moment your child is diagnosed, you are a "stranger in a strange land," both as you join the world of childhood cancer and then as you re-enter the "normal" world after treatment ends. Even long afterward, your frame of reference, your scope of experience, and your vision of the future may be unlike that of other people.

> Cami chose the color periwinkle for the walls of her room. Vincristine comes from periwinkles. Who else but a cancer parent would think of this?—*Robin*

Many families point out that the experience can lend poignancy and appreciation to life, a rearranging of priorities to give more importance to the intangibles and less worry about the "small stuff." Parents tell us that they are more tolerant of other people's problems or differences but less tolerant of trivial complaints. If you are more appreciative of what you have, you may be less driven to compete in some other areas. Your insight may make you more patient, more flexible, and more confident in your ability to handle life's ups and downs. The children, too, seem more resilient.

> I have noticed that my patience for nonsense is markedly less.—*Kirk*

* * *

> By this time, Nicky doesn't even cry when having his blood samples drawn. In fact, last week Nicky fell and skinned his knee. A neighborhood boy brought Nicky to Marcia with blood streaming down his leg and said, "Mrs. B., Nicky fell . . . and he didn't even cry!" —*Neil*

* * *

> I was changed profoundly. I used to be very ambitious and elitist. I have become a kinder, humbler person. During the years I spent in hospitals, I met parents from all walks of life, from all ethnic, educational, and religious backgrounds. Fear and pain do not know any of these boundaries. Anyone can get cancer. I try to live each day as if it might be my last. That attitude has to be tempered with common sense; as a middle-aged woman in good health, I probably have a long life expectancy. Also, I have young children for whom I need to plan and provide. Yet I anticipate death at every turn. I have every conceivable type of insurance policy, I update my will regularly, I have advance directives. When someone calls

me and says they have bad news, I always think someone has died. I try hard to be realistic about possible calamities. One part of me wants to control every variable to keep my family as safe as possible, and another part of me knows that disaster can always strike anytime no matter what I do. I go out of my way to talk to people with problems. I purposely made a mid-life career change because I needed a challenge. Nothing that happens at work can possibly scare me. At some level I enjoy navigating a crisis, because I know I am good at it. —*Naomi*

* * *

Childhood cancer teaches us the depths of love and pain. Life is irrevocably changed. Like Plato's famous image—we were all like the cave dwellers before diagnosis, watching the fire-lit shadows play on the walls. But, after cancer, we were thrown out into the real world. And we can never go back into the cave again. People so often want to know is this good or bad, black or white. I say it's just like the rest of life—a jumble of feelings, thoughts, and actions. But, oh so different from what it was before.—*Nancy Keene, author, parent, and advocate cancer patient*

On the whole, the new perspective is not always welcome, because it is coupled with anxiety and painful memories. You may see danger where others see none. The future includes so much more and so much less. You may find yourself clipping newspaper articles or watching television programs about cancer, even when they upset you. Emotions surface at particular milestones or special events.

It hurts me deep inside that my 6-year-old daughter has been forced to learn so early in life about suffering and death. I sometimes feel she has lost the joyous innocence of childhood. A friend once told me that serious illness robs children of innocence, but replaces it with wisdom. Well, NO MORE wisdom please. Give us a little blissful ignorance for a change. —*Jane*

* * *

It's the Kodak moments that get to me. I cried my eyes out at the school holiday program. The children singing, the beaming smiles from all the other parents around me. A simple pleasure I had always enjoyed, but probably once took for granted. I was just so grateful we could be there, you know?—*Joan*

* * *

I can't listen to the song "Butterfly Kisses" by Bob Carlisle. It talks about the major events in his daughter's life—the prom, how she grows up and gets married. I suppose in the back of my mind is the fear that my own daughter will never get there and the hope that she will.—*Mina*

Some parents feel that the world has unrealistic expectations and perceptions of cancer families, putting them up on a pedestal:

> Was this supposed to make me a better person or something? I didn't have an epiphany. I didn't discover the meaning of life or some explain-all philosophy. I'm not noble or heroic. I still say stupid things or complain about trivialities. I hate it when people say I'm so strong, or they don't know how I did it. You know what? They would do whatever they had to do. There's no choice about it.—*Shirley*

Relationships, both existing and new ones, are altered. Many families feel alienated from other people, although this is usually temporary. In the world, there are indeed the haves and the have-nots. To cancer families, this translates to those who have had a child with cancer and those who have not. Even a supportive network of family and friends does not really understand it all. Often, people back away, uncertain about how to relate to you, leaving you feeling "marked."

> Sometimes I feel we have the plague. There is an incredible fear for most people, because even though they consciously know that their child can't catch it from your child, I think subconsciously they feel that if they know us or interact with us that it will jinx their child into getting cancer. Every time I walk into a room or people see me, I am a constant reminder to them that children get cancer—and that is so painful and scary for most people to have to even think about.—*Gabriela*

* * *

> I used to think being different was a good thing. Being creative, smart, unique, funky, or even a little weird set you apart from everybody else and made you special. But society doesn't like this kind of different; it makes people uncomfortable. You're scary . . . a downer at parties, or something.—*Leslie*

This is your life and you adjust yourself to it, but that is very difficult for others to comprehend. You mention something in passing, and the response is uncomfortable silence or a change in subject. Friends may get tired of hearing about it or may stop sharing their problems with you because they "can't compete." The ambivalence plays out through half of you wanting to shout out "Hey, look what he's been through, look what he can do! Look where we've been and how far we've come!" The other half just wants to enjoy normal life and not think about it all the time, to put it behind you and get on with life. Each side of the ambivalence is important but is not the whole picture.

> I am tired. Everyone's tired of my turmoil.
> Robert Traill Spence Lowell, *Eye and Tooth* (1964)

A stranger might look at you and see nothing amiss, yet innocent questions have weighted answers. Sometimes you omit the truth, either because it is easier or unnecessary in casual situations. At other times, you might find yourself brandishing it. The truth carries shock value.

> Both my children talk about cancer freely, because we've always done so in our house. It's not shameful, or a secret. It's fact. But I've come to realize that sometimes, they thoroughly enjoy the reaction they get when they spring it on someone.—*Elise*

It is a primal preservation instinct for human beings to compare themselves to others and to want to "fit in." Since the dawn of time, to be different has meant to be cast out, literally or figuratively. To be cast out is a threat. Many cancer families feel stigmatized. But it does not have to be that way. Altering our own perceptions first, we provide a model for the rest of the world. For our families, normal is not lost; it is just changed.

> We should banish the word "normal" from the English language. Is there any normal? I know kids with cerebral palsy, ADD, asthma, severe allergies, heart conditions, vision problems, Down's syndrome, not to mention all the couples I know with infertility. Why do we aspire to something that doesn't really exist? Everybody has something to deal with.—*Fay*

* * *

> Except for [having had] cancer, there's nothing else wrong with him.—*Barbara*

Loss of Innocence

Cancer families know, as Rabbi Harold Kushner (see Bibliography) expressed so well, that bad things happen to good people. They tell us they no longer have a naïve, rose-colored view of the world where everything goes according to plan. Childhood cancer families are pushed out of the safety and ignorance of the world before cancer, eyes opened to pain as part of the human condition. This knowledge is unwanted, unbidden, and undeserved.

> We can never be the same, can we? We went to Disney World, courtesy of the Make-A-Wish Foundation, while Scott was still on treatment. We were in the cable car (up in the air) and I sat up there in tears, looking around, thinking the world isn't so wonderful now, and it never will be.—*Maggie*

* * *

> Even though Cordelia and Simeon are the same age, she looks older . . . not so much wiser or more mature, just older. She certainly does not have that "pre-cancer innocence" that Simeon does. If we think this disease robs us of all our innocence and hopes and dreams, imagine how they must feel.—*Tamara*

* * *

> Last Thursday, after we got the good news about Susie's counts, I took her out to lunch to celebrate. There we were, sitting at the table, doodling and talking about our day and the events of the past week. As she colored things, she would ask me questions like, "Mommy . . . will Jared die like Lindsey?" and "Mom . . . I hate bluekemia, don't you?" As I listened to her, I couldn't help but see the irony of what was going on all around us. Business lunches, "networking," people with their cell phones, palm organizers, and day planners discussing profits and sales and other important business matters. And here I sit with my little girl, while she asks me questions about life and death. I was smiling on the outside, but inside, I was screaming.— *Wendy*

Relapse anxiety robs parents of innocence. Parents find it difficult to revert to their former belief that all will be well, and so they become anxious whenever their child gets sick. Living with chronic fears of recurrence is widely known as the "Damocles syndrome" (psychologists Gerald Koocher and John O'Malley, see the Bibliography), an allusion to a mythical Greek figure. The title metaphor of the book, which discusses the landmark study of 103 long-term survivors of childhood cancer, refers to the experience of living with the threat of a sword that hangs by a slender thread over one's head.

> They sicken of the calm, who know the storm.
> Dorothy Parker, "Fair Weather," *Sunset Gun* (1928)

It is steadying to note that most parents agree the intensity of the fears does fade over time. As one mother put it, every year another thread is tied around that famous sword, keeping it from crashing down on you.

> Tomorrow is the seventh anniversary of Chelsea's diagnosis. I can't speak for every long timer, but for me the panic mode does go away. Chelsea had an infected finger, and we went to the doctor. Since we were walk-ins, we saw the first doctor available, one we hadn't seen before. Believe it or not, I didn't even mention Chelsea's cancer history. I can deal with colds, fevers, infected fingers, and even a tummy flu without fearing relapse. It took a while for me to get here, but I don't live in fear of cancer.— *Rita*

Chronic Sorrow

The term "chronic sorrow" has been used to describe the families of children with mental and physical disabilities. It is also an apt description for some cancer families, particularly those whose children have severe long-term side effects.

> Even though we got through it and she survived, I still feel deflated sometimes. Just beaten down and sorrowful. Everything is a struggle. Fighting with the insurance company, nagging the school system for special testing and services, dealing with the effects of treatment. Making sure she gets what she needs. Researching all the options. There will always be something to deal with, and somebody resisting my efforts. It never ends. I'm tired of it. —*Elise*

Professor and clinical specialist in child and adolescent psychiatric nursing Penelope Buschman (see the Bibliography) described it this way:

> Chronic sorrow is the pervasive sadness experienced over a lifetime by a family with a chronically ill . . . child. This sorrow is experienced most acutely at the time of diagnosis of the child's illness in response to losing a healthy child; it is rekindled with each exacerbation of the disease, at each new developmental phase, and at other unexpected moments. Chronic sorrow is present to some degree in all families with chronically ill children—that is, it is a normal response. The way that a family deals with its chronic sorrow directly influences the family's adaptation and, in turn, the child's response to chronic illness. (pp. 40–41)

I can't go on . . .
I really can't go on
I swear I can't go on
So I guess
I'll get up
And go on
Dory Previn, *On My Way to Where* (1972)

She likens the emotion to mourning, except that the child's life continues and so do the demands.

The chronic sorrow of a cancer family has been variously described as a black cloud, a shadow, walking along a cliff blindfolded, or as background music that starts out blaring and gets quieter as the years pass. "Chronic presence" may be more accurate to describe this than chronic sorrow. It is not that you are always sad, although you are sometimes; it is that the specter is always there. The enduring nature of the change is what makes it so difficult. Know that your feelings of sorrow, anger, guilt, resignation, and resentment are not unusual.

> The other day he just had his first haircut. His blond hair is really cute, he looks like his older brother. He was getting his sneakers on, running outside, his coordination's all back. I had such joy in me. Then all of a sudden, a "black cloud" swung over my head. Tomorrow this could all change. People who don't go through something like this don't really know how fragile life is, for lack of a better word. In a second, your life could be different. I don't think it's going to happen, but I know that it can.—*Faith*

Healing

> You gain strength, courage and confidence by every experience in which you really stop to look fear in the face. You are able to say to yourself, "I lived through this horror. I can take the next thing that comes along." . . . You must do the thing you think you cannot do.
> Eleanor Roosevelt, *You Learn by Living* (1960)

You do not have to let the loss of innocence and the presence of a chronic sorrow consume your whole life. You can go on. You can think and talk about other things. You can regain your positive attitudes toward much of life. The chronic presence may pop into your conscious mind at inopportune moments, but with time and help, it will become less of a focus.

Trauma reactions are normal. Having them does not mean that you are defective. While long-term emotional effects are possible, we can mitigate their impact by dealing with the immediate trauma early and dealing with the issues of later phases (emotional as well as physical) as they arise. The lingering presence of painful experience does not mean that you are permanently traumatized and damaged. You are permanently different, because of your intimate knowledge of vulnerability. That is not the same thing.

The struggle for cancer families is between fervently wanting to be normal and unchanged and the reality that they are different and their future will be different. You have to find the comfortable middle ground for your own family. It can take many forms. For example, attend survivors' rallies, volunteer at the hospital, keep up with medical advances, or commiserate with other cancer parents. Go back to school or work, or sign your child up for art class, soccer league, or dance or music lessons. Embrace the differences and celebrate the normalcy, because both will be present.

> I've been wrestling with incorporating the whole cancer experience into my life and moving on with it instead of always comparing NOW with time B.C. I suppose the best advice is to stop wrestling and just DO IT!—*Camille*

* * *

> The anesthesiologist laughed when she came to get Shannon. She said, "I have to share something with you. We were told all our patients today were completely normal, no risk or special concerns. We checked our list, and thought Shannon's name looked familiar. We opened her chart and remembered exactly who she was and laughed that anyone could consider Shannon 'normal.' We thought you'd enjoy hearing Shannon and normal in the same sentence at least once in her life!" I got a kick out of this and thanked her for making my day!—*Doreen*

* * *

Our future is unknown with cancer, but for now we forget. Nicky makes us forget, for he does not know the fear of a relapse as we do. He lives each day to the fullest and makes us do the same. That is such a blessing. We don't know how long Nicky's life will be, but I do know that he has it in great abundance now.—*Marcia and Neil*

CHAPTER 8

Recognizing Special Risks for Stress and Trauma

You can't prevent the birds of sorrow from flying overhead,
but you can keep them from building nests in your hair.
—Chinese proverb

When you set out to cross the sea, you want to be on a sturdy ocean liner, not in a leaky rowboat. The same principle applies to families who are making the cancer voyage. There is so much stormy weather along the way that you cannot control. You just batten down the hatches and hope that the tempest passes soon. While under way, it makes sense to prevent leaks whenever possible and to quickly repair any leaks that do occur. When a family is under great stress, the weakest parts are the most vulnerable, just as they are in a boat.

This chapter alerts you to the factors that may put your family at greater risk for suffering stress and trauma above and beyond what would normally be expected. There are some known trouble spots that may help you to recognize signs of danger early. These may occur in the child with cancer or in a parent or other family member. These troublesome signs, which are discussed later in this chapter, are

- difficulty managing the essential coping tasks, such as misunderstanding the realities of diagnosis, treatment, and survival; not being able to develop skills to accomplish health care responsibilities; having emotional reactions and distress that are out of control; not being able to maintain a basic sense of personal worth; not being able to maintain good relationships with others; and not being able to use helping resources to meet tasks

- difficulty handling medical treatment procedures, when the parent or child is highly anxious or fearful or the child has a difficult temperament (is not good at adapting to new people or situations)
- reliance on alcohol or drugs (this applies to adults and some teenagers)
- depression
- previous or coexisting family problems, such as a family crisis apart from the child's cancer, inability or unwillingness to support each other, or rigid family functioning.

No themes are so human as those that reflect for us, out of the confusion of life, the close connection of bliss and bale, of the things that help with the things that hurt, so dangling before us forever that bright hard medal, of so strange an alloy, one face of which is somebody's right and ease and the other somebody's pain and wrong.
Henry James, Prefaces, *What Maisie Knew* (1908)

Certain medical factors can also contribute: a poor prognosis or a high risk, a particularly rare or aggressive cancer (for which there is little research or support because there are so few families who have had to deal with it), prolonged or severe treatment, visibility of the disease (such as amputations or permanent tubes), and extent and severity of the late effects. These circumstances do not imply that you cannot cope, only that your boat is being rocked by big waves.

Difficulty With Coping

Almost any strategy used to cope can be adaptive, although some attempts might be problematic. This is an area in which common sense helps a lot. A child who gets anxious before needle sticks and cries when in pain or a parent who is discouraged by a child's symptoms or has an angry reaction to a insensitive staff member is not having a major coping failure. Ups and downs and tough moments are normal. However, if any one kind of response becomes extreme, it may shut out options rather than enhance them. Here are some signs of poor coping:

- Paralysis—inability to make decisions, to provide care, or to comply with treatment
- Persistent denial of reality—interference with constructive plans
- Emotional isolation—family or child withdrawal from support and relationships
- Persistent physical symptoms in other family members—being a hypochondriac or identification with the child through physical signs

- Unremitting negative emotions under poor control—anger, hostility—or unawareness of strong emotions while projecting them onto others
- Inappropriate demands for attention—poor self-control, lack of respect for others' needs
- Chronic regression to earlier stages of development—adults faltering on responsibilities or children reverting to babyish ways
- Caretaker burnout or overload—signs of burden, absence of respite, unremitting worry, inability to focus on anything but the illness or treatment.

Poor coping does not have to be permanent, but often it is deeply ingrained. It takes work to change it. You can improve and add to your repertoire of strategies. Coping is the focus of chapter 3; refer to the areas that touch on your family's situation. When the storm is unrelenting and the engines are faltering, good sailors know to send out a Mayday to the Coast Guard. Call in the professionals if the waves are washing over you.

Difficulty Handling Medical Procedures

Generally children handle difficult procedures such as spinal taps better when a parent is present and helps throughout it. An exception occurs, however, if the parent gets too upset. We know that children take their emotional cues from their parents. If the parent telegraphs great fear, panic, agitation, or fury, it is grossly upsetting to the child. When a parent is not able to withstand a child's procedure and be a secure container for his or her own feeling and the child's, then it is better for the child if the parent is not in the room.

Another signal for help occurs when a child is adequately prepared and a parent is able to be supportive, but the child is still not able to withstand a procedure emotionally and regroup readily afterward. Under those circumstances, it is not helpful to assume that the child will get used to it over time or will improve on his or her own. In fact, researchers Edith Chen, Lonnie Zeltzer, Michelle Craske, and Ernest Katz (see the Bibliography) found that even very young children have surprisingly clear memories of procedures. Having a bad experience with the first one generally means that the next one will be even more upsetting. This is a clear signal that the child needs special psychological and medical assistance to pinpoint the problem and find more workable solutions. A therapist can work with your child to examine his or her memories, re-evaluate his or her reactions, and enhance his or her perception of his or her own ability to cope, along with correcting any misconceptions or exaggerations. Bring the problem to the attention of your child's medical team, and ask for a consult to help your child and you prepare for and cope better with the procedures. Refer to chapters 6, 7, and 9 for specific suggestions on how to work with trauma, pain, and distress.

> I cringe when I think about the [bone marrow] aspirations. I can still see it on his face. For his first one, he was not sedated. He was in a great deal of pain, because the marrow was so sticky. Every time the doctor drew back, Anthony would let out a yell that literally went through me. It was the most painful thing I have ever seen in my life, ever. He's very anxious because he knows he has to have an aspiration done at the end of his treatment, even though the hospital now uses sedation. Because he remembers.—*Lynn*

Reliance on Alcohol or Drugs

Many parents have told us about the seduction of alcohol or pills when searching for a way to ease their distress. There is certainly nothing alarming about an occasional glass of wine with a friend nor with a few days of a sleeping pill prescribed by your physician to break a bout of protracted insomnia. Alcohol and drugs become a problem only under certain conditions—as a habit, a crutch for calming yourself, or an interference when you need to be available and functioning at your best or when associated with a teenager's experimental acting out while he or she is on treatment.

> Things were really getting to me, and I found that I was drinking. I stopped myself, because I was afraid that my son would need me in the middle of the night and I wouldn't be able to get up. I needed some sort of outlet, a way to get away. The hospital offered an exercise class, so I signed up for that.—*Joellen*

Another danger occurs when alcohol or drug reliance preceded the cancer diagnosis. All in all, substance abuse and dependence compounds the risks to coping. Habitual or binge use clouds your judgment and function. It often leads to family arguments and strains relationship bonds.

The simplest test for your own or a family member's situation may be to ask if you are in charge of yourself or if your need for a drink or a pill is in charge of you. Then answer the question honestly. When you are in charge of yourself, you are able to eliminate alcohol or drugs for the duration of this important period of your family's life. If you are not in charge of your alcohol or drug use, seek help. It is hurtful to you and your child to tough it out unsuccessfully and alone. If you want help and are not sure where to turn, start with the screening section of this chapter. You may refer also to chapter 2 for the section on choosing help. The first page of most telephone books contains state and local numbers for alcohol and drug hotlines and services.

Depression

Depression is no stranger in the cancer world, but for the most part it is temporary and can be relieved. Most children with cancer and survivors of cancer do well. A minority of them develops problems such as depression and anxiety that deserve assessment and treatment by a mental health professional. Children and teenagers taking steroid medication may be at a higher risk for depression and so may warrant observation and intervention.

As a parent you may use duration and intensity as your guide for concern. In other words, how long does it last and how deep does it go? Sadness, in response to dropping out of the school play for treatment or missing summer camp, does not equal a depressive episode. Three months of increasing withdrawal from favored activities is very likely to be a significant sign. If you think your child is depressed, it is worth raising the issue with your child, family, and treatment team. If your treatment team does not have mental health professionals, ask for the added consultation. Symptoms of depression usually come in clusters and include

- Sadness—tearfulness, "the blues," or down mood that is sustained
- Apathy—little or no energy, interest, or motivation for the normal pleasurable activities
- Disturbances—in sleeping, eating, and concentration
- Irritability—moodiness and refusals
- Beating up on self—self-criticism, guilt, or lowered self-esteem
- Impairment—to school performance and relationships with family and peers.

You are right to be concerned if your child is having what you would consider to be a global or large problem with adjustment and development or a noticeable cluster of symptoms. The most succinct description was given to us by a mother, who said that she knew her son was depressed when he had "draggy child syndrome."

Adults get depressed more often than children do. Essentially the symptoms are the same: sadness, disturbances, irritability or anger, beating up on one's self, impaired work performance, and social withdrawal. Adults are more likely to self-treat depression with alcohol or pills and more often believe that they must be stoic and ignore their depression.

> Depression is scary. I had a previous bout with depression. I was terrible to the kids and crying all the time. And yet I had no idea why. What was wrong with me? Friends were recommending therapy. I had a doctor set to prescribe medication and church leaders reassuring me it was ok to take it. I was sure it would mean I was weak. I felt so alone. I don't think I would have made as many positive changes in my behavior if I hadn't had the therapy along with the medication. This was about two years before my daughter was di-

agnosed with cancer. Little did I realize that the things I learned then would help me keep it together for as long as I did during her treatment. I learned to recognize anxiety attacks and take control of my emotions so that my thoughts wouldn't race. However, life doesn't stop just because your child has cancer. After my husband's mother died of cancer, I awoke on Mother's Day in a full-blown attack. I knew I needed to talk to someone. I could feel myself slipping farther and farther. So I found a therapist and began sessions. I needed medication once again. I felt like a failure. I'd told myself that I wasn't ever going on medication again. But I also knew that I was losing . . . me. I kept looking inside, and I couldn't find me. I was empty. Or rather I was hiding. Therapy was a way that I could look at those things I was hiding from in a protected way. Once they aren't so scary, I can come out of hiding and live again.—*Sheila*

For both adults and children, depression is highly treatable. Treatment may be psychotherapy, medication, or a combination of the two. There is no reason to suffer unnecessarily. There is no reason to listen to anyone who tells you to "just pull up your socks and get on with life." If you could be doing that, you would be doing that. Instead, use some of your cancer-facing courage to face depression. Use your resources and get help. See the choosing psychological help section of chapter 2, or refer to the screening part of this chapter.

Previous and Ongoing Family Problems

Any family or support problem that was already a source of distress before cancer will be exacerbated by the additional strain. Have you been thinking of divorce? Are you a single parent without nearby relatives? Does one of your children have a disability requiring special attention? Is your teenager in the midst of a major rebellion phase? Does he or she have an eating disorder? Is one of your parents ill? Are you in debt and without good health insurance coverage? Are you barely meeting expenses now and worried about meeting extras? Is the family's main breadwinner in a precarious job situation? Does your spouse have chronic emotional problems? Is the best medical care far away from your home? Extra support will be necessary when the demands of cancer are added to these sorts of demands.

When families, big or small, live in unresolved crisis. they become hampered by rigid, inflexible functioning. If you get stuck in a loop of despair and dysfunction, you can't be effective for your child's care. The biggest danger sign is a lasting and overall sense of being overwhelmed and unable to reach out for assistance. The biggest aid is to recognize the rigid noncoping pattern and take positive action to get help. As with the previously described trouble spots, you may want to refer to the section on choosing help in chapter 2. In addition, talk to someone you trust about generating some positive alternatives: ways and people who can support you and help you resolve the problems you are facing. You might be surprised but relieved to learn that if you reach out to someone, that person can often give you more options than you would think of on your own.

Screening

By searching the Internet you will find many sites that offer questionnaires to screen for depression, anxiety, alcohol problems, and eating disorders. The quality of these sites varies; they range from university mental health and government sites to frank entrepreneur sites that are not scientifically based.

A useful example of an accessible Web site is the one posted by a nonprofit organization, Screening for Mental Health, Inc. (http://www.nmisp.org). This site explains the National Screening Day Project, which has widely publicized screening days for the problems listed earlier all across the country in many communities. Among the numerous professional organizations serving as sponsors for the screening programs on this site are the American Psychological Association, the American Psychiatric Association, and the National Institute of Mental Health. You can find your local screening date and place through the national site.

Parents who do not have access to the Internet at home or work might use the hookups at your public library or in the family resource center at the hospital. National screening days are also widely advertised in your local media as a public service.

Parents who need person-to-person psychological screening for an assessment of your or your child's situation may get it at your hospital or clinic. For times after treatment or if you live far away from the treatment center, you will want to obtain local resources in your community.

You Are Not Alone

In reviewing important factors that put families at greater risk we did not want to dwell on painful psychological problems. Rather, we are responding to the feedback of many parents who told us of the need to make this kind of information available. The topics covered are the ones most often hidden from view, a source of shame. We have included this chapter in our book in the belief that it is less isolating to know what you are facing and that you are not alone. If you find yourself reflected in this chapter, seek a consultation with a mental health professional who understands both cancer and the kind of problem you are experiencing. Every problem in coping can be addressed and at least partially eased. Sometimes, even a 10% improvement tips the balance for an entire family's ability to cope.

CHAPTER 9

Relieving Pain and Side Effects

Fall seven times, stand up eight.
—Japanese proverb

For his procedures, I brought a tape recorder with lullaby music. He had conscious sedation with two medicines. I had constant skin and eye contact with him. He was seeing my face, hearing my voice; I was constantly keeping my hands on him. When he got a little bit older, reading a story helped. We still had music, but he liked me to read one particular book to him, over and over again. He would reach out and point to the pages and try to talk, keeping his mind off what was going on. Because they went so well for him when he was younger, he didn't panic. He got very relaxed. He didn't have a lot of pain. We tried to be relaxed for him so that he wouldn't sense from us that there was something stressful coming up.—*Debra*

The first obligation a parent instinctively accepts is to protect one's child from harm, from pain, and from fear. Cancer complicates that job. You strive to stave off feeling frantic and helpless and to fulfill the roles of protector and soother. One mother told us that her child's oncologist described her as a lioness fiercely guarding her cub—an apt image for many of us.

The best way to deal with any child's pain and distress is to prevent it. Absent total prevention, you can minimize painful experiences and maximize your child's ability to cope with them. Cancer and its treatments may trigger pain, nausea, vomiting, and anxiety in anticipation of difficult procedures. If distress over medical procedures becomes entrenched, it becomes harder with each new event to treat it. Fortunately, there is broad agreement about the approaches that provide relief and set the stage for children to handle their experiences and recover.

In this chapter, we concentrate on making a medical plan, identifying and assessing your child's pain and distress, and using particular methods to reduce his or her pain and distress. In the second half of the chapter we give practical coping tips that apply to any symptoms or side effects, as well as a specific discussion of nutritional issues, including steroid effects.

Making a Pain Plan

Every child and parent should be prepared before a procedure rather than trying to remedy trauma responses after the fact. A little preparation goes a long way to avoiding problems. Discuss both behavioral and pharmaceutical options with your child's physicians and nurses, as well as with any special pain team. Know who is in charge of your child's pain plan and who will make decisions in that person's absence. You need clear-cut, written instructions that describe

- How, when, and by whom the pain will be assessed and controlled
- Drug options and how they work, their side effects, methods of delivery, and how often they will be administered
- Contingency plans, such as how much time is given to see if something is working, what prompts moving to the next step, what obstacles might arise, and who will make the decisions? If one thing does not work, there is usually something else that will.

Fear of addiction sometimes keeps parents from using medications to their full advantage. Medications used for pain relief will not cause addiction when used properly. More damage is done by not properly controlling pain. Pain can escalate quickly. If you wait for a situation to go from bad to worse, making your child comfortable will be much harder. Pain is like a wave: It is very difficult to contain once it has started to break and easier to control if you put up a barrier to blunt its force. Untreated pain can be traumatic and can interfere with cooperation, coping, and recovery.

Nearly all of the families and professionals we spoke with recommended using a topical anesthetic, such as ethyl chloride, or EMLA cream, before needle procedures. One parent put it, "EMLA is the next best thing to sliced bread." However, some children do not like it, and some creams may constrict blood vessels, making a blood draw difficult. New alternatives are developed from time to time. The point is, a child should not be denied the option of this form of help.

For more invasive procedures, conscious sedation is prescribed for the child. It is a relief for both parent and child to avoid a stressful experience by allowing the child to "sleep through it." Sedation decreases the short and long-term stress and trauma and eases the cancer treatment routine. Sedatives usually provide some amnesiac function, that is, the child may remember little or nothing of what happened, even if he or she cries or feels some pain during the procedure.

Every child reacts differently to sedation drugs, and some reactions can be frightening to both you and your child. Through trial and error, you will come to know what works best for your child—and this may change over time. Be sure to inform the anesthesiologist of your experience before future procedures. There are many options available. The drugs used in the family stories are likely to change with pharmaceutical advances; the lesson about individual differences is likely to remain the same.

> When my daughter was a baby, we had a lot of trouble finding something to effectively sedate her. Versed didn't work at all; instead of going to sleep, she became agitated and cried. At the age of 3, when she needed dental work, she was given Versed again. This time she had a different reaction. It made her very woozy and sleepy, and she didn't even realize when they took her out of my arms.—*Elise*

* * *

> He had anesthesia twice a day during radiation treatments. He always came out of anesthesia really badly, except when propyphol was used. It's the wonder drug that works wonders. He fell asleep saying, "Oh, this is good." He can still get a laugh out of me with that. With other anesthesia he would come out of it crying and screaming and scaring the nurses. But I stood there and told them it was okay and they didn't have to hold him down, 'cause I know my kid. And I like it when they respect that.—*Bridget*

There are many children who prefer behavioral techniques to sedation. There are also occasions when sedation might not be feasible.

> The calming medications made him angry. He didn't like feeling out of control. It was more valuable for him to be told what was happening and to focus and relax. It really works. At night when he'd be in pain, we'd start the relaxation exercise and go down the whole body and make everything limp.—*Augusta*

* * *

> Spinal taps never bothered me. Everyone is amazed that I say that. The nurses were wonderful. I still remember one nurse who was very personable. She held my hand, stood in front of me, asked me how things were going to distract me. The only thing I ever felt was pressure.—*Elaine, young adult survivor*

It is beyond the scope of this book to further discuss medical approaches to pain and distress symptoms. Historically, children's pain has been underestimated and undertreated, but many cancer treatment centers now have valuable pain teams who specialize in helping children through arduous times. Consult with your own medical team about the available services for your child locally. The rest of the chapter focuses on psychological approaches to pain and distress and the practical experiences of parents.

Identifying Pain and Distress

There are several signs of distress you are likely to have to face with your child. Be assured that any of these may be a target for an individualized plan to treat it. Chronic, persistent, or episodic pain (such as leukemic pain, phantom limb pain, chemotherapy-induced pain, and headaches) is different from the acute but short-term pain felt in a procedure. It is harder for a patient to cope with and requires an advanced combination of the medical and behavioral relief methods but can always be relieved to some extent.

Perhaps the most common reaction is the pain and fright that happens during a treatment procedure, such as a bone marrow aspiration. The reaction might be triggered by acute pain or by pressure and can be exacerbated by scary sights and sounds. Many children struggle with anxiety in anticipation of a procedure. For example, they worry about an upcoming surgery or spinal tap or about having a nasogastric (ng) tube inserted for the first time.

Children, just like adults, may develop a conditioned response, such as an automatic nausea response to chemotherapy. Anticipatory nausea and vomiting related to chemotherapy are upsetting. Many people hoped the problem would be eliminated with the availability of drugs like ondansetron. However, the majority of children and teenagers still have at least mild symptoms. Expectations have a big impact. The more a child expects vomiting and is distressed by it, the more likely he or she is to experience it.

Phobic reactions, such as those to needles or equipment, also may develop. Distressing memories of previous procedures can heighten your child's fears. Children may believe that they can die from the procedure or that they are being punished.

> Melanie was really phobic about seeing blood, which made transfusions tricky. If she could see the blood in the hanging bag or in the tube, she would become very agitated. We hung a sheet over the IV pole and covered up the tubing. It looked like a ghost going down the hall, but it worked for her.—*Peggy*

Your own knowledge of both the procedure your child is to undergo and the ways to help him or her cope will reduce your anxiety. When you have a support "job" to focus on during a procedure it makes you feel less helpless and more involved. That is important, because your child takes cues from you; distress begets distress, and coping begets coping.

Children report that it really helps to have a parent present. You can help most if you are able to stay calm and steady.

If your child is highly phobic and filled with fear about a procedure, insist on a consult with a professional. Ask for someone who knows how to help your child reduce the anxiety and handle the procedure better. This person might be a specialist on your hospital's pain team—a medical, nursing, or mental health professional. It is better to act early in your child's course of treatment, because distress levels rise as the level of overload rises. Nip it swiftly, so the child can feel safe and able to manage the treatment demands again. If you are anxious or fearful yourself, get help. Work with a counselor to improve your own coping strategies so you can help your child by providing a good model.

The age and style of your child influence how pain and other suffering are communicated. It is important to both ask a child about symptoms and observe the child's behavior, especially changes in behavior. If a child who is not able to eat, play, relax, or sleep comfortably receives pain medication and afterward is able to do those things, the behavior change indicates that the child was in pain.

It may be helpful for you to know that, according to pediatrician and pain specialist Lonnie Zeltzer (see the Bibliography),

- Children as young as ages 3–5 may be able to give useful self-reports of pain.
- Children younger than age 7 give more reliable pain ratings with a vertical picture scale of happy and sad faces (descriptions follow).
- Teenagers show pain (such as clenching or muscle tension) in ways that may not show up on measures designed for younger children.
- Close to 99% of children report that the most helpful factor during a painful experience was a parent's presence, even though they show more distress when a parent is present.
- Effective strategies to decrease pain and distress must take into account two parts, the child's anticipation of an event and his or her actual encounter with it.

A child is the best indicator of his or her own pain. Young children respond well to the Wong–Baker FACES Pain Rating Scale (see the Bibliography and Resources), which is available in most treatment settings. Ask the child to choose the face that best describes how he or she feels: a happy face represents no hurt and a sad face means a little hurt, with the faces getting sadder as the pain increases. Other scales rate pain using poker chips, colors, or photographs. Older children can use descriptive words, a ruler, or a simple 1–10 number system to rate pain. It is not important which scale you use, but to explain the concept of different levels thoroughly and use the same one consistently to get the most accurate assessment.

Young children can point to themselves, a doll, or a picture of a child to pinpoint where the pain is. Children's answers can be creative but also rather accurate. For example, a child

Children's Pain Behaviors, Expressions, Fears, and Sources of Comfort

Pain Behaviors	Modes of Expression	Predominant Fears	Sources of Comfort
Infant, ages 0–12 months			
Total body movements Lack of responsiveness to feeding Changes in alertness Lack of contentment Sleep disturbances Poor responsiveness to caregivers Withdrawal, unusual stillness	Loud crying or whimpering Facial expression (brows knitted, eyes tightly closed, mouth open)	Separation from parents Fear of strangers	Presence of primary caregiver or consistent nurses Sucking, self-comforting (soother, blanket, etc.) Holding, rocking Favorite toy, object, photograph Medication
Toddler, ages 1–3 years			
Clinging to caregiver Restless, irritable Rejection of all others Refusing food, toileting Regression to infant behaviors Decreased exploration of environment Flailing arms and legs Holding body rigid Touching hurt body part	Crying (whimpering to screaming) Refusal of everything Withdrawal Anxious facial expression or hiding face Describing pain as "hurt" or "owie" (location not specified) Pushing cause of pain away before or after procedure	Separation from parents or primary caregivers Fear of immobility and restraint	Presence of primary caregiver or consistent nurses Special toys or objects Rocking, holding Distraction activities: stories, TV, music Self-comforting: sucking, holding on to special blanket Medication

Preschoolers, ages 3–5 years			
Immobility, rigidity Clinging to anyone Crying, kicking Regression to previous stages (loss of bowel and bladder control) Disinterest in normal play and tasks Anxiety Uncooperative, requires restraint	Crying, screaming Shrieking without tears Withdrawal Concerned only with how pain affects him/her Able to describe pain's location and intensity: "Bad tummy ache" or "legs hurt" Fearful of pain-relieving interventions and incessantly questions, "What are you doing?" and "Why?" Pushing cause of pain away before or after procedure Asking to stop procedure Verbal expressions: "ow," "ouch," "it hurts"	Separation from parents, siblings, home environment Fear that pain is punishment Fear of body mutilation	Presence of family Consistent staff Familiar toys, books Games and play activities (distraction) Regular caregivers performing painful procedures Fantasy Increased mobility (going to the playroom) Asking child what has helped relieve pain in the past and using child's suggestions and simple participation Simple routines and explanations Medication
School-age children, ages 6–12 years			
Hyperactivity, extreme passivity Body language: clenched fists, gritted teeth, stiff body Moody, temperamental Demanding, aggressive Angry; temper outbursts Withdrawal, extreme quietness; lying with eyes closed, "tuning out," not caring for self Regression to earlier behaviors, panic attacks, bedwetting Impulsiveness Anxious facial expressions and poor eye contact	Able to more accurately describe location and intensity of pain May groan, wince, scream, but try to hold back tears and "be brave" May deny any pain in presence of peers Demand scientific explanations of how pain treatments and procedures affect body functioning May ask for pain medications as long as they are *not* injections Stalling: "Wait a minute," "I'm not ready"	Fear of feeling inferior Separation from peers Fear of mutilation Fear of rejection Fear of loss of self-control	Relationships with peers Ability to engage in task Presence of supportive understanding adult Explanations at a level child can understand Encourage participation in care Hypnosis and biofeedback Medication

Box continues next page

Children's Pain Behaviors, Expressions, Fears, and Sources of Comfort (*Continued*)

Pain Behaviors	Modes of Expression	Predominant Fears	Sources of Comfort
Adolescents, ages 13 and older			
Wide range of behaviors	Able to describe pain: location, intensity, duration	Fear of losing control	Relationships with peers and friends
Regression to previous stages	May verbalize desire for pain medications	Fear of changes in self-concept, body image	Consistent roommates
Withdrawal, depression	May refuse pain interventions in presence of peers	Fear of loss of independence	Consistent caregivers
Aggressiveness, teasing	Less vocal protest but more expressions: "You're hurting me," "That hurts"	Separation from peers	Interests, hobbies
Manipulation		Concerns about future: relationships, sexual competency, fertility	Family members; may prefer siblings to parents at times
Poor eating and hygiene			Self-hypnosis
Refusal of care			Self-relaxation
Less motor activity			Control over the situation
Increased muscle tension and body control			Solitude
			Medication

Adapted from: Craig, K. D. 1984. Developmental changes in infant pain expression during immunization injections. *Social Science and Medicine* 19(12): 1331–1337, with permission of Elsevier Science; Katz, E. R., J. Kellerman, and S. E. Siegel. 1980. Behavioral distress in children with cancer undergoing medical procedures: Developmental considerations. *Journal of Counseling and Clinical Psychology* 48(3):356–365, with permission of the American Psychological Association; and Stevens, B. 1989. "Nursing management of pain in children." In *Family-centered nursing care of children*, 882–914, edited by R. L. Foster, M. M. Hunsberger, and J. J. Tackett-Anderson, with permission of W.B. Saunders.

who told his mother "my hair hurts" had a headache. Keep in mind that a child who is playing a game or reading but who says she's in a lot of pain is not exaggerating. She is instinctively practicing distraction activities to relieve her pain. In fact, children are much more likely to underreport their pain, often because they are afraid pain relief medication will be in the form of an injection, or their friends are present, or they simply want to please the person asking.

Adults often misinterpret the behavior of a child in pain. The preceding charts, based on multiple sources, show you some of the ways children express that they are in pain.

Reducing Your Child's Pain and Distress

There is an array of useful strategies for pain and symptom management. It pays to familiarize yourself with the approaches, so that you know the "menu" of choices. Then you will be able to try out the techniques that seem most suited to your child and situation. Some of these ideas are common sense. You have the knowledge of your child and the sensitivity to try most of them. Other strategies are likely to have the most impact when put into practice by a professional with clinical experience and creativity.

Preparation

Let your child know what to expect. Remember, the unknown is more fearful than the known. Fear and anxiety can make pain more acute. Anticipate misunderstandings; explain, for example, that a technician won't take all of a child's blood in a blood draw and the child will wake up from "sleepy medicine." Remind your child of a past experience in which he or she coped well. It is helpful to make it clear that the procedure is not optional; if a child senses any hesitation or room on your part for a way out, he or she will latch on to it. Avoid tacking on "okay?" at the end of an explanation. In parent language, this means, "Do you understand," or "Did you hear me?" To a child, this means, "You don't have to do this if you don't want to," which is a cruel falsehood.

Children need to hear the following messages:

- What will happen; how long it will take; what it might feel, look, sound, and smell like; and what the side effects might be—ask for written or picture materials, videos, or a "walk-through" from staff.
- What is expected of him or her—such as holding still or drinking contrast fluid for imaging.
- The purpose or benefits of the treatment or procedure—why it is necessary and that it is not a punishment.

- Whether something will hurt or not and what will be used to make the pain go away—what form the pain medication will take, such as by mouth or through an IV tube; the prospect of another shot can be worrisome to a child.
- That it's okay to be scared or to cry.
- That it's okay to ask questions—if Mom or Dad doesn't have the answer, he or she will find someone who does.
- That Mom, Dad, or another loved one will be there to help him or her through it—it'll be okay.

Two important things to keep in mind are first, that procedures should always be carried out in a treatment room and not in the child's hospital room or bed. The child needs to know that his or her bed is a safe haven. Second, give the child as much control as possible: choosing which arm for needles; choosing whether to take pills before or after a TV show; choosing breathing exercises, imagery, or both; or choosing to sit on mom's lap or by oneself. Choices give a child control, power, and a boost for self-esteem and independence.

In general, nurses have an excellent understanding of how to tell children about procedures. Parents can learn from them, as well as physicians, child life specialists, and other parents about practical guidelines and considerations. Parents often become expert at gauging their child's preferences for how information is handled, the timing (giving notice a day or two before a procedure or just an hour before, for example), and how much or little they can absorb. Avoiding explanations because your child gets nervous or upset is an easy pattern to fall into, but it is doing your child a disservice. Children deserve to know what is going to happen to them.

Prepare for nonpainful procedures, too. Parents are often surprised when a child "overreacts" to what a parent sees as an "easy" event. Your child may be frightened by the dim lights, strange machines, or cold jelly of an ultrasound. The child may have to drink a chalky substance, be alone in a room, be strapped to a table, or let a scanner come close to his or her face, any of which can be distressing. Preparation, combined with reassurance and distraction, will relieve this distress.

Motivation and Messages

One way to motivate is to encourage your child with rewards. A reward may be praise for any coping attempt, no matter how small or short-lived. A reward also may be a little treat from the hospital gift shop, lunch at a favorite fast food restaurant, or a fun activity. Most pediatric labs have prizes to distribute, such as character BandAids, stickers, temporary tattoos, and bracelets. One girl kept track of the really hard things she went through and earned "credits" at the Disney store from her family and their friends. One creative hospital uses colorful beads to acknowledge difficult events and procedures in a child's treatment, and these serve both as a conversation starter and a memento. After a course of chemotherapy or radiation, a trip to the emergency room, a test, a scan, a spinal tap, a blood draw, a transfusion, a week's hospital stay, a surgery, a transplant, or just a bad day, the child receives a particular color or shape of bead to add to his or her growing necklace. Anything positive that can be paired with the procedure experience adds to the child's coping arsenal. Be careful not to overuse the reward system by giving large gifts for every procedure. Use your judgment.

> As Jimmy got older, it was harder for us to take him to clinic, because he didn't want to go. His grandmother told him if he went to the clinic and behaved, she would take him to the train store and he could pick out one thing. It was out-and-out bribery. After awhile we thought this was not right, because he would think that whenever he behaves he will get a reward. But she said, it's just for a while, whatever it takes. So every week we'd go to the train store and pick out an engine. Now he's got a whole room full. They don't all fit on the train track. But it worked.—*Carly*

A note about negative reinforcement: It is never helpful to punish or threaten your child to get compliance with a procedure. Punishment does not work, and it sets up a destructive cycle for the next procedure. Deriding your child for expressing his fears (by crying, kicking, screaming, or trying to avoid a procedure) is also destructive. It tells the child that his or her feelings are wrong, and it does not help him or her to manage better.

Using personal messages is a great coping strategy. With a little advance help from adults, children can develop reassuring statements to make during difficult times. Examples are, "I can do this," "I know what this is," "The first step is done, only two more steps to go," "I know what to do next (squeeze Mom's hand, do my counting)," or "It will be over soon. I am okay." Any simple positive coping statement selected by a child, as long as it doesn't promise more than the child can manage, is fine.

Parents can motivate with words, as well. Focus your attention on your child, and use positive, reassuring words. Speak in a soothing voice. Talk about what the child can do ("you can do it," "squeeze my hand," or "tell me what comes next in the story"), what the child is doing well (focusing on breathing or describing a movie), and positives ahead ("it will get better," "only one more step," or "by tomorrow you'll be up and around"). Engage your child by giving him or her a job, including him or her in the process: "Can you help me count?" "Will you help me remember the story?" Like you, your child will feel less helpless if he or she has something to focus on.

Distraction and Hypnosis Imagery

The goal with any distraction technique is to focus the child's attention away from the distressing procedure to reduce the perception of pain or distress. Many hospital procedure rooms have "comfort boxes" with items to distract your child, but you can bring your own things, if necessary.

Norm sang "Amazing Grace" to his son during spinal taps. Robin kept her daughter laughing through a half-hour ultrasound by making her Barbie doll walk around and repeatedly fall off the bed. The title of the parents' Web site The Never-Ending Squirrel Tale was chosen in honor of a story that cofounder Colleen O'Brien told during a three-hour marathon imaging procedure to keep her daughter occupied. The story starred her daughter's stuffed squirrel companion.

Distraction Ideas

- Counting backwards from 100 or saying multiplication tables
- Looking at pictures
- Singing songs
- Reading or listening to stories (parents can tell a story through an intercom, if he or she can't stay in the room with the child; pop-up books are very engaging)
- Playing electronic or video games
- Watching a videotape
- Listening to music (try nature sounds, new age, Celtic, or Native American)
- Playing with visual puzzles and books that require concentration (such as *I Spy, Where's Waldo,* and optical illusions)
- Playing with Illusions in Art cards (artists such as Escher, Magritte, Del Prete, and Dali; available from Y&B Associates or at museum shops)
- Putting on a puppet show with favorite stuffed animals, dolls, or puppets
- Making a collage or booklet with pictures of beautiful places to visit on an imaginary trip or your own alphabet book with pictures cut from magazines
- Playing with a penlight or small flashlight in a dim room (two people could have a "duel" or "draw" with the light)
- Playing with removable stickers or Colorforms (placed, with a technician's permission, on a scanning machine)
- Playing with glitter-filled tubes (make one out of a small plastic bottle or lab tube; fill halfway with mineral oil and add glitter, sequins, sparkles, and food coloring; fill with water, leaving space at the top so the contents can shift; secure the top on with duct tape)
- Playing thinking or guessing games (such as 20 Questions or alphabet games)

Distraction really works. Psychologist William Redd found a 50% decrease in nausea among children who played video games before the beginning of chemotherapy rather than focusing on the intravenous infusion (see the Bibliography). Researchers Selwyn Mason, Malcolm Johnson, and Sheryl Woolley conducted a different study of distraction techniques, for children age 2–4, and found the use of short stories involving interaction between parent and child was a most successful way to relieve distress (see the Bibliography). Refer back to the opening story in this chapter for a good example. Art can work well, too.

> I use art to help children relax and also to distract them from procedures and pain. Once a nurse came into the playroom to do a procedure on a young child. This procedure usually caused hysterics and necessitated several nurses holding her down. The nurse warned me we would probably have a scene. The child was extremely involved in her art-making with her father. I said maybe the art would distract the girl, but the nurse was very doubtful. The child flinched during the procedure, but never stopped doing her art.—*Janet Ruffin, art therapist*

Hypnosis and the use of imagery provide powerful, effective distractions for children. In fact, they are widely researched distraction techniques and work especially well with children. Children are open to fantasy and are less hampered by reality constraints than adults.

Hypnosis is not hocus-pocus. It is merely the formal name for any of the processes that lead to altered states of consciousness. Another way to understand it would be as a focused state of attention. Everyone has the experience of a "trance" state; for example, when you are driving a car and suddenly realize you have not paid attention to how you got to your location because you were deep in thought, it could be called a self-hypnosis experience. Your mind was focused on your inner imagined world instead of the driving experience, although your body went through all the correct "autopilot" motions of driving the car.

Hypnosis experiences are known as guided imagery, directed fantasy, visualization, and emotive imagery. There are many opportunities to use imagery to distract children from pain and anxiety.

Let the soul banish all that disturbs.
Let the Body that envelopes it be still.
And all the frettings of the body,
And all that surrounds it.
Let Earth and sea and air be still
And Heaven itself.
And then let the body think
Of the Spirit as streaming, pouring,
Rushing and shining into it from
All sides while it stands quiet.
Plotinus (205 A.D.)

> The pain doctor taught Noah self-hypnosis to control his pain. He also showed him a picture of the spine, and explained how you can stop the pain going in, and what makes you feel better. He gave him chemical explanations: epinephrine in your body is the same as morphine. Noah had a good image of this and was able to put himself under to get rid of a lot of the pain. We did a lot of visual imagery. He liked images of walking on the beach, taking long hikes, trees. The other fantasy was dragons, and clouds. That kind of stuff. That helped an enormous amount. If he knew a procedure was coming up, we'd do the imagery in conjunction with massaging his arms and legs.—*Andrea*

Fantasy works best when it reflects the child's personality and level of development. The younger the child, the more help is needed, in terms of guidance, cues, sharing, and interaction. Teenagers may prefer to engage in imagery techniques by themselves or with a tape.

There is a well-known technique called the "magic glove" or "magic boot" that is used protectively to simulate the sense of numbness at the pain site. Other sensory images that may be used similarly are a "magic liquid" or sensation of snow. Cold images counteract pain sensations that are hot.

Another strategy makes use of superheroes, which are viewed by children as powerful and possessing the ability to rescue and help them. Superheroes act as support and protection. The child may also imagine that he or she is wearing a superhero costume, which offers him or her some protection.

Some children prefer images of animals, which they endow with magical qualities. Even without the magic element, a child who is attached to a pet (or who wishes for a dinosaur or a wild animal as a pet) can be guided through a lively befriending, feeding, and grooming experience with the imagined wild animal or beloved pet. Smaller children like the familiarity of routine and repetition.

The action of sports or playing music may be appealing to older children. They are often able to enter into the sequence of what they will do and how it feels to be on the soccer field or sitting at the piano playing a favorite tune, with all the sights and sounds and sensations. Almost any activity could be used: skiing, sunning on the beach, skateboarding, visiting Disneyland, sailing, or painting.

The goal of the distracting exercise is to absorb the child's attention and draw it away from the distress. Even partial distraction, for part of the distressing experience, reduces the negative intensity and aids coping abilities. To be most effective, these techniques take time to learn and practice. Ask about hypnosis and guided-imagery resources at your child's treatment center or near your home. At the major cancer centers, there are always experts in these techniques available for consultation. Even if you are not near one of these centers, there are psychologists and social workers and other professionals trained in these techniques in most communities. Another good source about pain and how to use these techniques is psychologist Leora Kuttner's *A Child in Pain* (see the Bibliography) and *No Fears, No Tears* (videotape, see the Resources).

> I used to do "make-up stories" about a family of little people who lived in a magic land. To get there you had to go in a hot air balloon, flying through the clouds. In one story, the family helped the Easter bunny color eggs by dipping them in the end of a rainbow. All the characters had goofy names, and my children were always incorporated into the story. It wasn't very original; I borrowed heavily from classic stories. But my son didn't seem to mind. You don't have to be Hans Christian Andersen. Just keep talking about things they like. —*Joan*

Breathing

Relaxation training is one of the primary anxiety-reducing techniques for adults in cancer treatment. It can be used with older children, who have longer attention spans and can maintain the focus and proceed through the steps successfully. Often it does not work for very young children. Simple breathing exercises do work with young children and may be combined with imagery. For example, with guidance and modeling your child can put a hand over his or her abdomen and feel the gentle rise and fall of breath while doing a few slow deep breaths. Then you can begin a story or a fantasy experience. The breathing may become the cue, the entry point for fantasy exercises.

Blowing activities are useful in helping a child get through a procedure or episode of pain. Blowing distracts and forces the child to stop crying long enough to take big, deep, relaxing breaths. After a minor procedure, that old stand-by "blow the hurt away" can still work. Some useful tools are bubbles, a pinwheel, a kazoo, a harmonica, bubble gum, or an old-fashioned toy "pipe" with a string that loops when you blow through the pipe. Fun activities can be used, such as painting by blowing paint around on paper with a straw; making music by blowing over the tops of glass bottles containing varying amounts of liquid; or playing tabletop "football" or "hockey" using a balloon, cottonball, or crumpled piece of paper. Many parents report success in adapting Lamaze breathing techniques for their children.

> I'm very good at Lamaze-type relaxation. A lot of it was common sense. I had older brothers and sisters, most of whom had children. So I'd heard about Lamaze and breathing. My mother worked on it with me, using the techniques to relax and to concentrate on something else. Even now, when I have to have blood drawn, I put my arm out straight away, and then I go into my own little world. I concentrate on something else, I start my breathing, and I don't even feel the needle.—*Shoshana, long-term survivor*

Modeling and Practicing

Modeling just means demonstration. It is "show and tell" that demonstrates active coping strategies. For example, a child may view a videotape of a similar-aged child undergoing a procedure and visibly using coping strategies. A parent may watch a nurse role-play a helpful parent's actions during a procedure.

Practicing is the rehearsal of the techniques that have been demonstrated. Children, as well as adults, do much better if they are familiar with what to do and how to do it before entering a situation that might make them anxious. They are more likely to be able to follow through if they have a little experience first. Practice techniques might make use of dolls as surrogates in younger children or the kinds of techniques described earlier such as breathing and imagery for any age. For children who have reached phobic levels in their dread and fear of a procedure, modeling and rehearsal techniques are taken to a higher level and used by mental health professionals to desensitize a child to the dreaded experience. The goal in these situations is to take away the child's panic and helplessness and to replace them by giving the child a measure of control through active coping strategies.

Physical Contact and Exercises

Physical contact can be soothing to a child of any age: rhythmic, gentle stroking of an arm or head; giving a back rub or a foot massage; alternating heat and ice compresses; bathing; patting; hugging and holding; rapid rocking or swaying; holding hands; changing your child's position; or letting your child squeeze your hand. Add humming or singing, and you have a powerful combination. One child asked her mother to stroke one finger vertically across her wrist and down her palm gently and repeatedly; it relaxed and calmed her. Another preferred peppermint lotion foot rubs. A father traces letters on his daughter's back, forming "secret" messages for her. Hugging teddy bears, dolls, or blankets is an old familiar standby.

There are some instances when touch is painful to the child. Work around this by addressing a small body area that does not hurt by giving a foot massage, perhaps. Swinging in a hammock, rocking in a rocking chair, and being pushed in a stroller are rhythmic motions that do not require being held. An electric fan provides a soothing breeze, a hypnotic object to focus on, and a quiet hum, all of which might soothe some children. Using heat or cold, depending on the nature of the pain, can provide some relief as well.

Holding your child during a procedure is a natural action that makes you both feel better. A hug and a cozy lap offer great comfort, keeping both parent and child involved and engaged with each other. This is not the same as holding a protesting child down while a painful procedure is performed. While a parent should not have to be the one to restrain a child, it is not always avoidable. This is a major source of stress for parent and child alike.

> Once I had to hold him when we couldn't wait for help to arrive. That was one of the hardest things I ever had to do. He said, "Why are you letting them do this to me, why are you hurting me, why do you want him [the doctor] to do this?" I said, "I don't want him to hurt you, but we have to do this." I never wanted to be that person. It's one thing to say you need to have this done, and another to be his vise grip.—*Rosamund*

Slow, smooth, rhythmic exercises can release tension, increase flexibility, and have a hypnotic effect, all of which can help a child cope with pain. Swinging or circling the arms or legs and shoulder shrugs are good examples. A physical therapist can help your child with exercises and therapeutic massage.

Debriefing

Give a child an opportunity to "debrief" after a procedure. Praise the child for going through it and for sitting still, even though he or she was scared. Being brave does not mean not being scared. It means doing something difficult even when you are scared. Try to avoid saying things like, "That wasn't so bad" or "You don't have to think about it anymore." Encourage the child to express his or her feelings, worries, and self-congratulations. Hours after even a relatively easy event, such as a blood draw, a child will want to talk about it; show off a Band-Aid, poke-site, or prize; and tell about his or her bravery, about the person who did it, or the trip to McDonald's or the gift shop afterward. Talking about a painful experience helps a child gain control over the situation and himself or herself, process the event and his or her feelings, and will make it easier next time.

Your Participation

The key strategies of preparation, motivation and messages, distraction and hypnosis, breathing, modeling and practicing, and debriefing are all worth trying. The right strategy at the right time will make a significant difference for your child's comfort. Even more important than the particular strategy is your participation. The gift you give your child is to be as present, calm, soothing, and matter-of-fact throughout these difficult times, as is realistically possible.

Gentle Reminders for Coping With Pain

- Make a pain plan.
- Teach your child how to assess his or her pain.
- Learn your child's distress signals.
- Identify and address your child's phobias (stumbling blocks or freeze points) and your own.
- Give your child options, choices, and control whenever possible.
- Motivate your child with positive messages and small rewards.
- Prepare your child for procedures; build in opportunities for practicing and modeling.
- Inform the staff of your child's special needs or preferences.
- Make use of distraction, imagery, and breathing techniques.
- Allow your child time to wind down and to talk about fears, thoughts, and experiences.
- Give yourself and your child the gift of knowing that you can get through these painful times intact.

Dealing With Side Effects and Symptoms

The side effects of cancer treatment range from mild to severe, temporary to permanent, inconvenient to life-altering. Looking over the laundry list of potential problems can be disquieting to parents. Older children and family members, who understand the implications, may get discouraged, too. Specific effects may be anticipated with great trepidation—something that just sounds like more than you can handle. These fears are often unfounded, based on misconceptions or lack of knowledge. Elise told us she dreaded her daughter getting mouth sores, recoiling from the thought of nursing the baby, but said that the reality was not as bad as her fantasy. A parent's apprehension can temper the ability to deal with effects and can rub off on a child, especially when verbal or body language tells the child that something awful is going to happen.

The sum total of effects does not happen all at once but is piecemeal. During active treatment, relief seems short-lived. No sooner does your child start to feel better than he or she is hit with another round. With each additional treatment, more bodily systems are affected. At each step, your family girds itself to cope. But the effects are cumulative, and your child is sicker. The growing "pile-up" may overload child and family, particularly if any effects are known to be permanent. To a parent, even a small inconvenience, when added to the pile, seems wholly unfair—one more thing the child must endure or one more thing he or she won't be able to do.

Parents may be glad, secretly, for the arrival of some limited side effects, because it means that the treatment is "working." Also, children sometimes think of vomiting as getting rid of the "bad stuff."

Strong effects can be repellent to both child and parents. Idiosyncratic reactions—special reactions or allergies that only your child seems to have—are impossible to predict, complicate treatment, and make the family feel "put-upon." Long-term effects require ongoing medical intervention and your advocacy as a parent. Rare and more serious effects give the family a new and separate condition with which to cope. Indirect effects are not attributable to a specific treatment. As a father wisely noted, it doesn't matter what caused an effect, you still have to deal with it.

Treatment is full of surprises, some which are dangerous, some merely inconvenient. You do not know which it is until after you have dropped everything and raced to the hospital. Fevers invariably seem to show up in the middle of the night, necessitating a hurried trip to the hospital. Nosebleeds, a response to low platelets or dryness, usually happen without warning and sometimes require a platelet infusion. Another surprise waiting at the end of treatment may be symptoms that occur from the discontinuation of chemotherapy agents, which differ from drug to drug.

Our purpose here does not include listing side effects. There are resources that do so quite well, but probably the most up-to-date information will come from your child's doctor. Our aim is to help you cope well with your child's side effects so that your child can cope well also. Here are some suggestions.

Know What to Expect But Don't Obsess

Read the materials given to you by your child's doctor on the potential side effects carefully, but make no assumptions. The doctors have an obligation to tell you every possibility, but that does not mean that your child will experience all of them. Two children with the same diagnosis and the same treatment protocol can have very different side effects. Parents, adolescents, and children can needlessly use time and energy worrying about something that may never happen. Knowing the time frame of a potential effect (when it might happen and how long it will last), the symptoms to watch for, and what can be done to prevent or lessen the effect can all be reassuring. Keep in mind that other cancer parents are a wonderful source of information and tips, but your experiences may not be the same.

Don't Panic

For every effect, there is something that can make it better. Talk to nurses and other parents about what they have done that works well, and try to adapt their ideas to your needs. If you cannot carry out your caretaker duties properly because of your own negative reactions, you may put your child at higher risk for infection, affect his or her ability to tolerate treatment, or increase his or her stress level. Work with the nurses to educate yourself, practice home care, and relieve your medical questions and worries. Arrange for visiting nurses to come to your home to help you if you are overwhelmed. Parents advise, "You can do it. It's not easy, but you won't believe what you can do." Many parents express profound pride in their newly learned skills.

Put Yourself in Your Child's Shoes

As compassionate as we are and as involved as we are, the cancer and its treatment are not happening to our bodies. We do not know what it feels like. Some adults report a rude awakening when they have a bad bout with the flu or seasickness. It dawns on them that this is what their child feels like all the time. One mother we spoke with was diagnosed with breast cancer herself after her son's treatment ended. She reflected that it took her focus of worry away from her son and helped her to understand some of the effects he had suffered. In particular, she mentioned that she felt a burning sensation in her esophagus after one particular medication, for which her doctor prescribed an antacid. When she described it to her son, he agreed that he had felt the same sensation. His symptom went untreated because he could not communicate what was happening at the time. In another example, a grandmother stated that the steroids she had received for her asthma produced upsetting emotional swings. She understood how much scarier those feelings would be for her granddaughter, who was on steroids, too.

Be Prepared

Pack a bag with clothes, toys, and trial-sized toiletries for emergency trips to the hospital. Keep with you any medications your child might need. Make your child's bed with three sets of sheets, one on top of the other, including pads or "chuks" (disposable plastic-backed pads) in between each layer. In the middle of the night if your child wets the bed or vomits, you can quickly and easily strip off one layer and put your child right back into a fresh bed, even in the dark.

Have a contingency plan in case of unexpected events: Who will pick up siblings if a trip to the day clinic turns into an overnighter? Who will dispense medications if the school nurse is absent? Know your child and anticipate reactions before they happen. Does your child need blood two days after chemotherapy? Arrange for a baby-sitter for the siblings, leave leftovers in the fridge, and have a free day if you are wrong.

Be Creative

Avail yourself of a variety of resources; there is an expert or an organization for nearly any problem that might arise. When one mother was unable to find age-appropriate clothes because her child's growth was delayed, a call to Little People of America brought a list of clothing and product resources. Another family sought out adult cancer patients for their tips, when they did not get sufficient teaching from their hospital about giving G-CSF injections. For other ideas about where to find expertise, turn to the Resources at the back of this book.

Be open to alternative ways to ease side effects or perform care. One imaginative parent used a peri bottle (from a maternity unit or any small plastic squirt bottle) to wash gently instead of using baby wipes on her infant daughter's treatment-related diaper rash. A father discovered that a garlic press crushed pills efficiently. Trying to gauge the effect of the "magic mouthwash" for easing the discomfort of her child's mouth care, one mother tried it on herself. She realized that it wore off quickly, and she changed the way she used it, no longer waiting for it to "take effect." Some parents find that if the child smells something strong (such as perfume, mint, cherry, cloves, or lemons) as the chemotherapy takes effect, the nausea is somewhat lessened. Put the strong-smelling item in a clean, plastic spice jar (the kind with holes in the top and an additional cap, to make it portable and mess-free). Replace it often to keep the strong smell.

Use the Skills You Already Have

A teacher used her skills to make innovative lesson plans that helped her child work with learning disabilities. A scientist used her technical research abilities to inform herself about her child's illness. Another parent used special education experience to understand neurological effects. Organizational skills were used by an aunt and uncle team to keep track of blood and platelet donors for a child who needed frequent transfusions.

Not all parents have résumés that match side effects, but you do know how to comfort your child. You know your child's likes, dislikes, fears, modes of expression, and level of normal activity. Many of the parenting skills you have used all along work just fine: a cool cloth on a fevered head; clear liquids for a child who has been vomiting; or sunscreen, sunglasses, and hats for a child with sun-sensitive skin. The best skill you possess is that you know your child better than anyone else. The rest will come.

Be Proactive

Know what is coming and try to mitigate it. A teenage boy directed his sister to shave his head, in a gesture of control, before his hair fell out in the shower or on the pillow. A mother shaved her own head when she shaved her son's. There are numerous stories of classmates wearing hats on a cancer child's first day back at school. Communal support bolsters a child's self-esteem and feeling of belonging.

Basic common sense comes in handy. If your child's skin is tape sensitive, use alternative methods to keep a central line or ng tube in place. If your son wakes up with joint pain on day 3 after receiving the drug vincristine, medicate him on night 2 and do not make any plans for the next day. If sedation or anesthesia is planned for one procedure, arrange for other necessary uncomfortable procedures at the same time. Initiate physical therapy before a child's muscles are atrophied. Have braces removed before treatment starts to avoid infection or minor injury to gums. Start hydrating your child with drinks before a round of chemotherapy, so you do not have to wait for the staff to do it intravenously. When your child's platelets are low, use a humidifier in his or her room to help prevent nosebleeds and avoid strenuous activities where he or she might fall. Avoid substances that inhibit platelet function, such as guafenesin (in cough syrup), large amounts of purple grape juice, or ibuprofen.

If a certain drug constipates your child, prepare a day before the treatment. Talk to your child's doctor about laxatives or stool softeners. Avoid constipating drugs or food. Instead, give your child plenty of water, fruit juice, fruits and vegetables, and whole grains. Exercise helps, too. The opposite problem, diarrhea, can be lessened by offering rice, bananas, apples or applesauce, yogurt, toast, crackers, pasta, and cooked cereals.

Practice Infection Control

Parents tell us they can get a little "crazed" about infection control, observing the child closely for signs of infection. Low blood counts are worrisome, marked visually by lethargy, paleness, bruising, or the presence of petechiae (tiny red dots indicating leaking blood vessels). Fever is a worry also, as that is sometimes the only indication of an infection. Nevertheless, you cannot isolate your child in a bubble. Your house is full of germs; family members are, too. Hospitals harbor germs everywhere. In their upset and in a well-meaning effort to protect their children, parents can go a little overboard.

> When we first got our dog, she was nervous and had frequent diarrhea. I was freaking out, crying, thinking we would have to have to get rid of this beautiful dog, or Max would catch a horrible germ and get fatally ill. I ran out to the store to rent a rug-steaming machine. At midnight we were steaming our carpets, cleaning the floors, and giving our dog a bath. It was all incredibly stressful at the time, especially after having spent the entire day at the clinic getting chemo. But when I look back on it now, I am able to laugh.—*Gail*

Even if you could keep your child completely isolated in a germ-free environment, opportunistic infections could still arise from microorganisms normally carried within the child's own body. While there is no need to lapse into compulsive behavior, many infections can be avoided by practicing standard infection control, the most important of which is hand-washing (for a minimum 20 seconds with warm water and soap). This goes for *all* the family members. Teenagers with cancer may need extra reminders to keep their hands and underneath their fingernails clean and to avoid touching acne, as it may be an entrance point for germs. Talk to your doctor about whether it is necessary to use HEPA filters, send pets away, step up house cleaning routines, give children separate baths, or do any other infection control measures.

Avoiding anyone who has cold or flu symptoms, recent live-virus immunizations, or chicken pox can mean missing social contacts. As one father put it, "Your family and friends may be offended, but that's too bad. Your child's life is at stake, here. It's only temporary." Aside from the medical dangers, exposure to disease mandates isolation. Your child cannot play in the playroom or be with other children on the unit if he or she has been exposed to chicken pox.

Hospital staff sometimes send conflicting messages about the need for vigilant infection control. For instance, a neutropenic child may be placed in a room with a roommate who is obviously suffering from something contagious, in the theory that most of the infection danger comes from within his or her own body. Parents who are uncomfortable with this arrangement usually take this up with the charge nurse and request a change. Unless the floor is completely full, they should be willing to accommodate you. Many families also expressed concern about staff not washing their hands. While most professionals will tell you that they may not be allowed to use a patient's sink and have used one in the hall prior to entering the room, it is an issue that worries many parents.

> We had a problem with a roommate's nurse. She had a cough and congestion. Her patient had just relapsed. I said, "You're touching his tubing, you're examining him, you have your hands all over him, and you're not wearing a mask or gloves." She said, "I'm going home in an hour, and the masks don't really work anyway." I was furious. Not only was she putting her patient at risk, she was putting my child at risk. We had a meeting with our doctor, the infection control nurse, and the nursing manager. Hospital policy states you must wash your hands before patient contact, but they can't enforce it. They did nothing. So, if my son's counts were down, we put a little sign on the door that read, "Please wash your hands before you examine me," so we didn't have to say it every time. If it's there in someone's face, how can they deny seeing it, and how can they not be reminded to wash their hands?—*Marisa*

Gentle Reminders for Coping With Side Effects

- Identify and address your child's fears and misconceptions as well as your own.
- Inform the staff of your child's allergies and idiosyncrasies.
- Inquire about ways to prevent and lessen side effects.
- Monitor for predicted side effects.
- Be prepared, proactive, and creative.
- Practice infection control.
- Remember to be compassionate.

Dealing With Nutrition Issues

Like protecting your child from harm, feeding your child is one of the most instinctive, elemental roles you have as a parent. When a dietician or nutritionist tells you that your child is not thriving, is not getting enough food, it feels like an assault on the most basic of your parenting abilities. It puts you on the defensive, despite the nutritionist's best intentions. The problem is that, too often, a nutritionist is not called in until there is a crisis, and the child has stopped growing and developing. Parents are upset about the implications and put off by the thought of intrusive interventions. At this point, the child has more trouble tolerating assistance also. Prevention and the early use of simple strategies are much more effective.

Your child should be assessed by a registered dietician at the time of diagnosis, to get a baseline record of your child's nutritional status, preferably one with experience in oncology. Dietician Nancy Sacks and physician Faith Ottery (see the Bibliography) advise that the best course is to prevent complications as well as treat them.

Nutrition alone will not cure your child of cancer. However, it can have a major impact on your child's health. It is extremely important for your child's growing and developing body and brain to have the proper nutrition. The treatments for childhood cancer can cause malnutrition, which contributes to weight loss, fatigue, muscle weakness, susceptibility to infection, dental problems, and delays or interruptions in normal physical and mental development. Researchers Alvin Maurer, Juliene Burgess, Sarah Donaldson, Karyl Rickard, Virginia Stallings, Jan van Eys, and Myron Winick found that sufficient nutrition can help a child tolerate treatment, metabolize medications, reduce complications, and improve the feeling of well-being and the quality of life (see the Bibliography).

In the following section we have separated nutritional support into three levels. They progress from the least intrusive, level 1, to the highest grade of assistance, level 3.

Nutritional Support Level 1

The first level involves nutritional counseling. A registered dietician works with you and your child to encourage voluntary intake of nutritious food, working around your child's likes and dislikes. Children on treatment tend not to like sweet things, because the chemotherapy makes them taste metallic. Instead, they prefer salty or spicy things. Many a cancer parent wishes he or she owned stock in the company that makes Cheetos, a very common food preference. However, while a child has mouth sores, or mucositis, a bland diet of soft foods is better tolerated. Gloria, a teenager, lived on broth, liquid shakes, and baby food. Food preferences and taste alterations can last long after treatment ends.

> I learned after a very short while to listen to her. She was really good at knowing what her body could tolerate and what it couldn't. If she was hungry or thirsty for something really ridiculous, it was usually fine. Tortillas with Cheez Whiz or melted Velveeta was a staple, ice pops were a biggie—we'd even take those to the hospital and leave them in the freezer to have them there, Italian ice was a fave of hers.—*Pam*

Liz reported her oncologist's directive: "Protein and calories! Protein and calories! Protein and calories!" High-fat foods are desirable, such as whole milk, cream, cheese sauce, butter, peanuts, and peanut butter. The nutritionist can help you alter recipes and recommend supplements to include specific nutrients your child is lacking, such as lipids or phosphates.

> To encourage my son to eat healthily, I hung a food guide on the fridge. Get a standard food pyramid from your pediatrician or hospital dietician that divides the food groups into color-coded sections, and gives recommended daily portions, with pictures of typical foods in each category. Opposite the food guide, I have a rainbow with matching colors. I use corresponding color magnets (from an office supply store) to count the portions he eats. My son likes to choose the foods and move the magnets himself.—*Krystle*

Dealing with food aversions

Foods consumed either right before or right after chemotherapy can become lasting learned food aversions, because the child associates the food with nausea and vomiting. Try to avoid giving your child his or her favorite foods at that time or using them as bribery for compliance with a painful procedure, or else they may lose their preferred status. Judith's son Bobby still cannot eat potato chips or peanut butter and jelly sandwiches, because that is what he ate during treatment.

Frequent, small meals, timed around therapy, seem to be what everyone recommends. Space meals a couple of hours before and after chemotherapy. One parent waited two hours after radiation therapy to feed her son. An adolescent girl arranged her day schedule around feeling nauseated in the morning; she slept late and ate her biggest meal in the late afternoon.

> I went to the health food store and got gingerroot. I would give him a syringeful when he felt sick. That worked better than any medication. It didn't make the nausea go away, but it helped.—*Darlene*

Your child may be ultrasensitive to smells. If so, do not serve his or her meals in the kitchen, where smells linger. Let him or her eat in the dining room, or spread out a plastic-backed tablecloth and have a picnic on the living room floor. If other members of the family join him or her, meal times will remain social, positive occasions, which may make them more palatable.

> I was nauseated, but what can you do. "Enjoy it while it lasts," is what I would say as I ate my Big Mac, shortly before it made its way back up.—*Hayley, survivor*

Other ways to avoid nausea include serving food room temperature or cold. Encourage lots of fluids and avoid activity for an hour after eating. Encourage the child to sit up (gravity helps) in a chair or at a table. Keep clothing loose. If a child is vomiting, use a cool cloth on his or her forehead; let him or her rinse his or her mouth; wait an hour or so and then try little sips of flat ginger ale, water, or weak tea (no milk or fruit juice). Try a trick pregnant mothers use: Have the child eat crackers before even lifting his or her head off the pillow in the morning. Antinausea agents are commonly used in pediatric oncology. Take full advantage, but remember that they have side effects, including drowsiness and decreased absorption of nutrients.

Dealing with food fights

Feeding your child gets more complicated when it becomes a control issue. The adult mind sees a child wasting away and worries. The more a frantic parent nags, the less a child wants to eat. Ultimately, the child may refuse food altogether. The parent, struggling with failure, becomes more frantic. It is a vicious circle. This problem may call for a variety of strategies, including referral to a counselor familiar with both cancer issues and eating disorders. A grandmother described how that worked for her daughter and granddaughter:

> The eating disorders clinic is wonderful for us. Delia (age 6) is stubborn and has used food and eating as her power, to the point of her destruction. The clinic offers a day service in their rapid treatment program. Delia and her Mom go daily and stay there until Delia has consumed (eaten or been tube fed) a set number of calories, as prescribed in her personalized contract. There are two rooms—the playroom and the feeding room. Parents are not allowed into the feeding room when their child is fed. The hospital has the "bad guy" role so Delia and her Mom can stop fighting about food at home.—*Dorothy*

Oral aversion issues are not uncommon and can be physiological or psychological in origin. If your child is unable to put anything in his or her mouth and has a particularly strong gag reflex, the problem may be oral aversion. Ask for a referral to a speech therapist, who will help your child work through it. It may seem odd, but speech therapists are trained in this area.

Flex all your creative muscles to foster a younger child's voluntary intake. Put a star on a calendar every time he or she eats something. Make award certificates for taking medications or gaining a pound. Dredge up your old college "drinking" games and adapt them to your child, using very small amounts of fluid to play quarters, guessing games, or board games. Make ice cubes or popsicles with juice, punch, or yogurt. Freeze grapes. Soak raisins in water or juice to make them soft and plump. Use your blender to make snow cones and fruit shakes. Let your child play with messy foods like whipped cream, pudding, frosting, ice cream, pasta, or yogurt. Add food coloring. Finger-sized cereals with a hole like Cheerios, Apple Jacks, or Fruit Loops can be strung as beads on a string to make an edible necklace or bracelet or used as betting money for poker. Snacks are more fun if they are speared with colorful hors d'oeuvre picks. Foods may be more edible with dipping sauces like ketchup, ranch dressing, yogurt, sour cream dips, or commercial sauces. Serve meals with nothing but finger foods or foods of all one color (such as carrots, macaroni and cheese, oranges, and orange soda), or serve meals backward (offering dessert first).

Parents may be shaking their heads, thinking, "Yeah, right, my child just won't eat anything." It is very difficult to get enough food into a sick child to maintain weight, let alone enough to continue growth and development. The problem is further complicated if the child has allergies, is lactose intolerant, or has diarrhea or constipation. Help is available, but it requires moving up a level to a more intensive plan.

Nutritional Support Level 2

The second level of support involves enteral feeds: giving nutritional supplements through a gastronomy tube or an ng tube when a child is unable to take in enough nutrition by mouth. As long as the child's gastrointestinal tract is functioning, he or she can still receive feedings that will be absorbed by his or her body in the normal way. Usually with these methods, the child can continue to take foods by mouth as well.

Most parents are troubled at first by the idea of the ng tube: It looks uncomfortable, it triggers the gag reflex, and it gives them the "heebie-jeebies." However, the use of the tube releases all the stress and control issues over food. Your anxiety is relieved; your child gets what he or she needs.

> We always used to laugh in the day hospital at the idiotic people on the TV talk shows, because they had no clue what real problems are. One show happened to be about piercing, with a teenager who put a chain up her nose, out her mouth, and over to her earring. Here I was, wishing I didn't have to put a tube in my child's nose to feed her, and this chick did it for fun. Ugh. How did she get a floppy chain to go through?—*Susan*

Parents of children who have had an ng tube compare it to the central line; they have an initial worry about taking care of it, followed by relief when it makes life easier. You can usually give medications through it without disturbing the child, without fighting, and without worrying that he or she will spit it out. Feedings can be given while the child is sleeping, playing, watching television, or being pushed in a stroller.

Older children can do the placement of the tube by themselves, giving them a sense of control. Usually, they opt to use it only at home, at night, so that they do not have to wear it to school in front of their classmates.

For longer term use or if the child cannot tolerate the ng tube, he or she may need a gastronomy or jejunostomy tube. Should your child be a candidate for either of these tubes, your child's physician will discuss it with you. These tubes require surgical placement but are not permanent. They can easily be hidden under the clothes and are thus less of a social issue.

Nutritional Support Level 3

Parenteral support is feeding the child through the veins. Parenteral support can be used in conjunction with tube feeding or used alone when the child's gastrointestinal tract simply cannot function. There are many names for this program: central venous alimentation, hyperalimentation (HAL), total parenteral nutrition, and peripheral parenteral nutrition (through a vein other than the central access line, usually only short-term use).

Parents seem to have many worries about these feeding options. Discuss your concerns freely with your child's oncologist and nutritionist. One parent told us of her experience with HAL feedings. Although they helped her son greatly, she had a chronic worry concerning "whether we were feeding him or the tumor." An open consultation with her hospital team allayed her fears.

Other Considerations

There are occasions when your child is not allowed to take anything by mouth, which is called being NPO (*nil per ora,* a Latin phrase meaning nothing by mouth). A child who will be under general anesthesia is not permitted to eat or drink for several hours prior to a procedure. For some scans it is also necessary that the child's bladder or bowels be empty. Being NPO is particularly difficult for the youngest of children. Grumbling tummies add to their anxiety and irritability. As the clock ticks on and the child begins to complain, a parent's veneer of control wears thin. Try to schedule the event for the time you think your child would best cope—not the time they normally need a big snack or meal. Check with the person performing the procedure or the anesthesiologist to see if it is possible to allow your child to suck on a lollipop or hard candy. Distraction is key to handling this situation. Keep the child as busy as possible. Bring something special for the child to have immediately afterward, but keep it out of sight and as a surprise.

Long after treatment is over, vestiges of nutritional issues can continue. Tastes and preferences can last; learned food aversions remain. Parents still equate feeding their children with taking care of them. Eating disorders and weight problems can occur or a combination of physical and emotional effects. Children who have been constantly cajoled to eat whether they are hungry or not, or who were allowed unbalanced diets because that's all they could eat, may have trouble shaking these habits. Counselors trained in eating disorders can give you some good ideas about how to reteach your child healthy eating habits. Some parents work very hard to insure that survivors, siblings, and family members stick to diets recommended by the American Cancer Society. Others take another route:

> My kids had never had junk food before. They were raised on organic vegetables and whole grains. They didn't eat anything with artificial colors or flavors. They were both breast-fed

for a very long time. And still Timmy got all the things a healthy diet is supposed to insure you from getting: allergies, asthma, and cancer. So food is not magic to me. During his treatment, he didn't feel like eating much. When he felt like eating, he got what he wanted. When he wanted hot dogs three times a day, we were eating hot dogs three times a day. We got him to eat, just not a lot. You do the best you can and don't sweat it.—*Zoe*

Gentle Reminders for Coping With Nutrition

- Nutrition issues and difficulties are not your fault or your child's.
- Good nutrition helps your tolerate treatment and improves his or her quality of life.
- Consult early with a registered dietician or nutritionist who is experienced in pediatric oncology.
- Prevent and lessen problems wherever you can.
- Work with child's likes, dislikes, and ability to tolerate food; be creative and flexible.
- Take advantage of any supplements or strategies that might work for your child.
- Reteach good eating habits when treatment ends.

Dealing With Steroid Effects

There's no way to sugarcoat it: The effects of steroid medication regimens are difficult to manage.

He slept one hour a day, and usually it was from 1–2 in the afternoon, and then he was up ALL night long. We took turns staying up all night with him. And I was pregnant.—*Faith*

It can be alarming to witness the behavior and personality changes that occur in a child taking steroids. The child himself may feel wildly out of control of his or her body and emotions and have no idea what to do about it. These feelings can be frightening. The hyperactivity, anger, and depression sets an entire family on edge. Everyone gets upset. Siblings have a hard time because they often cannot separate the brother or sister they know from the strange one who is yelling and hitting them. Siblings often bear the brunt of the child's worst behavior.

He has become hypersensitive about everything—physically and emotionally. When he has five days of steroids, he cries a lot. One minute he's happy, then he crashes and he's sobbing.

> He opened the milk the wrong way, he put it in the wrong glass, it's a dramatic crisis. He sobbed himself to sleep last night crying for an hour. He kept saying it's not fair. I'm the only one in this family with cancer, I'm the only one that has to take needles, I'm the only one that has to take medicine every night. It's just not fair. And it broke my heart. I said you're right, it's not fair. If I could take this from you, I would do it in a heartbeat, but I can't and it isn't fair, but we'll get through this.—*Gina*

The physical effects of a child taking steroids include weight gain, a moon-shaped face, and fluid retention. The result is that the child looks "fat." Peers and schoolmates may tease him or her. Children get discouraged when they feel fat, conspicuous, and unattractive. Even parents, who know that weight gain is a side effect of a drug, are uncomfortable with their child's appearance.

Side Effects in Children Taking Steroids for Cancer Treatment as Described by Parents

- Agitation
- Mood swings
- Depression symptoms
- Moody, teary
- Vivid dreams, nightmares
- Lethargy, fatigue
- Hyperactivity
- Weight gain
- Insatiable appetite
- Out of control
- Panic attacks
- Fearfulness
- Demanding but don't always know what they want
- Never satisfied
- Inability to be soothed or reasoned with
- Stomach upset
- Drug takes over, not yourself
- Insomnia (up 20–22 hours a day)
- Irritable, frustrated
- Nasty, picking fights
- Back-talking
- Manic, depressive
- "Devil child"
- Screaming for hours
- Stressed, miserable

It may be a small comfort to parents and children to know that these effects are exactly that: effects from a drug. Caused by the medication, they are temporary. It is extremely important that you also get this message across to your child, repeatedly. It is not his or her fault. It is temporary. You still love and will help him or her. Counseling is an effective option for helping the child and parents to cope with the physical and emotional turmoil.

In some cases, the dose can be lowered, or a substitution made, although on some protocols, that is not possible. There is not a lot you can do to prevent the effects of steroids, but parents and professionals do have some suggestions for coping with them.

Coping Strategies for Steroid Effects

> Do not mistake a child for his symptom.
> Erik Erikson

Above all, parents need breaks. Take turns; have other family members and friends help take care of the child for an hour or two while you take a walk, take a shower, go shopping, take a nap, or get out of the house. If you can do it all day, they can do it for an hour or two. This is the time to call in all your helping hands.

Decrease stimulation; do not make big plans, move slower, lower the lights, allow no loud noises or music, buffer your child from crowds of people, and give him or her time alone if he or she wants it. Speak in a calming voice, and try not to match his or her behavior with similar levels of intensity. If your level of agitation is stepped up, he or she will react and get worse. Control the environment.

Allow your child to rant and rave in a kid-proof area; let him or her punch pillows, scream, and run around. Let the child "zone out" on computer games or Nintendo. If he or she is up all night, let him or her watch a lengthy videotape while the adults take turns sleeping on the couch for an hour or two at a time. Offer food choices: If you put something out, he or she will eat it. Put out healthy snacks, but sometimes give in to cravings. Keep a well-stocked pantry and refrigerator, including some prepared or frozen meals, to make it simpler for you to pop something in the microwave at 2:00 a.m.

Ask for a psychological or psychiatric consult. When symptoms are severe, talk to your doctor about antianxiety medications, psychotropic medications, or sedation.

> Even 10 minutes in the garden taking some deep breaths of fresh air and looking at the sky can be so restorative. I found that really helped me break the stress build-up, and in the garden the screams and kicks would be at least muffled if not inaudible!—*Camille*

Using What You Already Know

Of all the strategies for alleviating distress, the best one is the most obvious one: Match the technique to the child. As a parent, you are the mediator between your child and the treatment team. Your role includes asking for the best available alternatives for your child's relief. The alternatives include distress-reducing techniques, medications, and the practicalities of advocating for experienced professionals who carry out the mechanics of procedures well and smoothly. The effectiveness of any strategy is measured by how well it eases your child's discomfort.

We have suggested a variety of strategies for coping with pain, distress, and side effects. Which combination of medical and psychological techniques works best will depend on your child's age, personality, and needs. The combination may vary from day to day or over time. We hope that we have given you some ideas to work with and add to your arsenal.

CHAPTER 10

Encouraging Child Development

I learn by going where I have to go.
—*Theodore Roethke,* The Waking (1953)

Hannah had a complete shutdown of physical development. She was very weak and had no muscle tone. After treatment ended, she wasn't catching up. She was 18 months old and didn't even crawl. For so long, she had been either on my hip or in the bed. As a result, her hip flexors were so tight, she was stuck in the sitting position. She used to scootch around on her bottom, pulling herself along with her hands to get where she wanted to go. We took her to a physical therapist. Hannah was anxious, and I had to stay with her the whole time. We had to bribe her with bites of Nutri-Grain bar to get her to do anything. She held things between her feet in order to play with them. Her physical therapist said she'd never seen any child who wasn't an amputee do that! It took more than seven months of physical therapy before she started to walk and even longer for her to catch up. Now she's almost 6 years old, and she's doing great.—*Irene*

One of the most important effects of childhood cancer is the disruption to normal child development and family function. Cancer affects a child in different ways than adults, because a child's mind and body have not yet reached maturity. The good news is the impact is neither inevitable nor permanent.

This chapter starts with cancer's potential impact on development, followed by a discussion of the factors that build your child's strengths and positive achievements, including specific ideas for attainable goals. The middle section focuses on specific age levels, with suggestions for each age group. The last part presents fun ideas for children that nurture development.

The two essential goals related to development are to lessen the impact as much as possible and to prevent dysfunction. By fostering a sense of safety, security, regularity, and predictability of life, natural growth and healthy development of the self can occur. We want our children to survive and to flourish.

Impact of Cancer on Development

The first step toward reaching those goals is recognizing the potential disruptions. Your child is an individual and will react and respond in an individual manner, depending on his or her age, developmental stage, coping skills, personality, and temperament. The following is a list of the inherent aspects of cancer that have the potential to disrupt your child's normal development. Not all of them will apply to every child. All of them can be assuaged. Many of the coping skills and suggestions in other chapters address these stresses.

Stresses that may affect development include

- Medical treatment—surgery, drugs, radiation, and transplants
- Changes to self- and body image, daily activities and routines, and long- and short-term goals
- Physical restrictions
- Painful or upsetting experiences
- Loss of control related to procedures, diet, feelings, and bodily function
- Separations from parents, siblings, and friends
- Decreased independence
- Isolation or lack of cognitive and motor stimulation
- Inconsistency or tension in the environment (in family, school, or the medical setting)
- Rejection or alienation from peers or authority figures
- Diminished opportunity to practice normal skills
- Poor understanding of medical information (involving distortions or fantasies)
- Treatment effects, either physical or cognitive
- Distressed parents, leading to overprotection, inconsistent discipline, or lowered expectations.

Unrealistic expectations will add stress to your child and to you as well. Anticipate some regression or delay in physical, cognitive, and emotional development. A toddler will likely lose recently learned toilet-training skills. A 10-year-old might wet the bed because of chemotherapy effects, altered sleep schedules, or emotional regression. A teenager may need reassurance about skills he or she once took for granted. Baby talk, whining, temper tantrums, and demanding attention can manifest at almost any age. Everybody wants a mommy when they're sick.

> Lili (age 9) regressed to a lot of childish things when she was on chemo: sucking her thumb and having bad dreams for a week before an appointment. All those behaviors went away when she felt better.—*Camille*

Fears long assumed to be conquered might reappear, such as the fear of being alone, of the dark, of being abandoned, or of strangers. Skills such as walking, talking, doing things for oneself, social skills, self-control, and academic skills may be interrupted, delayed, or hindered. A few parents reported changes in survivors' personalities; some became more outgoing, others became more skittish. Physical development, too, can be affected. Puberty can be accelerated or arrested. Adult teeth may take longer to come in. Growth may be slowed or halted. Older children and adolescents are often embarrassed or worried by these effects, particularly if younger siblings "pass them by." Even as they continue to develop physically, children may retreat backward emotionally and act younger than their age as a mechanism for coping and self-preservation.

> My husband and I were just talking about Jorge's lack of growth. Jorge keeps asking when he is going to get bigger. He has only grown a tiny bit, and I feel so sad for him. His little sister is passing him by, and he tells me it isn't fair. I am so blessed to have Jorge with us . . . size shouldn't matter, and it doesn't to me, but he has been through enough, darn it! —*Fernanda*

The causes of developmental effects are not always obvious. Some are directly related to treatment, some indirectly. Some effects are temporary. For example, Billy became a "couch potato" after treatment ended, lying around and watching television all day. Then, two new boys moved into the neighborhood and were the catalyst for him to resume bike riding and outdoor play. Some effects are longer lasting. For example, it is well known that intrathecal (administered into spinal fluid) chemotherapies and cranial radiation can cause learning disabilities. Other developmental effects may occur without such a clear origin. Parents want acknowledgment of the effects on their child, whatever the cause. Parents need an accurate understanding of a problem to cope and develop a game plan for addressing it.

Building on Strengths

There are certain major developmental tasks that cross cultural and community lines, which means they apply to children across the board. While cancer makes these tasks more difficult or may prolong or delay their accomplishment, helping your child achieve these basics can pre-empt long-term problems.

The primary tasks from infancy to preschool are becoming attached to the parent or caregiver, developing language, and learning self-control and compliance. The primary tasks for school-age children are adjusting to school and achieving academically (such as learning to read and do math), getting along with other children, and learning and following rules of social conduct. The primary tasks for an adolescent are academic achievement, involvement in extracurricular activities, forming close friendships (including those with the opposite sex), and forming a sense of identity. Your child may not have access to the usual avenues to accomplishing these goals, but there is more than one way to get there. And remember, good adaptation is a success—it does not have to be superb achievement.

There are also some characteristics that can make a child more resilient. A child with good intellectual functioning; who is sociable and easy-going; and who has high self-esteem, talents, or a strong faith has an advantage. A child has an advantage if he or she has a close relationship with a caring parent, support from extended family and friends, socioeconomic advantages, or parents who are warm but firm disciplinarians who continue to have expectations of and for the child. Cooperative and supportive schools, connections to outside support, and good relationships with adults outside the family are also advantages. Possession of even a few of these positives can put you ahead of the game.

Children can succeed in the face of adversity. Researchers Ann Masten and J. Douglas Coatsworth (see the Bibliography) report that

> successful children remind us that children grow up in multiple contexts—in families, schools, peer groups, baseball teams, religious organizations, and many other groups—and each context is a potential source of protective factors as well as risks. These children demonstrate that children are protected not only by the self-righting nature of development, but also by the actions of adults, by their own actions, by the nurturing of their assets, by opportunities to succeed, and by the experience of success. (p. 216)

* * *

> I met a man in his 30s who had retinoblastoma when he was 2 or 3. He had the right eye removed. He lost his peripheral vision, so he wasn't able to drive. Yet he was so optimistic. He played every sport that had a stick: hockey, baseball. He said, "I was batting lefty because that's the way I could see the ball; I compensated on my own without any kind of inter-

> vention. When you're a little kid and you can't see out of one eye, you just deal with it because you don't know any different." Meeting him made me feel more optimistic for my son's future.—*Sonia*

* * *

> We were starting to notice some learning problems. We'd give her instructions, and she would have a blank look on her face, as if our words made no sense. The hardest part was explaining to the school officials so that they'd understand Brianna needed help. She's a 7-year-old who has trouble counting objects beyond 5. She spells her name right most of the time, and she can write it. She reads pretty well, but I don't know about her comprehension. She is so good at memorization that I have to make sure her teachers ask her questions or test her skills under different circumstances and with the questions rephrased, otherwise they think she's mastered the skill when what she's done is memorize the "right" answer. She progressed a lot this past year. This time last year, we couldn't even hold a conversation with Brianna because her responses weren't appropriate for what you had said. Now we can't get her to be quiet. I love it!—*Perri*

Psychologist Anne Kazak (see the Bibliography) highlights the importance of focusing on the ways to help your child adjust rather than the more limiting considerations of disease and treatment. As a child and family proceed with life after treatment, the need to integrate the cancer experience and the developmental influences become more intertwined.

> She started kindergarten. I didn't expect her to make much progress, but I knew I couldn't provide the one element I felt she needed the most . . . socialization. Plus, by getting her in the system we could find out just how far behind she was. She started off loving school. Although she was shy, she enjoyed being in class. Then she got sick again, with an infection, and was rehospitalized. She was old enough to realize that something very scary was happening. After that she didn't want to leave the hospital and certainly didn't want to return to school. I made her go, and she was absolutely miserable for a while. If I hadn't felt it so important to teach my children to never give up no matter how scared you are, I would have just given in and said, "Fine, stay home." This past year has been wonderful though. Watching her in an environment that suits her, making friends, it's amazing and thrilling to listen to her giggle.—*Kathryn*

Children's brains are profoundly responsive to experience. Both the way the brain grows and how it works are affected by experience. This is known as *plasticity.* The brain is adaptable, stretchable; it may stop going in one direction and start going in another. It is comforting to know that plasticity works both ways. Interventions (steps taken to avoid or lessen or get around effects) depend on that plasticity. Just as your child's brain is affected by the experiences of cancer treatments, so, too, will his or her brain have the capacity to adapt favorably to most circumstances that occur after cancer.

Common Needs at All Age Levels

No one age is the worst or best. There are advantages and disadvantages to each. Most parents say that they feel "lucky" that their child went through treatment at his or her age, finding some positive aspect on which to focus. Remember that the following information is applicable to siblings, too. Also, unless you start out with an adolescent in treatment, you will be coping with the effects through each of the subsequent stages as a survivor.

Children of all ages have some common needs to allow or enhance social, emotional, and cognitive growth. Some attainable goals are to

- normalize the abnormal and balance your focus between cancer-related issues and other aspects of life
- combine pharmacological and behavioral techniques to reduce side effects (see chapter 9)
- be understanding and patient with regressive behavior
- give the child as much control as possible
- limit separations from family and friends, and encourage visits
- make no promises that you cannot keep
- give the child privacy (such as having exams in private room and limiting the number of observers)
- maintain discipline, house rules, and chores as much as possible
- stimulate language and symbolic communication
- encourage exploration of environment
- mentor in basic cognitive and social skills
- praise the child's abilities and successes
- rehearse, expand, and celebrate new skills
- protect from punishment or ridicule for developmental delays.

Maintaining discipline lets the child know that he or she is a normal, responsible, and capable individual whose life goes on. It also heads off sibling resentment.

> Find that really fine line between overcompensating and belittling what they're going through. We gave Sam the extra care and attention he needed but also let him know that he's going to be okay and we won't give in to every whim. He got away with a lot more than he would have. You know, it's really not that big a deal if the kids drop potato chips in the family room. But he was still responsible for doing the right thing. Just because you're sick doesn't mean you can be mean to people. Everybody else is struggling, too.—*Barbara*

Children with cancer disruptions or after-effects may need special help to make sure that all the attainable elements listed earlier are present. Special technology, tutoring, programs, and individual schooling attention may all be added successfully to a child's life. Such boosters minimize the deficits and allow children to be and feel successful.

Special Issues at Each Age Level

Infants

Cancer parents often talk about cancer in terms of "we:" "we have an appointment," "our oncologist," and so on. This is readily apparent when the sick child is an infant. A baby is rarely separated from the mother or caregiver for more than brief periods. Many mothers of infants talk about an event as though it were happening to themselves. The mother's talk of "we" reflects that early life level of attachment, before a baby has a sense of self apart from the mother. The bond between mother and baby is strengthened during this time, frequently to the detriment of the father and siblings, who are left out undeliberately.

Parents of new babies have not had much time to practice their roles as parents and may feel lost, guilty, or inadequate. They may not even fully realize their importance to their baby's care.

Parents of infants express relief that they do not have to explain cancer or treatment or death to their child. You hold them, rock them, and soothe them. Babies do not seem to mind being bald; they are not subject to peer approval. As they grow up, these children accept their illness and long-term effects as inherent, because they have never known anything different. Many families also take comfort in the idea that the treatment period will not be remembered consciously by a child who experiences it at such a young age.

> Mandy (9 months) didn't suck her thumb or hug a baby doll or a blanket when she was upset. The only thing that calmed her was breast-feeding. I nursed her through procedures. There was no room for shyness on my part. Sometimes, to save my back, I'd get up in the crib with her so I could lie down instead of sitting in those uncomfortable chairs. The look on the faces of the residents when they walked in the room was priceless! About a year after treatment ended, my husband was awarded a five-day Caribbean vacation by his employer. I weaned her then so I could go, too. It was the first time I'd been away from her for more than an hour. What's interesting is that since she didn't have nursing any more, Mandy needed a way to soothe herself. She started playing with her belly button. She still does it, as a way to relax.—*Elise*

On the other hand, infants do not go to cancer camps, get wishes granted, or have support groups. As a result, their siblings may also miss out on those opportunities. Infants cannot learn relaxation techniques or do imagery. They can not verbalize their wants, their fears, and their symptoms, so parents must figure those out. In addition, as these children grow up, once-avoided explanations have to be done after the fact. And while they may not be able to verbalize their memories, they do have impressionable minds, on which cancer leaves a mark.

Gentle Reminders for Helping Infants

- Parents are best able to interpret an infant's cues; look for distress.
- Soothe and minimize distress by cradling, holding, touch, rocking, swinging, humming, singing, or giving opportunities for sucking (this is not the time to take away a pacifier or wean from the bottle or breast-feeding).
- Babies take cues from mother about how to react; be calm.
- Prevent separation from parents; make sure the nonprimary caregiver also spends time with the baby.
- Ask for a primary nurse to keep caregiving consistent.
- Do not do all tests and procedures at once, even if you want to get them over with. Babies cannot regulate stimulation. Give the baby a chance to recover.
- Give the baby (from age 9 months and older) a comfort object such as a blanket, stuffed animal, or doll.
- Give the baby things to play with; provide positive stimulation with toys, board books, books or toys with varying textures, colorful mobiles, noisemakers, music, and soft lighting; try keeping a separate bag of toys for the hospital and rotate items so that the baby does not get bored.
- Hang pictures in crib or make mini-photo album of family members (including siblings, parents, grandparents, pets, and the home) and look through them often, identifying each photo.
- Do all the normal physical tasks and play you would have done anyway (such as peekaboo, "so big," clapping games, and walking in the stroller).
- Talk to the baby in both normal and baby-talk voices, and encourage babbling by repeating sounds that the baby makes.
- Encourage skills such as crawling, standing, and feeding self.

If for some reason you must have a significant period of separation from your child, be aware that your child may react with indifference and detachment when you return. In that case, do not be bowled over by your own feelings of rejection. Instead, allow the child to revive his or her attachment to you in a gradual way. Become a consistent, accepting, and loving presence again.

Toddlers and Preschoolers

As parents attest, this age group may prove a particularly trying time for the child and the parent to go through treatment. Toddlers continue to be very attached to and dependent on parents, especially the mother. At this age, children need a firm base of safety and security as they branch out into development of autonomy and self-control. Toddlers and preschoolers see the world as revolving around their needs and cannot see another's point of view. This is the "no" stage, the "mine" stage, the "I'll do it myself" stage that can be exasperating for parents. The explosion of language is the other key process in motion for this age group. It can be amazing to hear a 3-year-old use extensive medical terminology, although he or she may mangle the delivery. For example, leukemia becomes "bluekemia," petechiae becomes "tiki-tiki-eye."

Magical and immature thinking influences their interpretations and reactions. They might think that adults can read their minds, that bad thoughts can make bad things happen, and that two things that happen at or near the same time are connected (that one caused the other). These thoughts can trigger guilt, anxiety, or confusion.

> One night, Chloe said, "Remember last summer when I ran Troy over in Sally's driveway with my bike? I ran right over his head. If I didn't do that, he wouldn't have gotten a brain tumor." I told her it was an accident and did not cause his cancer. She said, "But whenever I ride my bike he runs away." I said, "Well he doesn't want to get hit by your bike again!" I called the counselor, and she said it's a normal reaction for her to feel responsible, and I did the right thing to correct her belief. I was relieved to hear it.—*Darlene*

Toddlers and preschoolers also see inanimate objects as being "alive"—machinery might swallow them up and syringes can poke all by themselves. Toddlers and preschoolers often think that a simple exam will hurt; that an arm or leg can "fall off"; or that losing blood, urine, or feces is losing a part of themselves. These thoughts magnify their fears, causing children at this age to be hyperreactive, even to a painless or non-cancer-related incident. On the other hand, sometimes the magical beliefs of children are a comfort to them and are a source of fun.

> I tried to keep things normal, even at the hospital. As soon as he woke up, we would start the day just as we would have at home. We got dressed. I'd open the shades. We'd have breakfast and then get out of the room as much as possible. Whatever programs were being

done in the playroom that day, we'd do. Most of the time, no matter how lousy he felt, he wanted to be on the go. I found that made the time go quicker, and my son didn't get as bored or cranky (and neither did I).—*Joan*

Gentle Reminders for Helping Toddlers and Preschoolers

- Give frequent reassurance.
- Keep consistent discipline and rules; limits will make them feel secure, protected, and loved.
- Maintain routines, schedules, and rituals (such as bedtime, baths, sleeping, and eating).
- Allow the child to make small choices to foster independence and self-assertion.
- Have patience with typical reactions, such as temper tantrums, dawdling, physical aggressiveness, hostility, and manipulative behavior; don't take these personally; view them as an emotional release.
- Interpret your child's communication, and explain his or her needs and routines to the staff.
- Encourage verbal and physical outlets for emotion, such as banging pots, yelling, screaming, crying, punching a pillow, talking, or using a noisemaker.
- Avoid physical restraint or restriction.
- Allow movement and independence as much as possible.
- Old familiar toys bring security: Now is not the time to give up the "Velveteen Rabbit."
- Give opportunities to accomplish new skills.
- Brief separations are better tolerated than longer ones; Give the child something of yours (such as keys, purse, or a jacket) as a symbol that you will return.

During this age period, a child widens his world of relationships to include people other than the mother, forming meaningful connections. Doing so is not easy if the mother is always the one with the child at the hospital or if low counts preclude visitors. Within those restrictions, give as many opportunities as you can for the child to foster ties with his or her father, siblings, and grandparents. Do not be surprised if your child develops a close connection to a special staff member. Several children we know developed comfortable relationships with the cleaning staff; they were friendly and upbeat and never performed anything painful!

School-Age Children

This is the age of growing mastery and accomplishment. New skills are added all the time. New experiences and knowledge are welcomed. Self-esteem tends to increase as children become increasingly independent. School relationships and peer approval become very important. Separation from peers or visible differences from peers may be problematic. Your child's friends and their reactions can have a big effect on your child's morale. Most children benefit greatly from maintaining friendships, although sometimes the emotions can be ambivalent.

> Once a week, his friends did a video for him of all the things happening in school. In the beginning, he really enjoyed it. But the more treatment went on, the less he wanted to watch. When his friends brought in a tape of the school play, he started watching with them, but then he said, "Turn this off, I don't want to watch." It became more a reminder of what he was missing.—*Hallie*

It is a good idea to prepare your child's friends (see the explanation guidelines in chapter 1, which are applicable to friends). Educate them about your child's illness; invite them to ask questions so that you can correct misconceptions; arrange for them to visit your child; and above all, let them know that your child is still the same person and wants to be treated as normally as possible. By "sticking around," the friends send a message to your child that he or she is still a normal and valuable person, not just a cancer kid to be pitied. With younger children, you may need to network with their parents as well to avoid misinformation.

Children in this age group come to understand that adults are not all-powerful or all-knowing and cannot always protect them from pain and illness. They begin to develop logical thought processes and can understand what is happening to them better than younger children. Yet they still take comfort from sleeping with a teddy bear. They have a beginning sense of morality and are quick to tell you something is not fair. The younger children in this group know the rules but do not always comprehend the reasons behind them. Older children take into account intent and context. Regarding their bodies, most school-age children take a strong interest in their condition but are embarrassed by body exposure and intrusion.

School-age children may seesaw back and forth between dependence and independence, which can be confusing to parents. It takes patience for parents to let go a little while simultaneously keeping their children safe and cared for. Parents may feel conflicted about allowing independent activity, particularly if they blame themselves for not noticing signs of illness sooner or think that only a bad parent would let a child on treatment visit with friends, spend a couple of hours alone at the hospital, or go alone to cancer camp.

There was a school bus evacuation drill scheduled. When the buses arrive at the school, the driver opens up the emergency door in the back, and the kids jump from the ledge to the ground. It's a long jump, and Charlotte is the smallest child in the school, due to treatment effects. She was so anxious about it, she cried and said she didn't want to go to school. She said, "I want to be late on purpose so we miss the bus and you have to drive me." I tried praising her previous success and told her she could do it. I told her she had "girl power." She wasn't convinced. So I told her the story of *The Little Engine That Could* with its theme of "I think I can." She spontaneously decided to "jump" off the chair she was sitting on. Together we ran around the house jumping off chair arms and boxes, and she really felt confident. She still looked a little nervous when the bus was leaving, but she did it! When she came home that day, she said it was no big deal. Whew!—*Marta*

Gentle Reminders for Helping School-Age Children

- Maintain connection with the family and siblings: Let the child know that he or she is still an integral part of the family.
- Arrange for visits, letters, calls, and messages from friends whenever possible.
- Ask his or her teacher or class to send cards and letters.
- Foster relationships with other children at hospital by attending formal and informal support groups and playing in the playroom.
- Be flexible with homework: Some children will be comforted by the fact that they can still do homework. or take pride in not only keeping up, but making the honor roll; others need freedom from the stress of schoolwork. Children who can't do homework can learn new things on their own, with you, or with the hospital tutor (even if it's just reading about goldfish, polar bears, or fire trucks).
- Make a smooth transition back to school (see chapter 2).
- Appreciate the child's need for independence; he or she may want parents to leave the room during procedures.
- Encourage personal responsibility and empowerment.
- Insist on social conduct rules.
- Let the child participate in planning and care.
- Allow for explorations of faith, both positive and negative.
- Offer books, story-telling, word games, competitive games, collecting things, and daydreaming.

Lili was diagnosed at 9 years old, and we saw lots of kids of all ages undergoing their treatment. She decided that she was really happy that she wasn't any younger because, even though it was hard knowing the seriousness of it all, she was able to understand the reasons

> for all the unpleasant and painful things being done to her and to cooperate. Whenever we heard a little one crying, she would say she was happy she was older and I could explain to her what was happening.—*Camille*

While school-age children do understand more than younger children, they still can misinterpret information. They often act like they understand, even when they do not, because they are embarrassed or mistakenly believe they know it already. You might check on your child's understanding by asking him or her to explain it to someone else or to draw a picture. Use human figure outlines and informational videos, and ask medical staff to help in teaching your child medical information.

Teenagers

The issues for teenagers are remarkably similar to those of toddlers: They are preoccupied with their bodies, they want independence, they do not want to do anything their parents tell them to, they think the world revolves around them and their concerns, and they often appear to be fighting for autonomy and self-control. It is a process of separation and individuation at a more mature level. As with toddlers, teenagers may be in a particularly trying period in which to undergo treatment.

Teenagers get conflicting messages from the adults around them. They are often expected to act like adults—to endure painful procedures stoically or to understand complicated medical information. Yet they are sometimes treated as much younger—being talked down to or passed over as staff speaks to parents directly. Intellectually, they can understand what is going on and be scared by the implications. But they do not have the emotional maturity to cope with their situations like adults.

Normally, during this period, teenagers become increasingly self-sufficient. They practice adult roles involving work and romance. Cancer treatment goes against the developmental grain. As they stand on the edge of adulthood, they are thrown back into the need for help, with a lack of privacy, control, power, and choices. Like all adolescents, they vacillate between the "perks" of childhood and those of adulthood, alternately pushing you away or hanging on. The trick is to recognize what your child needs or wants in a given situation and let him or her guide the choice.

> When Ebony (age 14) was first diagnosed, she lay in her hospital bed surrounded by our family. She kept crying and repeating she didn't want to lose her hair. She didn't want to look sick. We tried to comfort her by offers of buying a wig, by saying that it was the least of the problem and only temporary. But for Ebony, only how she would look at school mattered at the moment. She was inconsolable that night.—*Vanessa*

Forming an identity is a major goal of adolescence. A teenager's sense of self encompasses both present and future: Who am I? What group do I fit into? What am I going to do or be? Adolescents care very much how the world perceives them and work very hard to project an image that represents their own sense of self. Acceptance from their chosen peer group is of paramount importance. Cancer throws a giant wrench into the job of identity formation.

> There are lines that need to be respected everywhere. With any teen, you struggle to let them know you love them and yet let them have their own space. Throw in a cancer diagnosis, and those lines become very blurred. Just as he should have been pulling away, he was thrown back toward us. As he was making another break, going off to college, he relapsed and needed to stay close to us again. Yet, when I look at him I see a young man who is independent, yet considerate of his family. Maybe he's just missed the "bad" parts of adolescent rebellion. Who's to say?—*Lucille*

The role of cancer patient or cancer survivor is not easy to incorporate. Physical effects leave teenagers feeling insecure and unattractive at precisely the time they wish to attract someone and in a society that idolizes health and beauty. Missing school, sports, clubs, or social activities robs teenagers of important opportunities to explore and expand themselves and their world. Teenagers have long-term concerns, too, involving possible changes in college or career plans, dating, marriage, and the ability to have children. With an adolescent's healthy fantasy life, the roles of hero and martyr can hold some appeal. Some teenagers also enjoy the role of expert (about their condition) or mentor (to other kids with cancer). Mostly, they want to be seen and treated as the same person they were before the diagnosis. They do not want pity from parents, staff, teachers, or peers. If they perceive pity, they may withdraw from those relationships.

Some teenagers see only the losses incurred, at least temporarily, and are ashamed and resentful. They may refuse to be seen by friends during treatment, be angry at their limitations, or refuse to work toward future plans for fear of relapse. Others take the changes in stride and become proud of, or at least comfortable with, how to handle their cancer experience. Having cancer usually is not the sum total of their identity but is an important part of what makes them who they are.

One of the more disturbing possibilities of cancer treatment during the adolescent period is risk-taking. Adolescents are already testing their limits, but risks taken during cancer treatment are much more dangerous. As a way to deny the cancer and assert their "normal" selves, they may participate in activities that put their health in danger, such as drinking or contact sports. A more subtle rebellion might take the form of uncooperativeness, "forgetting" to take medications, or being late for appointments. In panic or in a mistaken assertion of control, they may try to quit treatment, run away, or even make a suicide gesture. Teenagers often see things as black or white. They may falsely believe there is no point in trying because they are going to die or be disabled anyway. This not a typical or frequent reaction. Most teenagers are quite health-conscious and careful. If you observe risk-taking behavior, get professional help immediately.

Many teenagers and their families report positive changes in outlook. Teenagers describe themselves as more considerate of other people, closer to family, having a better perspective on life's problems, and being more aware of the good things in life.

> When I found out in 8th grade I was to lose my leg, I was devastated. Field hockey was a huge part of my life. I knew the amputation was a necessity and life would go on, but having been the leading scorer and captain of my middle school team, it was difficult for me to accept. The first season of high school, I tried to stay connected as the manager of the team. I found it frustrating and was not ready to be there as a spectator. I often spent time in my best friend's yard, hitting the hockey ball back and forth. With the support of my friend and my old coach, I decided to go out for the team. I knew I could stand for long periods of time without my crutches. I also was able to hop for steady periods (this being the way I get around at home). I remember the first practice. It was not like it used to be. Playing on one leg was harder than I ever imagined. I was no longer the fastest player or the leading scorer. I was not the team leader, and I did not want it that way. Remembering how it was to play with two legs intimidated me. I wanted to quit. I lay awake thinking that night, and I finally realized that I am not the same person. I will never be able to play at the ability as I did before. But I need to stand up and play the best of my ability now. I told the coach I wanted another chance. I practiced day in and day out until our first game day. It was an amazing feeling just to be in uniform with all my friends: a member of the team. I was afraid my emotions would run me away, but I didn't allow them to. One leg or two, I was a hockey player. The outpouring of fans was unbelievable. Teachers, students, friends, family, media . . . it was amazing. I played sweeper (the defensive player right before the goalie). It did not require tons of running, but I did have to be able to get around and help my goalie defensively. It felt awesome the first time I hit the ball. I was playing hockey again! I like to look back and see how much of a hurdle I had to get over in order to pursue what I wanted. It made me realize I did not have a disability, I still had the ABILITY. It was a battle well worth winning. I was honored that year by the regional Field Hockey Association with a prestigious award at a banquet in front of my peers. From the people I played with, and the people I played against, I received much respect. It was amazing to see how much I helped others by what I did for myself.—*Monica*

Parents of teenagers report several common themes. Peer support groups are generally more available for this age group. However, some parents lamented that their older teenager was the only adolescent on a pediatric ward full of young children, leaving little or no chance for peer support and isolating both the teenager and his parents.

Gentle Reminders for Helping Teenagers

- Keep consistent limits and expectations; treat them as "normal."
- Invite participation in planning treatment and choosing options; avoid overprotecting them.
- Encourage continued participation in academics and activities.
- Encourage goal-setting—something to look forward to, to live for, to fight for, or to work toward.
- Help maintain connections with friends with visits, calls, and cards.
- Foster new connections at the hospital: bond with other patients, do unit activities (such as programs, newspaper, radio, closed circuit TV, and art or music therapy), join support groups, and participate in Internet programs (see Resources)
- Practice tact and timing; the way you impart medical information, suggest interventions, or communicate expectations is as important as the information itself. Avoid authoritative or condescending tones.
- Acknowledge what your teenager cares about, even when it seems trivial to you.
- Recognize typical reactions, such as emotional retreat, acting out aggressively, uncontrolled temper, frustration, attention-seeking, regression, or panic.
- Promote temporary escapes (such as daydreaming, watching movies, doing hobbies, visiting with friends, having time alone, and listening to music and other meaningful stimulation.
- Encourage emotional outlets (such as the punching bag, distractions, writing in a diary, or sharing feelings with an adult, who does not have to be the parent).
- Permit the teenager to vent without passing judgment or trying to "take charge" or "fix" it.
- Introduce the topics of fertility testing and sperm banking.
- Do not rebuff the teenager's expressions of thoughts and fears of dying; Reassure him or her with medical facts and examples of other patients doing well (a grandparent or famous person); explore religious beliefs; and even allow for the making of a will, which can help an adolescent regain a sense of control and peace.

My son's 15, and all the other kids on the unit are little. The programs are geared for them. He doesn't want a prize from the treasure chest. A guy with a guitar, or the Easter bunny comes around singing songs. His nurses get a kick out of that. I don't mingle much with the moms, partly because I'm a dad, and partly because their kids are little. I just try to keep my son company. Once we were watching an action movie. The nurse walked in on a racy scene, and she started kidding that we were watching an X-rated movie. Now it's a running joke.—*Maurice*

Many teenagers can handle a good part of their own care, slightly easing the parents' burden. While most teenagers' parents insist on staying with their children, they do feel more able to leave them alone in the hospital for short periods (so that they can eat, shower, run errands, or go home) than they would with a younger child. At an age when most children want nothing to do with their parents, parents and teenagers with cancer sometimes find an unusual opportunity to grow closer. On the down side, parents feel that they have less control, worrying that a son or daughter will not take all his or her medication or that a survivor will not maintain follow-up care while off at college or on his or her own. Disagreements or arguments that preceded the diagnosis can make parents feel guilty or add to their worry.

Complicated issues may arise during adolescence for a child who went through treatment at a younger age. Old emotional issues, long-term effects, and disabilities that have been coped with all along suddenly take on new dimensions for the emerging adult. Long-term implications become clearer. With continuing support, the adolescent can incorporate his or her experience into his developing persona.

Follow-up Care for All Ages

After treatment ends, there are additional steps to take to encourage your child's healthy development.

- Maintain an image of the future; make plans and reach for the stars.
- Monitor growth and development.
- Get baseline assessments of physical and cognitive abilities.
- Educate yourself about possible late effects, and know when they might occur. Share this information with whoever needs to know it (such as the pediatrician or family practitioner, the child, family members, and teachers).
- Insist on periodic exams for whichever systems were affected by your child's treatment—vision and hearing, neuropsychological, cardiac, liver, kidney, or cognitive—to assess function and the need for interventions.
- Rehabilitate or remediate to gain needed skills.
- Use every available resource, such as tutoring, special education, and physical accommodations in school.
- Monitor psychosocial as well as physical functioning.

Fun Ideas to Nurture Your Child's Development

Any skill can be learned through some sort of game. In fact, that is probably the origin of games—for children to learn and adults to practice life skills in an appealing way. Some activities may have to be put off until your child is feeling up to them, but even a bed-ridden child can benefit from stimulation. Taking into account your child's developmental age and needs, choose from or adapt any of the following to help your child along his or her developmental way. You will need all your creativity, and that takes a lot of energy, especially when you may not have much in reserve. Ask for assistance from a physical therapist, an occupational therapist, a child life specialist, or a teacher (special education experience helps) for help in assessing your child's abilities and needs or for additional ideas. Enlist family members and friends to play.

- Have the child make a door sign for the hospital room to identify him or her, request privacy, or write messages.
- Have autograph or guest books that everyone who comes into the room has to sign with a message. The child can choose a daily theme, such as a joke, favorite food, or pet story.
- Let the child earn certificates or small prizes for successes.
- Help the child learn new academic, physical, or recreational skills.
- Invite the child to keep a journal in a blank or spiral notebook, calendar, or a tape recorder if child has trouble writing.
- Encourage the child to write a declaration of independence, bill of rights or "we the people" letter to the doctor or anyone else about their feelings and needs; correspond with a pen pal (such as a friend of the family, classmate, or another patient or through pen-pal organizations).
- Participate in group activities with other patients on the ward, such as a "progressive" drawing or story that travels from room to room or is kept in a hallway for the children to write or draw on board game or card tournaments; a tea party in the playroom; parties for made-up holidays; or musical instrument "band" or "parade."
- Play "No Peeking"/"What's in the Bag"—fill a pillowcase with various small items, the child closes his or her eyes, picks an item, and tries to guess what it is.
- Have a beanbag toss (into an emesis basin, baby basketball hoop, or cardboard target) or ring toss, play wastepaper basketball or velcro darts, go fishing (use a

dowel or pencil with string and magnet on one end as a rod, with colorful paper fish with metal paper clip on end).

- Use old-fashioned toys to help with hand-eye coordination, such as a paddleball, ball and cup, jacks, and magic tricks.
- Make a homemade "obstacle course" for the child to traverse.
- Have the child create a "fort" or secret place; put a blanket over a card table or over the backs of a few chairs or even in bed.
- Do art projects, such as painting (with sponges, stamps, pasta, watercolors, or oils); making collages with any small nature, craft, or household items; making wire or thumbprint art; making jewelry; macramé and other craft kits; playing with Etch-a-Sketch or Spirograph; or drawing and cartooning.
- Take an imaginary trip: Use magazine pictures, food, and music from a place the child wants to go, remembers, or imagines. Glue a picture of the child into the collage to help him or her visualize the place and what he or she can do there.
- Give the child a noisemaker, toy microphone (one that amplifies the child's voice), karaoke machine, or a water pistol to use as a means to "be heard."
- Use a washable play, exercise, or nap mat to provide space for the child to play, exercise, or nap.
- To foster big muscle skills, use light fabric scarves, hula hoops, water toys, ribbon dancers (10–15 foot ribbons attached to a stick), big giant balls (to roll on, kick, or punch), and "reachers" (long, narrow devices whose "mouth" opens and closes to pick something up when you squeeze the handle, often in shape of a shark or other animal; keep putting the object reached for farther away, so child has to stretch).
- To increase tactile stimulation, play with clay, sand, a "noodle" box (fill a box or plastic bowl with uncooked pasta of various shapes), water (in cups, utensils, containers with holes so water pours out, and dolls), "oobleck" (which is corn starch, food coloring, and water), and other soft substances (such as whipped cream, shaving cream, "Gak," Jello, cornmeal, or flour). Use messy cooking (such as mixing ingredients by hand or kneading bread) or nature items (such as snow, leaves, or rocks).
- Play with sewing cards, puzzles, shape sorters, stacking blocks, peg boards, Lite-Brite, pick-up sticks, tangrams, geoboards, dominoes, and cat's cradle.
- Do crossword puzzles, Mad Libs, word games, guessing games, matching games, and memory games (such as concentration). Make up stories, invent mythical animals, play with magnetic poetry (use a cookie sheet for the board), solve a Rubik's Cube, or do spatial puzzle games.
- Play games like Simon Says, Follow the Leader, Hear and Do game (give a

sequence of directions to follow), Mastermind, chess, and flashlight games (make shapes on the wall or ceiling, use colored saran wrap over the head of a flashlight to make different colors, or make hand shadows).

- Use small candies, beads, cookies, tiddly-winks, counters, coins, and little rubber or plastic critters to make math problems visible or tangible.
- Grow plants or keep goldfish.
- Alter surroundings and sensory input by changing lighting, playing different types of music, rearranging the furniture, putting posters on the ceiling, and decorating the room to be visually stimulating (try teacher or party supply stores for decorations).

After treatment is over, your child may need extra boosting, particularly if there are cognitive effects that slow down the learning process. Howard Gardner (see the Bibliography) described multiple intelligences: linguistic (verbal), logical (mathematical), spatial (visual orientation), musical, kinesthetic (body movement), interpersonal, intrapersonal, and naturalist. Each child has a style combination that suits him or her best and may need more than one way to grasp a new concept. Discuss your child's needs with his or her teacher, and ask your school principal for a child study team to outline an individualized education plan for your child (see chapter 2). Use computer learning programs, repetition, and one-on-one tutoring. Give the child extra time to do homework or to finish classwork at home, and ask for separate, untimed testing at school. Praise any success, and make sure your child knows the cause of the problem: He or she is not stupid, it is not his or her fault, but he or she does have to get around the challenge. Give your child plenty of opportunities to do the things that he or she is good at so that he or she feels successful.

Your child's development may not progress as you had expected before the cancer. There are likely to be some setbacks. But children are not limited by the norms. Instead, they find their own pathways to development—over, under, around, and through obstacles. As one child said, when asked how far he expected to get with behavior that was exasperating his father, "all the way."

For a more comprehensive discussion, see the work of psychology professor Laura E. Berk (see the Bibliography). She does an excellent job of surveying the research and presenting child development in a readable style. Her textbook is now in its fifth edition and is available in many libraries.

CHAPTER 11

Building Self-Esteem in Your Child

If a child is to keep alive his inborn sense of wonder, he needs the companionship of at least one adult who can share it, rediscovering with him the joy, excitement, and mystery of the world we live in.
—*Rachel Carson,* The Sense of Wonder (1965)

Life introduces plenty of opportunities for successes and failures. The question is what we make of them—and what we teach our children to make of them. Self-esteem gives us a vital sense of who we are and what we think of ourselves. It is our set of beliefs, judgments, attitudes, and feelings about our worth. Childhood cancer introduces special challenges to families who want to foster self-esteem.

In this chapter, we offer positive steps that you can take to help your child grow to the fullest possible potential. To do that, we fill in the background on how self-esteem forms and what goes into building a healthy sense of self. We alert you to some of the ways cancer treatments can have a negative impact on that. Finally, we end with 10 strategies to foster your child's self-esteem.

High self-esteem is a wonderful inoculation against the stresses of living with cancer and its aftermath. It gives children and parents alike a core of self-acceptance, self-respect, and realistic attitudes about individual characteristics and abilities. It is powerful medicine indeed, because it is one of the most important factors affecting behavior and mental health. If you understand how self-esteem is created and what the ingredients are, you will be better able to select ways to help yourself and your child.

How Self-Esteem Forms

Self-esteem does not exist apart from the social fabric of our lives. Parents are the mirrors that show a baby who he or she is. By responsiveness, acceptance, and admiration, parents hold up an image for the baby to see. The baby gets messages about himself or herself and information about differences from parents and other close caretakers. Just think for a moment of the pleasure sparked when a baby takes her first step or utters his first word. The baby revels in the family's delight.

With developing language, a 2-year-old is able to make categories. He knows about differences (baby, man, big, small) and about judgments (good dog, bad dog). By age 3, the child makes clear self-evaluations. She beams with pride at riding a tricycle successfully or looks stricken when embarrassed by spilling juice. Children learn about failure and frustration, too. Think of the many practice attempts a child makes before learning to tie a shoelace and the encouragement they need to keep trying.

By about age 7, the child has developed self-esteem in three distinct areas: academic, physical, and social. The sense of self in all of these areas gets honed and shaped as the child grows older and progresses through the school years. Gradually, a child learns to combine the many self-evaluations into a whole picture. Acceptance by others plays a big role in the self-view she forms. As an adolescent moves toward adulthood, he makes active choices about whom to turn to for acceptance and validation. Teenagers want to be "cool" in the eyes of friends, as any parent who has wrestled with requests for the newest expensive sports shoes, pierced body parts, or tattoos knows. Nevertheless, they continue to be influenced by what their parents think and value, even when they don't say so directly.

Ingredients of Self-Esteem

You will recall that many of the stories throughout this book illustrate children building worth about how they look, how they succeed, how they relate to family and friends, and how they come to terms with being "good enough." These are the key issues to consider in self-esteem.

Physical Appearance

Looks matter to children. They want to fit in and be accepted by others. Across all ages of children, physical appearance is more closely tied to self-worth than any other individual factor. It influences how others see a child and how a child comes to see him- or herself. Unfortunately, the current popular culture of the United States is obsessed with appearance fads and unrealistic ideals. This phenomenon only makes it harder for anyone who does not fit the cultural standard for reed-thin beauty or who does not have the right sneakers. Guidance and reassurance by family and friends can help children accept their physical reality and make the most of their appearance. A child's looks may change a lot as a result of cancer treatments. When children are able to make friends in the treatment center and through support groups, they realize that there are many other children out there who are like them. They pick up tips from peers about how to handle the reactions to their appearance in the wider world.

> I find that people aren't rude, but they look. Troy always looks like he's tired. He has days, geez, does he have blood in him? His eyes are droopy. He's got a big scar down the back of his head. That's pretty obvious. Some people will say, "Is he okay, what happened?" I find that little kids are very accepting. No big deal. The older kids, around 10, 11, they stand and stare. I say, "What's the matter." The kid will say, "What's wrong with him?" I blurt it out. "If you want to ask a question, you're going to hear the answer. If you don't want to hear the answer, go away."—*Darlene*

* * *

> There was one boy at our hospital, he had the right attitude. Every time he was in-patient, he'd wear this white t-shirt that said, "Cancer sucks." I think his family made it with iron-on letters. Plus, he'd get somebody to draw things on the back of his head, like extra eyes. He was a riot. He always made the other kids laugh.—*Susan*

Mastery

Success matters to children. Learning new skills is often hard work, and children make judgments about their reasons for success and failure. Some children are mastery oriented: They believe they have the ability to be successful, and they use that stance as their guiding compass in facing problems. When they fail, they maintain a good sense of self by deciding the task is hard or they need to try harder. They persist. They have a step-by-step view of their ability. Other children, however, believe that success only happens by luck but that failure is a reflection of their ability. They feel bad about themselves and tend to give up. They have an all-or-nothing view of their ability.

Parents and teachers can help a child by supporting a mastery-oriented approach to learning and problem solving. You can teach your child to persist (because many tasks are difficult at first and trying can lead to increased successes) and to view success as a product of both ability and persistent effort. This kind of approach is especially helpful for children with late effects and disabilities, because they are climbing a steeper hill than they were before the cancer. It takes a lot of patience to learn a hard skill, but when they do they feel great. That success gives them confidence to climb over the next challenge.

Social Acceptance

Being liked matters to children. It starts at home in your circle of family relationships. Later, as soon as they are old enough, children move beyond home into a school setting. They begin to find their place in that world. Acceptance by other children has a major impact on adjustment and self-esteem. Likable children are generally sociable and cooperative, although they may range from the outgoing class leader to the somewhat shy and self-contained student. Rejected children lack social skills in general and are either overly aggressive or overly awkward and anxious. Parents and teachers can help children with social skills, such as reaching out and going with the flow of a group of peers, or with self-regulation skills, such as impulse control or managing feelings.

> My son was sort of a-social before treatment, and he still is. He's never liked to talk about how he feels. He'll discuss philosophy, religion, science, anything but how his cancer effects his life. He just trudges along and takes his meds and relies on science to cure him. I have sometimes thought that he was holding back starting new relationships until he is done with treatment. What a burden it could be: "Want to date me? Oh, by the way, I'm undergoing cancer chemotherapy. I can't drink or party, and I might die." Maybe he has fewer relationships, but those relationships are true and good ones.—*Anita*

* * *

> Chris' friends were so phenomenal. They were so happy when he was in school; they would carry his books. His best friend had a hard time. Chris was elsewhere, but he was still in the same situation. He pulled away some. His mom was concerned. He would come see Chris, they spent a lot of time on phone. A lot of the girls were great, they'd send him cards, call him, send pictures. That he enjoyed, being in middle school. There were three or four friends he wanted to be with, mostly. It really became a closed group. They'd sit, and Chris would say, "Excuse me I have to throw up." They'd say, "Do it quick, we're in the middle of Nintendo. Are you done yet?" It used to crack us up because they couldn't care less. Same thing with losing hair. There was a group of friends who wanted to shave their heads, whose parents said, "I don't think so."—*Simone*

Belief in "Good Enough"

Feeling good about themselves matters to children. How can we teach our children to accept their limitations and still feel good about themselves? The answer lies in accepting reality and working with compromise. No one is gifted in all areas of life. We cannot excel simultaneously at nuclear physics, quilting, writing the great American novel, public speaking, parenting, and have everyone we meet like us. Compromise is necessary. We have to learn to ground our self-esteem in the sense of "good enough."

D. W. Winnicott, the famous British psychoanalyst and pediatrician (see the Bibliography), coined the phrase "good-enough mothering." He recognized that no mother could respond to her infant perfectly, but that if she were reliable and responsive, the infant's physical and emotional needs would be met. As a result, development could proceed naturally and well. Different authors have since applied the concept to relationships beyond the mother–child bond, such as good-enough marriages. We believe it is useful to link it further, to childhood cancer families trying to foster self-esteem in their children. Your family cannot be perfect either, only good enough.

> She struggles with math and spatial concepts. She hates it. So, she'll never be a mathematician or make a million on Wall Street. And she might need help balancing her checkbook (so do I, and I didn't have cancer!). But you know, she's really good at lots of other things, like telling stories and riding horses.—*Trudy*

Competence and Resilience

Self-esteem is strongly related to competence and resilience. A competent child feels safe, functions well, and has many skills. A resilient child recovers from setbacks and less-than-optimal circumstances. Competence and resilience help children to feel good about themselves. Researchers Ann Masten and J. Douglas Coatsworth (see the Bibliography) have identified three powerful resource areas that play a central role for all children. These three areas nurture and protect children in both favorable and unfavorable situations. Because cancer can certainly be considered an unfavorable situation, you may find their results helpful. The three areas are

- quality in the parent–child relationship—the presence of adults who care for the child
- cognitive development—normal brain function
- self-regulation—the ability to manage his or her own attention, emotions, and behavior.

Children are at risk when any of three domains is threatened. During or after cancer treatment, your child may be especially vulnerable to separations from you, cognitive problems, or self-management difficulties. If a lack cannot be prevented, it is important to take remedial steps to bolster your child and restore his or her access to supportive help in any of the three areas. You may want to refer to chapter 2 for suggestions on working with the team, chapter 10 on child development, or the Resources for related information.

Blows to Self-Esteem

The assaults of cancer and its treatments can have a negative impact on a child's sense of self. Many effects are temporary, but some are long lasting. These include

- hospitalization—separation, isolation, and being in alien culture
- the body—temporary changes include hair loss, a steroid moon face, and weight gain or loss; permanent visible losses include amputation, scarring, mutilation, and stunted growth; and invisible losses include infertility and organ removal
- cognitive—learning problems and developmental delays
- social—dating, sports, peer rejection, and adults writing them off or not encouraging future plans.

Virtually every child will encounter one or more of these impacts. Beleaguered by repeated tests, procedures, and interventions during treatment and in follow-up, some children come to feel that there is something essentially wrong with them or that they can never "win." Fortunately, some effects are relieved with the ending of the treatment that caused them. A middle schooler, sensitive to how his peers perceived him, delighted in his new-found image after finishing steroid treatment. His mother described watching him emerge like a strong and beautiful butterfly from the cocoon of weight in which steroids had encased him.

Hair loss is a significant event in the lives of many children undergoing chemotherapy, especially to older children and teenagers. How people react can make a difference. Some family members or friends make a gesture of solidarity by shaving their heads also.

> My 10-year-old son went to a fair with his friends. He had his baseball hat on. I told him there was a chance the hat could fly off on the rides, but he said he was okay with that. Inevitably, that happened. He was embarrassed. Then one girl said, "What's wrong with you, Josh? Do you think we care that you're bald? You're the same person inside as you were before you got sick. Forget it." That broke the ice. The kids responded better than adults. The kids were fabulous. That made it easier.—*Karen*

* * *

> Seth (age 14) was trying hats on in a store. A woman came in and said something nasty about skinheads. A smile came over his face. He turned to her and said, "I'm not a skinhead; I have cancer. I'm losing my hair, and I thought this hat would be warm and look good.

> What do you think?" I thought this woman was going to die. The young kid at the checkout counter burst out laughing because he thought Seth was making it up. The woman apologized and walked out rattled. The kid asked Seth if he really had cancer. Seth said, "Absolutely. I'm on chemo." The kid said, "You can have the hat, just take it." At that moment, I realized that having cancer was part of Seth's identity now. That was the moment it clicked for me that my son accepted the fact that he had cancer.—*Mim*

Long-term or permanent effects can be harder to cope with. After treatment, a cancer survivor expressed her belief that she was not a whole woman because her cancer treatment left her unable to have babies. Therapy and a fulfilling career in the health field eventually helped her to regain her self-worth. Another young child had to shift her perspective and potential when treatment-related cognitive deficits forced her out of her school's gifted and talented program. She didn't feel special in a "good" way anymore and had to find another outlet where she could shine. Author and Ewing's sarcoma survivor Lucy Grealy's memoir "Autobiography of a Face" (see the Resources) focuses on her struggle to come to terms with the pain and fear that comes with looking different and feeling ugly.

Media images portray children with cancer as either heroes or as objects of pity. Although children are capable of heroic acts, the role of hero is an impossible one to live up to—it implies more power over the disease than they truly have. Parents and children often feel ambivalent about the victim role. No one likes to be pitied, but they do want the special treatment, compassion, and acknowledgment of the illness. Sometimes children find that they can manipulate others and use the disease to their advantage.

> I guess she'd heard me talk about it a lot lately, because I was setting up her IEP [individualized education plan] at school, and I had to explain everything. So she must have thought it was an excuse she could use. We were sitting at the dinner table one night, and the girls were quibbling over something. Jasmine said, "You have to be nice to me, 'cause I'm tired, and I had cancer." I looked at her sister, and we burst out laughing. I said, "That has nothing to do with this!"—*Winnie*

* * *

> J. C. can also play around with my emotions, knowing that he can get me going. It's not to say that he isn't feeling badly, but sometimes I think he plays it up a little. He doesn't want this dinner, or he can't do his homework, or his head doesn't feel right, he can't do chores. My daughter Kimmy (age 3) has watched this and learned that it's effective. Every now and then she'll say, "I can't do it, I don't feel good."—*Toni*

Children need realistic images for developing self-concepts, not extreme ones. The child with cancer must somehow incorporate the illness into his identity and self-image. The illness becomes a part of him or her—"my cancer." In a sense, the child may take possession of it—it doesn't belong to a parent or sibling. Teenagers and older children, especially, may prefer to answer questions from medical staff, family, or strangers themselves, resenting what they see as the parents "taking it over." Temporary and long-term changes in the body and abilities must be adjusted to. Children don't want to be defined entirely by their cancer experience, but to deny it is to deny a part of yourself, part of what makes you "you." With positive self-esteem, the child can "own" the cancer without the cancer owning him or her.

Tips for Enhancing Self-Esteem

Parents often are creative about finding ways to enhance their child's self-esteem. One family gave a 4-year-old a bald doll when she was bald. The mother of an amputee made bright decorative crutch covers for her son out of plastic shower curtain rod covers. Pretty earrings, bright colors, temporary tattoos, and t-shirts with slogans they might not normally be allowed to wear can make a child feel good about him- or herself. Hospital staffs frequently give nicknames to children, which they delight in, such as the "Wizard of Woz" or "Miracle on 34th Street." Please remember that the following strategies are also effective for your other children.

Gentle Reminders for Fostering Self-Esteem in Your Child

1. Listen and accept your child's feelings, point of view, differences, and uniqueness. When you offer this kind of loving respect, your child receives the message that he or she is worthy.
2. Praise your child's efforts, approximations, and progress rather than the outcome of attempts. For example, "You did a great job of holding still while getting that shot," praises the child for cooperating with a procedure, even if he or she cried and fussed. In the future, the child can build on that attempt and make further progress.
3. Give realistic feedback to your child, framed positively. You want to avoid negative, demeaning, critical feedback at one extreme (because it teaches shame, not self-respect) or exaggerated, gushy feedback at the other extreme (because the child will not believe you and will discount it as not meaningful).
4. Identify your child's strengths and abilities. This is part of recognizing the child's "specialness." Your child becomes confident of these strengths over time, and it

Box continues next page

Continued

gives him or her a strong foundation on which to build other life skills. It does not matter if the strength is a big talent or a small one. Your child might have a musical ear, a smooth swimming stroke, an aptitude for math, or an easy sociability. Your child might have a talent that might seem more eccentric. You and your child can capitalize on any strength.

5. Teach and encourage your child to build skills in many areas of life. Help him or her to forge new pathways for improvement if some traditional ways are blocked or limited by cancer consequences. This is an area with unlimited possibilities for any parent who is willing to not only be a child advocate but also a creative and problem-solving teacher, too. Most parents already have the common sense and tools to garner old and new ideas, try them, modify them, and build on every new gain that happens. Experts can help, but practical solutions can come from any quarter, including other children, so it helps to stay open to new information. Areas for your child to master include handling emotions; getting along comfortably with family, school peers, and authority figures; developing physical prowess and stamina according to potential; finding successful ways to learn language and academic school skills; and increasing problem-solving options.
6. Set reasonable standards and limits. Your child needs to know what you expect of him or her. The pitfalls are if you set standards too high for the child to meet, you convey that you don't really believe they will be met (a failure); if you set too few standards, you convey that you don't expect your child to have anything to contribute (a failure). But with loving clarity and a modicum of consistent discipline, your child will learn predictable consequences and acceptance by others. The important life lessons apply to cancer children as well as other children—do your best; be reliable and trustworthy; do your fair share; cooperate with others; do not be violent; and do not lie, cheat, or steal.
7. Offer your child choices, within appropriate limits. This gives your child the opportunity to gain comfort in making decisions. It fosters growth in autonomy and the chance to learn from mistakes. In one family, a 4-year-old girl insisted on wearing a ballerina tutu costume every day, even in the winter. Within the limits of laundry timeouts to clean it and wearing long pants and a long-sleeved shirt under the costume outside, she was allowed to choose the tutu for as long as she loved it. She felt spectacularly beautiful in her tutu. Now that she has become an adult, she is none the worse for wear and has a comfortable sense of her own autonomy.

Box continues next page

Continued

8. Create a family atmosphere in which your child can contribute. The ability to help others and to have something of value to offer others are part of a good self-concept. These give your child a sense of purpose and connection, while taking him or her beyond the role of a receiver to that of a donor. As long as the gifts are within their capacities, children are pleased to feel appreciated for doing a small favor (such as getting a diaper for mother when her hands are full with a wiggling baby); contributing to a family discussion (such as offering a schedule-juggling idea for the following day); or making a donation of time, a toy, or a portion of allowance to a good cause. It is especially important for children who have faced losses resulting in not being able to do things they once did to contribute on new levels or in new ways.
9. Look to your own behavior as a model for your child. You are teaching constantly by example. How do you react to frustration, when caught in traffic or the lawn mower breaks? How do you tackle learning new skills, such as figuring out that new computer program? How do you face disappointment and rejection, when you do not get the choir solo part for the holiday service or you lose a school board election? How do you respond to the visible tension between your father and mother, your child's grandparents? How do you handle your anxieties about your child's illness? How do you speak about your child when he or she is not present? What are your sources of support and acceptance? All of these reflections of your own self-esteem are conveyed to your child. Fortunately, children can learn that one doesn't have to do everything well, all the time, to be a worthy and lovable person.
10. Be realistic, truthful, kind, and undaunted by your child's limitations. Your child will absorb that attitude, and it will buffer him or her. It will help set a positive tone to go forward.

CHAPTER 12

Dying and Grieving

Give sorrow words; the grief that does not speak
Whispers the o'er-fraught heart and bids it break.
—*William Shakespeare,* Macbeth

The specter of death is every cancer parent's worst nightmare. Children are symbols of hope, of the future, and of our legacy and immortality. It feels unnatural to outlive our children. Coming to terms with our limits as parents, we realize that we cannot protect our children from everything.

For any parent facing the death of a child, we recommend strongly that you take advantage of specialized resources. Your hospital should offer one-on-one bereavement counseling or group support with other families. Many private therapists specialize in bereavement counseling. Get in-person support. In addition, local and national support organizations offer good and sustaining services. Many of them, along with numerous books for both adults and children, are listed in the Resources at the end of this book.

This chapter is meant as a primer of the grieving process. We explore the hallmarks of this phase: the time leading up to the death, including ending treatment, how to talk to children about death, and suggestions for ways to help your dying child; the period immediately after the death, including funerals; the process of working through grief, including symptoms of grief, acknowledging and accepting the loss, and adjusting to life without the child; how children grieve and how to help them; and re-investing in life. You will have your own ways of accomplishing these tasks. These are a good start, but you will need many resources during the most life-altering event you will ever face.

Leading Up to Death

> When you are sorrowful look again in your heart, and you shall see that in truth you are weeping for that which has been your delight.
> Kahlil Gibran, *The Prophet* (1923)

When it becomes clear that treatments are unsuccessful, you must come to terms with your child's impending death. You may feel resentful that the child had to suffer through treatment, only to have it fail. Some parents frantically search for alternative treatments or religious healings. Some direct anger at the "failure" of medical staff or themselves for being unable to save the child.

When the loss is inevitable, the family members begin to grieve in advance. This is anticipatory grief. In this phase, you are alternating between focusing on your child and focusing on your own anticipated loss and between raw pain and numbness. You may find yourself avoiding touching or talking to the child, either because the child is unresponsive or is physically unable to do much. Feeling guilty about leaving the child's bedside, parents often keep vigil. However, if the dying period is drawn out, you need to be able to take turns with another person to relieve you and have some time away to regroup. A certain amount of distancing is normal, as long as you continue to nurture and reassure your child.

The child, too, will turn inward. He or she is grieving the loss of himself or herself, the family, the things he or she will never get to do or see, and all the things that are important to him or her. Your child may not want to talk or may withdraw from your touch. This is painful if you feel rejected or not ready to let go yet. Know that he or she is pulling into himself or herself and not away from you. This is necessary for the child; don't let your own needs supersede those of your child. Give the child permission to wind down life at his or her own pace, according to bodily needs.

A dying child is a jumble of fear, anger, sadness, and anxiety about what is happening to his or her body and what will happen to him or her after death; worry about what will happen to the family afterward; and an awareness of having to face mortality alone. Your child may alternate between fantasies of a miracle cure and knowledge that there is no hope. It is vitally important to parents and child alike that the child will not be alone—make sure your child knows that you will not abandon him or her. Encourage your child to express feelings, both positive and negative. Allow for disagreements, without criticism or judgment. It is okay to express anger, disappointment, and to heal old wounds—unfinished business can make everyone uncomfortable and prey on survivors' minds a long time. However, it is better to do it with a hospice professional, clergy member, or therapist's guidance, so it's effective rather than hurtful.

Parents worry about the quantity and quality of the time they have left with their child and keeping the child pain free. Marital strain, differences in coping styles, spiritual distress, financial concerns, and siblings' issues may become heightened as the child's care becomes an unremitting focus.

> When the doctor got it through to us that he was going to die, I got stronger and Doug fell apart. Everything caught up with him. I'd been dealing with it all along, where he had been so sure Chris would not die.—*Simone*

Unfamiliar with the process of dying, parents do not know what to expect, physically, emotionally, or practically. They are distressed by the changes in their child and in their child's care.

> There are many ways that the child's body will change. For example, loss of appetite, changes in breathing patterns, decreased urination, increased heart rate, swelling, bleeding, etc. There will also be emotional changes. Many kids single out one person they want with them at all times, exhibit anger or depression, sleep during the day and stay up all night, want to sleep in a room other than their own. I tell parents that most parents are worried about going insane at the time of their child's death but the hardest time is usually before that. Many parents are actually relieved at the time of death.—*Cathy Chavez, pediatric oncology nurse*

* * *

> Upon her relapse, I was dismayed at the lack of continuity with her care. It seemed as if there wasn't one person who knew her well enough. I would verbalize how I thought she was deteriorating, and I was told that I was overreacting. I was furious at the lack of concern over her not eating. In retrospect, I suspect that everyone at the hospital knew it was highly unlikely she would recover. I wish they had told me.—*Rhonda*

* * *

> The intensive care unit was different from what we were used to. We no longer had control over taking care of our son. We weren't allowed to stay in the room all the time. I regret not knowing enough about the respirators. We weren't thinking that once he went on, he might not come off. For 10 days I didn't hold him, because if you knock the respirator out of whack, he can't breathe. Right before they put him on the respirator, the nurse said, "Come on give him a kiss, we're going to put him on." I had no idea that would be the last time I could hold him. I'm sure they didn't want to say that. But I might have savored that hug.—*Suzanne*

Emotional support and freedom from pain are of utmost importance to easing the dying process. Many families choose to have their child die at home. Home or hospice care is a valuable resource that offers medical, practical, and emotional support. Families and professionals report that parents and siblings cope better during and after the death when the child is allowed to die at home. Family members are less anxious, less depressed, have fewer irrational fears, and experience less marital strain. While some parents are initially nervous about being able to care for the child, dying at home is quieter, less hectic, less frightening, more familiar, more comfortable, and more peaceful. If you do not feel comfortable with this option, do not feel pressure to do so. It may not be suitable for your family's circumstances.

Gentle Reminders for Easing the Time Leading to Death

- Advocate for relief from pain and discomfort.
- Continue coping techniques such as imagery and relaxation.
- Know what will happen to the child.
- Know what your role can be.
- Make your and your child's wishes known to staff.
- Seek out a counselor.
- Encourage family involvement, especially the child's siblings.
- Plan and make funeral arrangements.
- Decide on a DNR (do not resuscitate) order; talk to the doctor about whether this is appropriate for your child.
- Decide whether to allow or ask for an autopsy.
- Find out whether hospital can accommodate your cultural or religious rituals, such as washing the body, anointing, and saying prayers. If not, consider a home care or hospice program.

Ending Treatment

As the treatment becomes an issue of comfort rather than cure, the goal is to keep the child free of pain. Emotions surrounding this decision can be ambivalent. To a parent, it feels like giving up, which is not easy when you have fought so long and hard. You may be torn about what will happen to your child. The feeling of responsibility for "allowing" the death of your child is overwhelming. At the same time, you may be relieved, in that the turmoil will end, the fighting is over, and the toxic treatments and their side effects will ease. Stopping treatment is an intensely private decision that must be made with input from your family members and medical team.

The decision is especially troubling when one person does not agree with how to proceed. One family had told their son that he would be part of that decision, but when the time came, they had the difficult task of explaining that the treatments were no longer working and therefore had to be stopped, because the son did not want to give up. In some cases, the family and the doctor are of differing opinions—one is ready to give up and the other isn't. Sometimes a doctor feels that stopping would be a failure on his or her part or wants to try yet another experimental drug, and the parents feel that the child has suffered enough and it isn't working anyway. Conversely, a doctor's experience and emotional detachment may give him or her the perspective to realize that treatment is not working sooner than emotionally involved family members are willing to admit. Discussion and examination of motives is crucial to resolving those differences.

> Early in my daughter's treatment, I overheard a mother who was opting to stop experimental treatment, rather than destroy what little time her daughter had left. I was horrified. I could not imagine giving up. I felt I would continue to grasp at every straw on the way down, but reminded myself I was in no position to judge the actions of another further along. Years later, I still remember that girl and her mother. When we ran out of options for treating my child, after years of difficult treatment and numerous close brushes with death, I was able to understand that she did the right thing. You reach a point where the best thing you can do for your child is to simply keep her comfortable and not grasp at any more straws.—*Naomi*

Helping the Dying Child

Dying children need help in special ways, too. Although you feel powerless to save your child, there are in fact many things you can do to ease your child's physical and emotional pain.

- Stick to routines the child feels comfortable with; advocate for consistent caregivers.
- Allow the child to hold onto goals, dreams (such as learning to read, finishing school or a project, or applying to college); goals get smaller and shorter term as death approaches.
- Allow independence (in personal care, being alone, or making decisions) while accepting growing dependence and regression.
- Encourage the child's end-of-life directives: creating a way to be remembered, leaving something behind (such as writings, artwork, belongings, or a legacy), or creating a will.
- Encourage contact with friends and extended family as long as is meaningful for the child.
- Provide diversions when the child is up to them, such as reading, playing card

games, listening to music, telling stories, and going for a walk (even if in a wagon, stroller, or wheelchair).

- Give as much privacy as possible, as the child's bodily changes can cause embarrassment.
- Take care of the child's physical comfort with back and footrubs, massages, feeding, rinsing the mouth, putting ointment on dry lips, dimming too-bright lights, and adding or removing blankets.
- Observe your child's needs and inform staff of them, such as an air mattress, clean sheets, more pain medication, suctioning, oxygen, and other physical comfort measures.
- Buffer your child from extraneous visitors or unnecessary intrusions.
- Seek help of a counselor to cope with behavioral and emotional extremes.

Talking to a Child About Death

Deciding when, what, and how to tell the child is hard for parents. Burdened with their own grief, many parents cannot bring themselves to broach the subject for fear they will break down and upset the child. Some believe that they can hide this information from their child. In all likelihood, the child already knows—from watching and listening to adults, observing other patients, and experiencing what is happening to his or her own body. Even if you think your child knows, remember that he or she needs time to assimilate the reality. Talking about it and expressing fears and questions make the child feel less anxious and alone and help the child come to his or her own terms with death. Admit that you do not know all the answers to all your child's questions, and do not be surprised if your child's beliefs about death and afterlife do not exactly match your own. Aside from a simple, honest explanation, what children need most is reassurance that they are loved and will not be left alone.

> The psychologist talked to him first, but I needed to be there in the corner of the room. He told Daniel things were not going well, there was a possibility he could die. Daniel looked at me, looked at the doctor, and said, "Can you tell me again?" He did. Daniel got a little teary and said, "I think I already knew. I don't think I want to live if I have to deal with this much longer." They talked a long time. Then we sat and looked at each other. I said, "Are you okay with this?" He said, "Yeah, but I don't want to talk about it anymore." I said, "Okay, but can we just do things the way we would normally do them? Is there anything you want me to do for you?" He said, "No, just be Mom." I said, "I can do that."
> —*Sarah*

* * *

> Your role as a parent is to protect your child. When you're told that your child's life is out of your hands, you have to relinquish that innate parental role. You need to be able to hold your child and say goodbye. I kind of explained things on my own. Giving permission to go, I told her, "Everything will be okay, Mommy will be okay." Her last words to me were, "I love you Mommy, Mommy, I love you." I will always cherish that. Of course, the moment she died I yelled, "I lied! It's not okay, I'm not going to be okay, come back!" My husband thought I really lost it. And I did.—*Lucia*

To help your child understand, talk about death—use the word. The use of different words and terms to evade it (such as "lost," "gone away," "sleeping," "on a trip," "taken by God," or "passed") are society's polite, emotion-avoiding terms, but they mislead children, who are very literal. Most experts advise describing death as a universal part of the cycle of nature, the circle of life. Further suggestions for talking about death to the child's grieving sibling follow later in the chapter.

Immediately After Death

In the moments immediately after a child's death, parents may experience shock, disbelief, denial, relief, confusion, dissociation, disorganization, and letdown. Leaving the hospital afterward is described by parents as a surreal experience: You are leaving without the child. You pack up and take home the child's belongings. There is no pressing reason to return. Your job has abruptly ended. "Now what?"

> When it happened, we looked at each other and said, "Oh my God, that's it." It's so final, that last breath. Another thing you're unprepared for is you're abruptly cut off. You leave the hospital, you have no more support, you can't lean on the doctors anymore.—*Patrice*

* * *

> You can't turn your relationship off. I wasn't ready to leave him. My daughter and I spent an hour with him. I needed to help wash him and take the IVs out. I almost see it in slow motion. We had music playing. I had brought in my own blankets, and the whole room was decorated. We packed up all the stuff, but I couldn't leave him with that bare white bed. So, I laid his Yankee jersey over him. I felt so much better.—*Simone*

It is helpful for each family member to have a memento of the child to keep. The "last" things—the last book he read, the last doll she held, the last clothes he wore, or the last pictures taken, take on special significance.

We each chose something we wanted to keep for him to sleep with towards the end. My husband thought it was morbid. He couldn't do it. But my daughter and I needed to have a connection to keep when he was gone. Kayla chose his Tickle Me Elmo doll. And I wanted his Peace Beanie Baby bear. That was one of the last things Travis touched. I find it helpful to have that piece of Travis with us.—*Hallie*

* * *

In the last four days before he died, I stayed in the same clothes. When I came home that night, I slept in them. The next morning, we had to deal with the funeral. My girlfriend said, "You need to shower, get out of these clothes." I said, "I'm not. I'm going to the funeral like this." She and my husband said, "No, you need to take the clothes off." It was the most painful thing, having to take off my last connection to him. Doug said, "I'll help you, we'll do this together." He undressed me and put me in the shower. I still have these clothes folded next to my bed in the drawer. Having them helps me.—*Simone*

Most hospitals will allow you to remain with the child for a time. Some hospitals will allow you to help wash and prepare the body or accompany the body to the morgue, if you so wish. You might ask permission for clergy or family to be there. There may be religious or personal rituals you wish to have performed. Performing these tasks and rituals has been a response to death since the dawn of civilization. They confirm for you that the life is gone. You demonstrate your love and care by performing the last, most intimate tasks you can for your child. You need to do what feels comfortable and right to you. If you respectfully and firmly inform the staff, you will most likely be accommodated.

Another little girl died right before Felicia, and I learned so much from what I overheard and saw and questions I asked. I heard a mother say to the grandmother, "It's not Kelly, Kelly's gone. It's only her body." And that statement stayed with me, and helped me to do things with Felicia I might not have been able to do otherwise. I asked the nurse a lot of questions, what's going to happen to this child, and what are my rights? She said, "You don't want to know this stuff." And I said, "You're wrong, I do. I do need to know it."—*Lucia*

* * *

When my baby died, the hospital took a picture. They asked me if I wanted a copy, but I thought that was really morbid. The nurse explained to me that they always take an extra, in case the parents change their minds. Sure enough, about two weeks later, I changed my mind. The hospital sent me the picture, and I put it away in a safe place where I always know it's there.—*Helene*

* * *

I'm glad we had an autopsy afterward. It helped a lot. I wasn't too keen on it at first. But I had to get something out of it: they might learn from him in order to help other kids. I

> had to realize it wasn't him, he was up in heaven. When you read that autopsy report, it's not nice. I started reading it, but when I saw the measurements of the brain, I put it away, I couldn't read that. About a year later, I got it out. Then it was more curiosity. I wanted to know.—*Suzanne*

It may come as some comfort to you to know that staff also grieves. Some of them have developed a warm and true bond with your child. However, in some instances a doctor may be concerned that you blame him or her for the inability to save your child. Some doctors feel a sense of failure. If a staff member is acting "weird" or standoffish, that person probably is upset and either does not want to show it to you or is "putting a lid on it" to protect himself or herself. Some parents report with surprise and bittersweet pleasure that their doctors or nurses cried with them, came to the funeral, or reached out in some other way. Almost always, parents are deeply gratified when staff members, by showing grief, demonstrate their caring and emotional investment in the child. This personalizes the often impersonal image of the medical profession. Some hospitals have formal memorial services that include parents.

> We have a quarterly memorial service to remember those children who have died. It gives an opportunity for both families and staff to grieve and acknowledge the loss. We show slides with the children's pictures (provided by the families) and play music. It is touching but sad to "see" the kids again. Sometimes it takes your breath away when you see what they used to look like before they got sick. We enjoy seeing the parents and families again, especially if we weren't there the day that the child actually died. Staff want to know "what happens" to the parents and families after the child dies. Sometimes our connection has been so long and so intense that we, too, feel a little lost when the connection is suddenly gone. Also, the Memorial Service is a way to ensure that all children get remembered and their lives acknowledged.—*Mary Choroszy, pediatric oncology nurse practitioner*

Funerals

A funeral service pays tribute to the deceased child, but it also serves an important purpose for the people left behind. A funeral is a formal good-bye, a ceremony to mark the cycle of life. It is an opportunity for those gathered to reflect on the meaning and significance of the child's life and to show support for the family. The service often combines tradition with the unique wishes of the family and the child and confirms the family's cultural or religious beliefs.

Make the funeral a celebration of your child's life. Little things can make it more personal, such as placing meaningful things in the casket, writing elegies or obituaries, or incorporating themes that were important to the child (favorite color or flowers, for example).

> I was very adamant that there would be children at his funeral. This would be a celebration of Drew's life. We played music. The eulogy was upbeat, about his strengths. I spoke, I knew there were things Drew wanted to say. If I didn't say them right then and there, no one would ever hear it. I wanted people to walk away saying this is an incredible child, and we have to do something to keep him alive.—*Maren*
>
> * * *
>
> In a Jewish burial tradition, everyone helps shovel a little bit of dirt. Everybody did so, then began walking away. Phil said, "I can't walk away with him unfinished." I said, "I'll help you." Then a friend picked up a shovel, then another. My daughter, Leah, and her friends helped. This was the last act we could do for him. It was incredible. Phil was making the grave look perfectly formed, to the point where he was smiling. In a way, I felt like I was tucking him in. Leah said, "We need to do something." So we put our handprints in the dirt. I walked away not feeling so empty. Look how many people love you honey. And everything's going to be okay now. That helped so much.—*Sarah*

Parents struggle with the question of allowing their surviving children to attend a funeral service. Like adults, children can benefit from attending a funeral, having a chance to see, in a concrete sense, that the sibling has died, and having a chance to say a last goodbye. Children who are not allowed to participate may have trouble believing the child is gone, which disrupts their grief process. There is a common thought that children will be upset by seeing the body, but it doesn't have to be that way. They need to know that the sibling may look different; have makeup on; and cannot hear, see, feel, breathe, eat, or move anymore. The key to a nontraumatic experience is information and explanation before and afterward. Explain what will happen in small practical detail: who will be there, what will happen in the service, what behavior is expected of the child, what the room looks like, whether the casket will be open or closed, what the deceased will be wearing, and so on. Funerals may be strange and unfamiliar to children, but if conducted sensitively, they can be understood as the natural and special ceremonies they are for a family and a community.

That said, you should never force a child to participate in any part they are afraid of. If, after reassurance and detailed explanation, the child is still afraid, don't push it. Be guided by your child's readiness.

Suggestions for Family and Friends

Here are some ideas for family and friends who wish to help. We suggest you make photocopies and distribute them to people in your circle.

- Help make funeral arrangements.
- Put up out-of-town relatives; transport them to the funeral or airport.

- Stay at the house during the funeral.
- Help make or get food, extra chairs, and paper goods for the reception at the house.
- Put together a photo album or collage of the child.
- Write down memories of the child in a letter.
- Collect memorial donations.
- Run errands or do chores.
- Talk to the bereaved family members (all of them), and call or write often. Avoid platitudes: You do not have to make it go away, make them feel better, be original, or tell them about your losses; just let them talk, cry, or go over and over what happened.
- Do not tell the family how or when to grieve or make judgments on their actions or reactions.
- Give them a hug and hold hands.
- Remember birthdays, anniversaries, and holidays.
- Take them for a walk, out to dinner, out for coffee, or to a movie or museum.
- Expect mood swings, physical reactions, and faith questioning.
- Do a memorial: plant a tree, hang a plaque, dedicate a garden, name a child, donate something, or create a scholarship in the child's name.
- Do not clean out the child's room or personal effects; do not put away photos in the child's home or those you have on your own wall or mantel.

Working Through Grief

Working through grief is a process neither finite nor linear but personal and individual. The common physical and emotional reactions to the grief process are described in the box on the next page.

> There's no safety zone. Nobody can fix this. In some ways this is liberating. Fear, a constant in the life of a mom with a child with cancer, is gone. Your fears have been realized, and now all that remains is numbness. You don't realize at the time how divine the shock stage is until the numbness begins to fade and the real pain emerges. There are times when the only time you can stop crying is to wretch. After a while you begin to let glimmers of happiness seep in . . . and it ain't easy. Pleasure can be a guilty task that requires fortitude.
> —*Rhonda*

Common Grief Responses

- Shock: feel numb, unreal, hysterical
- Anger at God, doctors, self, the deceased
- Guilt, self-doubt, blaming self or others
- Sadness
- Relief
- Fear, panic, anxiety, "going crazy"
- Physical symptoms: exhaustion, lower/higher sex drive, can't sleep/sleep too much, weight loss/gain, heart palpitations, feeling heavy, lump in throat, nausea, headache, diarrhea, sweating hands, backache, dry mouth, can't breathe, altered taste, weakness, shaking, sighing
- Regret: if-only, "shoulda-woulda-coulda"
- Thinking that you hear or see child, searching for child, dreaming about child, feeling presence
- Feeling restless, can't sit still or focus on tasks
- Throwing self into work or other endeavors
- Overprotection of other children
- Yearning for child, loneliness
- Feel like piece of you is missing, "empty arms"
- Bitter resentment
- Feeling vulnerable, powerless, hopeless
- Moody, irritable, extra sensitive
- Lack of concentration, can't make decisions
- Constantly thinking about or reviewing the circumstances of treatment or death
- Questioning faith, becoming more religious
- Searching for causes, how and why it occurred, how it will affect survivors
- Refusing help, driving away family and friends
- Picking up child's hobby or cause, acting like the child did
- If the relationship was troubled: only remembering the negative
- Cutting self off from emotions
- Loss of self-esteem, becoming passive
- Depression, lack of concern for self

Your emotions are a raw bundle. Panic attacks and phobias are not uncommon. Guilt and despair are powerful. There may be a feeling that you should have done something more to save your child or that you should not outlive your child. Decisions you made, how you acted in a bad situation, harsh words that were spoken, and "what ifs" can run around and around in your brain, and you keep thinking of alternate outcomes if you'd only done something differently. There is tremendous upset over any negative feelings toward your child. But people are not perfect, and neither are children. Acknowledging your negative feelings does not mean you don't love your child. It is more unreal to idealize the child.

Detaching yourself temporarily from others is a form of self-protection. You need all of your energies for your grief at first. You may have a sense that you do not have the will or strength to support others now. You may need to withdraw from painful encounters or reminders.

It is a basic part of the grief process to express your emotions. Feelings come out directly and indirectly, in symbols and plainness. Just as a torrent of water rushing down a hill may find more than one path, your torrent of grief will find many paths of expression, too. You may overreact to minor crises or experience physical symptoms (such as asthma episodes, aches and pains, vomiting, or diarrhea). You may create private rituals, such as making a shrine, smelling your child's clothes, sleeping with your child's teddy bear or blanket, or continually going through photo albums or watching home movies.

Families typically feel that the child's life was unfulfilled, that so much potential was wasted. In thinking and talking about events, the time the family spent together, the child's personality or accomplishments, the parent's role in the child's life and struggle, or the family's changes in priorities and outlook, parents can take comfort in the knowledge that the child's life has meaning.

> My daughter's life, her great joys, laughter, pain, and courage, taught us how we would continue to live without her in our life. She showed us how important it was to be in service, to smile when a butterfly lands upon your nose, to cry when it hurts, to ask for help when you need it.—*Mauritzia*

One mother was disheartened when she was told she would never get over the death of her child. She could not imagine living with such intense pain for the rest of her life. She needed hope, she needed to know that her life could go on. She sought out another perspective.

> I went to see my neighbor, whose son had died in an auto accident three years earlier. I completely fell apart in her arms. She let me cry. I said, "Tell me one thing. Do you enjoy life now?" She said, "Yes. It's not easy. You have to fight for your recovery as hard as you fight for your child's life." Not just personal recovery, but recovery of family, as well. That's a challenge. We took advantage of professionals—we needed them, we used them, all along the way. It made a huge difference.—*Marjorie*

Everyday life intervenes and forces you to carry on. However, even the smallest chore or most ingrained habit can bring you up short with a reminder of your loss.

> The funeral is the tip of the iceberg as far as bad days go. To me the bad day is the first time you do the laundry. You have one less pile of laundry, and you're hysterical crying. Or the first time you go to the supermarket. I'd put all his favorite things in the cart. To this day I buy four potatoes . . . , it's automatic. Or I'll say something to my daughter, and she'll say, "wrong kid." You do that when your kids are all alive, call the wrong name, or something. That part of you doesn't change. I don't think I want it to change.—*Eve*

Some parents feel resentful of people whose children survived or of those who have never experienced suffering. Others opt to maintain relationships with other cancer parents, who are linked to their experience, validate it, know and fully understand what happened to the child, and allow the bereaved parent to talk freely about their memories and feelings.

I think it is only natural to feel resentment toward parents whose children survived, though no one likes to admit to it. I try to cope with the feeling by not denying it; to let it wash over me and then set it aside. I guess that's a grief coping strategy: don't deny it, but don't wallow in it, just acknowledge it and move on. Another thing that helps me to accept the resentment is the realization that you never know what lies in store for another person. I always remind myself that some of the parents at the hospital, of whom I used to be very jealous for one reason or another, subsequently experienced a terrible tragedy. I learned not to be envious of people who appear better off than I am today, because no one knows what lies in store for them tomorrow. I think about that when I am jealous of anybody over anything.—*Rona*

* * *

I think of the people I met in the hospital as my friends. I have a bond with them because of the time we spent together that transcends whether your child lived or died. I can't get that from anyone else.—*Trudy*

One common thread that parents often experience is what author and parent Ann Finkbeiner calls "phantom child phenomenon" (see the Bibliography). That is, a parent thinks about how old the child would have been, what he or she would have been doing at this point in time had he or she lived. These thoughts are frequently prompted by anniversaries, birthdays, or community or worship milestones; by seeing the child's friends progress along their paths of life; or just by coming across a person born the same year.

People say, "Oh, you're so strong." I'm just trying to survive each day. People don't realize how hard it is. We were at a birthday party for one of my son's friends. I noticed all the kids were taller, their voices were changing, they're bigger, more mature. That is painful because my kid will always be a child. Twenty years from now I'll meet his friends and they'll be adults and I'll still have a 12-year-old. Seeing everybody else grow up is hard. I think that's pretty common.—*Hallie*

* * *

I've had trouble with the millennium. She should have been part of the celebration, of the turning of the century. It's so final. She was born in the 90s, and they're gone. The child I'm pregnant with now will be born in the year 2000. I'll have to say, your sister was born in 1988. That will seem so old. So removed.—*Estella*

Family members often maintain strong connections to the child after death. You may have dreams or experiences of "seeing" your child. They tend to be comforting, as though the child comes to say, "I'm okay."

> Peter wanted to be an astronaut. He used to get his brother Matthias out on the roof and talk to him about the stars. One night, a couple of weeks after Peter died, Matthias said, "I looked out in the stars, and I saw a P written in the stars. The stars in the P glowed very bright, like lights that were turned on and then got dimmer. I know my brother is in the stars, now. That is where heaven is. He's an astronaut." And from that moment on, everything was okay. He came to that closure. I've connected with Peter myself in dreams. It's a dream, but you know it's something different. Just a knowledge and awareness of presence that is comforting and yet an ache.—*Marjorie*

Misconceptions About the Time Frame for Grief

One of the more difficult aspects of the grieving process is that other people have opinions about how, when, and how long you should mourn. Generally, people are uncomfortable with grief. As a result, they tend to avoid it or make attempts to console you that only end up upsetting you. This may lead you to feel you must hide your feelings or reactions. At the other extreme are people who treat a bereaved parent like an emotional invalid, walking tentatively, as if on eggshells. Parents do not like to be reminded of the child's death or their loss, but they do like to be reminded of the child. We have found that parents truly appreciate opportunities to reminisce and need outlets to do so.

> I'm still me. You can talk to me. My best friend from high school called me. We'd always kept in touch, but she lived far away and had never even met Robbie. After he died, there was such a connection. It was not what she said, but that she talked to me like I was still me. I felt she really cared.—*Kelly*

* * *

> Too often, people wouldn't let me talk about him. I really cherish those people who let me remember him.—*Marjorie*

Grief is not resolved in a one-year mourning period. It is not unusual for parents to report strong grief feelings up to even seven years after the death. That does not mean that the wrenching emotions you feel when it first happens will be there that long. As time goes on, your perspective changes. The waves of pain become less frequent, less intense.

> You want to crawl into bed and say forget it, I can't survive this. This is way more than one person should have to endure. But you do it. I'm not sure when or how, but it happens. Moment to moment.—*Ellen*

* * *

> It's getting different. For years, I would cry, or I would pray. I got mentally exhausted, trying to figure it out. I gave up. I guess that's what you call accepting it. No matter how hard I cry, or pray, he's not coming back. Maybe around three years, that was when I had time to think.—*Alma*

* * *

> What I've learned is that death is not the end of life, it is a radical transformation of life. Your relationship with your loved one doesn't change the fundamental way that is most important. You still love each other, still care about each other, that connection never dies. —*Val*

How Men and Women Grieve Differently

When a child dies, the disparities between two parents' coping styles may become more apparent and cause a rift. Mothers and fathers express their feelings in different ways (see chapter 4). One father said there were times when he'd been having a good day and wasn't thinking about it, only to come home and find his wife in tears and wanting to talk. People in mourning may also cover one feeling with another. If tears are not "manly," then irritability can be a ready substitute. If anger is not "feminine," then turning it inward and becoming depressed can become an alternative. Gender role expectations are strong in many communities. Family members sometimes get upset with a parent who does not grieve in ways they expect, pushing for conformity.

According to psychologist Therese Rando (see the Bibliography),

> since each parent has a separate and individual relationship with the child, different things will constitute losses to each parent. Bereaved parents must recognize this and not expect their mate to be grieving the exact same losses as they are.

Parents may have little emotional energy to comfort each other, or they remind each other of the grief, which offers no respite from it. Anger, blame, and unrealistic expectations (such as your partner will grieve the same way, make the pain go away, or answer all the whys) drive a wedge between spouses. Involvement in your own grief makes you less empathic toward your spouse or your other children. Patience and acceptance of differences can go a long way toward easing this painful period. The effect on a marriage is profound. If the couple has a good history of communication and support, the relationship can be strengthened. See chapter 5 for suggestions on handling emotions and communicating well.

> When you are grieving, you become very selfish. You can't understand why another can't understand your point of view. I'll be making dinner, I'll think of some story about Brad and start talking. And my daughter will talk with me. And I see Jeff fading into his chair.

Karen and I feel uncomfortable because we can see he's uncomfortable. Karen has learned to talk about Brad with mom, not dad. We try to understand differing coping styles, but it looks like they're not caring about your feelings at all.—*Holly*

* * *

After Evan's death I sought the help of a support group, but my husband declined to go. I continued for about six months and stopped when I was confident I could say Evan's name without crying. I never denied or chose not to mention him. My husband Gabe was visibly upset, but he soon went back to work and had a lot of co-worker support, so for months things seemed fine. Then all of a sudden about six months after Evan's death he came home from work and broke down. It was as if we had buried Evan that morning. Here I was, "accepting" Evan's death, and Gabe was just acknowledging it. In the support groups I had attended a couple of the husbands said they had a delayed reaction. I had no idea what they meant until then.—*Roz*

* * *

I want to stay home, my husband wants to go away. He has a hard time coming home. There are too many painful memories. My husband and older son want things to remain the same. They don't like the furniture moved, because that is not how it was when Brian was alive.—*Bev*

* * *

My wife put it to me in an interesting way. She said you lost a son, and I lost a son. But I also lost a career. She felt I had a career outside the home, doing fulfilling things. Her career was taking care of the children. When Peter got sick, that was the priority of that career. She felt a sense of failure and loss that she didn't complete the project she had, as well as the fact that she lost a son.—*Carl*

* * *

He said that it was just as hard to watch me, this woman he loves so much, bear such an overwhelming ordeal. He doesn't like for me to be unhappy, he's always tried his hardest to make things wonderful for me. Losing Jenna, and watching me hold her as she died, nearly broke him. He was somehow able to treat me with tenderness and patience during the times following her death. Yes, he has really bad times, but somehow we manage to be strong for each other when one is really low.—*Nancy*

Special Family Concerns

Special concerns exist for single parents, divorced parents, and parents of an only child. As the parent who has lost an only child, you lose your identity as a parent, as a family. You lose the possibility of grandchildren and thus the dream of legacy. Strains on the marriage may be increased, and questions about the purpose of remaining married may be raised. There are specialized bereavement groups for parents who have lost an only child.

Single parents lack a partner with whom to share the loss. A single parent may also have a doubly heavy emotional involvement with the child. The parent–child relationship may have been your only very close relationship. You may have tried hard to be both mother and father to your child if the other parent was absent. Your child may have been the only connection to your earlier relationship with the other parent.

If you are a divorced parent, you and your ex-spouse may have trouble setting aside differences to cooperate with or support each other. Old wounds can be opened up. Divorced parents who lose an only child lose their connection; however contentious it may be, you may be losing the primary person who shares all the memories of the child's life.

Extended Family

Members of the extended family can be a vital source of support for bereaved parents, but they, too, need time and space to grieve in their own way.

> When my son died, I was in a blur. What had been going through my mind was I don't know how we did this. When I walked into my mother's house, I saw the collection of things from the hospital—boxes of cards, an afghan someone crocheted, a video his friends made, pictures, a basket of toiletries people brought us, and I realized how long we'd lived at the hospital. When I looked at that pile, I knew in a moment how we had gotten through it. We had been loved, too.— *Val*

Gentle Reminders for Working Through Grief

- Avoid extra stresses; don't take on any added activities, projects, or duties.
- Find someone who will let you talk about the child.
- Talk to your surviving children about their sibling and their feelings, fears, and hopes.
- Set aside time to think and grieve.
- Grieve your own way, and let others do the same.
- Express emotions constructively.
- Get support from other bereaved parents, family and friends, a group, or a professional.
- Acknowledge the negative aspects but focus on the positive ones.
- Appreciate the time you had with the child and quality of your own life.
- Avoid the overidealization of the deceased child and the overprotection of siblings.

* * *

> I don't think the grandparents will ever be the same. Watching your grown children bury their child has to be unbelievably difficult. Seeing the fathers cry breaks whatever is left of your heart. To this day, my dad can't look at pictures of her without breaking down. When we go to the cemetery, my dad practically falls over with grief.—*Julie*

Child Grieving

Siblings exhibit most of the same reactions as adults but have their own special issues. The first thought is a fearful one: "Someone like me can die." The world feels very unsafe. Siblings may feel that they caused the death or that the sick child died on purpose to abandon them, which makes them angry. Reverting back to behaviors of an earlier age is quite common. Fears may appear—of the dark, of illness and doctors, or of the possibility that someone else may die. Grieving siblings frequently have poor performance in school or desire to drop out of extracurricular activities for a time.

The death of a sibling causes a reorganization of the family: Birth order is thrown out of whack, and roles change. The sibling may now be an only child, cheated out of the experience of growing up with a brother or sister or of someday being an aunt or uncle. Siblings need time to try on and incorporate their new role. Siblings may feel that they must fill the role left open, such as being the "athletic one" or *A* student.

Children's grief is different and often misunderstood by adults. It may seem like children are not reacting, because they have such strong defenses. Or, they may blurt out facts or details to strangers, to see what they'll say. To the dismay of their parents, children often play funeral games. The child may pretend it did not happen or think that the child will come back. The child may ask about getting a new sibling. Normal, ambivalent feelings toward a sibling breed feelings of guilt, especially if they recently argued.

> The last time Kyle saw Jenna, they argued because she couldn't go home and he could. She was so mad that she told him she didn't love him. We told him she didn't mean it, but he was devastated. The tears stung in his eyes. I was so angry at her for saying that, and as it turned out it was the last thing she ever said to him. The day she died we came home before he got up. We climbed into the bed with him, told him she said she was sorry for being mean, and that she loved him. We also told him that she wanted him to have all her Beanie Babies forever. After holding our sweet 8-year-old for a long time, we somehow emerged and made all the arrangements for her funeral. Kyle was brave, strong, and sweet. He held up so well through the ordeal, even becoming more outgoing than ever before. Our support group brought him Nintendo 64, and the escape of video games has brought him great

> comfort. He grieves still, in his own way, and his face gets a "nauseous" look when he hears the word leukemia or cancer.—*Nancy*

Children do not detach from the deceased as quickly as adults do. Their grief process is kind of stop-and-go, and so reactions sometimes come out much later, especially at a time of a big or distressing event, like moving, changing schools, or another loss (big or small).

Siblings often grieve alone, in an attempt to protect the parents' feelings and "be strong," so as not to upset parents or other family members or because they are embarrassed to call attention to themselves. In a way, siblings also temporarily lose their parents at the same time, because the parents are so wrapped up in their own grief. Parents find themselves emotionally unavailable or yelling at the surviving siblings.

Siblings need a lot of support. Reassure them that your family will continue, that they are still loved, and that they will be taken care of. Some hospitals and communities have bereavement groups for them, as well as for parents. Not only are groups an opportunity to meet others who are in the same situation and outlets for emotions, but they also provide models of other siblings who are handling it.

> All these things you never would worry about before are now monumental. I can't make it monumental for her. One of our goals was to raise Jodi as normally as possible. We let her do what she needed to, to be her own person. That's something I worked on: to love her but let her go and grow in her own way. It is very difficult. I was concerned that she would feel guilty because she donated, that it was her marrow that killed her brother. But she felt no blame whatsoever. This was her brother's illness. Which is heartening, because we worked really hard for that.—*Ellen*

* * *

> We were very concerned with Matthias, he was only a year and a half younger. They were very close. Fortunately, he had a friend who lived just behind us, they spent a lot of time together afterwards. He helped somewhat to fill the void.—*Carl*

Talking to a Child About the Death of a Sibling

The explanations for children found earlier in this chapter apply here, but there are some additional things that siblings need to hear (not necessarily in this order or all at once): "It is okay to be sad. I'm sad, too"; "It's okay to cry"; "It's okay to talk about your sister/brother, and your feelings, even bad ones"; "If you don't want to talk to me, you can talk to (grandparent, aunt/uncle, clergy, family friend, or therapist)"; "It's okay to go play with your friends if you need a break"; "Dying is different from going to sleep, or going away, because in death the person doesn't come back, but in sleep or going away the person does"; "It's not your fault"; "There's a big difference between regular sick and dying sick (having a fever doesn't mean you have cancer, too)"; "This is what we think happens to a person after they die. What do you think happens?" or "I love you, and we'll all get through this together."

Repeated explanations and discussions help the child understand the finality of death and the emotions that come with it. They often ask the same distressing questions over and over. It's not that children don't know the answer but that they need to reinforce it. Repetitive play, talk, and drawing help make the grief more bearable for children. Check their understanding by asking them questions. The sibling may need a private place to cry or a third party to confide in.

Gentle Reminders for Helping Surviving Siblings

- Encourage the sibling to create memory book or photo album.
- Tell stories about the child to the sibling, and listen to the sibling's stories, too.
- Provide art supplies so that the sibling can express emotions by drawing pictures of the child, memories, fears, and feelings.
- Talk to the sibling's school; let teachers know what's going on and how they can help.
- Spend extra time with the sibling.
- Allow time for independence, distraction, other activities, and new opportunities to grow.
- Never compare the surviving sibling to the deceased child, and never expect the sibling to be a stand-in for the deceased child.
- Enlist professional support from bereavement counselors and child therapists.

Re-Investing in Life

Grief does not end cleanly—it comes and goes, and the pain gradually diminishes. Psychologist Mary Jo Kupst (see the Bibliography) found that

> Although it is a void that will remain with them throughout their lives, most are able to manage their emotional reactions, to gain a perspective on the death, and to proceed with life without the child. While no one would wish such an unfortunate experience upon anyone, it is true that several families showed positive adjustment and even growth in terms of closer family relationships, improved individual functioning, and appreciation of life.

A lively understandable spirit
Once entertained you.
It will come again.
Be still.
Wait.
Theodore Roethke, *The Lost Son* (1948)

Focus on what is possible—not what is impossible—and on what you have and what you can build.

Families eventually begin to feel more comfortable with their grief. They can talk about the child, the loss, their emotions, and others' emotions without falling apart. They have more good days than bad. They can remember the good times instead of only the illness.

The memories become more balanced over the years. I can remember the good times we shared without the searing pain that would come with it. Last week was his brother's birthday. We were sitting around the table, talking about some of the stuff they used to do. Peter was full of the hi-jinks; Dennis the Menace times two. We were having a wonderful time talking about the memories. We couldn't have done that a few years ago. It's wonderful for the one brother who never knew him. Simon says I have two brothers, one in heaven, the other on Earth. Peter's still a part of the family.—*Marjorie*

* * *

I think the best that we can hope for is that we find a special place for this emptiness and learn to live with it. We are surprised by how OK we are—that is not to say that we don't miss Christie terribly, because we do. We are often blind-sided by grief and pain—but there are good days too. In time, the wonderful memories will become stronger, and the memories of her as a patient will fade and become more tolerable. A friend wrote to me when Christie died [a quote from *Beside the Still Waters* by Patience Strong], "Slowly, patiently you draw the coloured threads out of the skeins of memory and work out something beautiful from what is left behind; another way of life to make, new hopes and joys to find." When it came time to put an announcement in the paper of Christie's death I closed with the following: "So many of you have asked what you could do. Nothing can heal our pain but maybe you can learn from it. Find the time to do something special with your loved ones. Christie would suggest the biggest, highest, fastest roller coaster you can find, a round of golf at Wonderland, or a batch of homemade cookies shared with someone special."—*Lenore*

* * *

As a general rule I don't bring up the subject. Sometimes I get trapped, how many kids do you have? Then you try to be cagey about it. How do you deny him? You can't. Finally, you let it out and they say, "Oh my God, I'm so sorry." I've learned after many years to quickly say, "Well, it's a long time ago. I've learned how to live with it." I think that's an important message to get out. You can live with this.—*Gillian*

Although the process is filled with ambivalent feelings, a survivor begins the process of healing by detaching from the focus on the child—no longer infusing every thought, every emotion, or every conversation with the child. At this stage, parents may feel better able to donate the child's toys and clothes or redecorate the child's room. Searching for a tangible way to memorialize their child, parents may start a scholarship fund in the child's name, plant a tree, dedicate a garden, or put together photo albums. Do something special for an anniversary of your child's death or birthday, but also leave yourself some time during that day to grieve.

> What I need to do and am still looking for is to get a comfortable space for Daniel to live in my body where he doesn't invade my space. There are places he doesn't belong. Sometimes Phil and I are having an intimate conversation, and he'll come into my head. Or times with my daughter, Leah, he'll come into my head. I need to put him in a square where he can live comfortably and I live comfortably. It is better now than a year ago, and it will be even better 5 years from now. There's a part of me that doesn't want it to happen because that means I'm losing pieces of Daniel, and I can't do that.—*Sarah*

Parents can re-invest in their own lives and in the lives of their other children, finding a way to incorporate the painful experience as an important but not all-encompassing part of their identity. Parents can even begin to enjoy life again.

> And time remembered is grief forgotten,
> And frosts are slain and flowers begotten
> And in green underwood and cover
> Blossom by blossom the spring begins.
> A. C. Swinburne, *Atalanta in Calydon* (1923)

> So, I went back to work. I am once again attempting to educate the wayward teenagers of the world. It's good to be back. I'm a better teacher now, more patient and thick-skinned. Every once in a while I'll take a student aside and show them a picture of Jenna, followed by a picture of her headstone. This has averted one suicide, prompted one run-away to return home, and a few kids have kicked drugs.—*Nancy*

Mourning is never completely over. Sadness, loss, and memories remain. But with hard work, you can heal, ease the painful symptoms, and find your own sense of peace. Pain should lessen with time.

Having Another Child

Though this topic is discussed in chapter 13 on survivorship, having another child takes on added dimensions when your child did not survive the cancer. Some parents have a strong desire for another child; it can become a powerful need to replace the child who died. Sometimes more children were in the family plan, anyway. Having a baby can be a means to begin again—another chance. Initially, some parents feel bad about being happy. Some feel disappointed and some relieved if the new child is a different sex than the first one.

Not everyone can or will choose to have another child, but for those who do, there are often fears about the health of the new baby. When a baby is born soon after the other child's death, it can complicate your grieving process, as your feelings for the two children become jumbled. If you do decide to have another child, many parents and professionals suggest that it is better to wait awhile, until you are ready to love the new baby for himself or herself.

> When Rae first died, I felt that I had no reason to go on living unless I could have another child. Now that I have a "replacement" child, and another on the way, I have thrown myself into their care. I keep my feelings about those times shoved into a dark closet at the back of my head, and I keep the door locked. There is no point in revisiting the pain. On the other hand, my entire life is changed because of Rae, and I want my living children to know about the sibling that went before them. It is hard to find a balance between honoring the past and functioning in the present.—*Naomi*

* * *

> I would never imagine that this is a replacement child. I could never replace Marisa. But I want to replace the experiences I would have had.—*Estella*

* * *

> I enjoyed "normal babyhood," since I didn't get that with my son. I would get so excited, almost overwhelmed, then feel guilty: you can't be happy, because your son's not here. I have to keep myself together for my daughters. They are a riot. The first time I took Ashley to school, she told the teacher her brother's in heaven. She can't grasp the concepts: Can Robbie come back down here for a little while, and can I go up there (to heaven)? NO! One day, we were driving by the cemetery and I heard one of the girls say, "There's Robbie's house." Amy asked me does Robbie have feet? Do they hang from the sky? Does he walk in heaven? Is he still a baby, or is he growing in heaven? Am I going to have a baby in heaven? They really get me going with questions.—*Sandy*

* * *

> We waited a full year after Peter died. You want to do it immediately, but you need to have the child for its own right. This kid brought so much healing into this family. The day I heard Simon's heartbeat was the unknotting of so much pain. A heart had stopped beating, and here there was a new heartbeat. The day the kids came into see Simon, who is the image of his brother Peter, the look on their faces made me think, "Oh thank you God for this moment." I also went back to the hospital and brought the baby to show the staff. They see you at your down moment, and then they see you with new life in your arms. It was a very healing thing to do.—*Marjorie*

Carrying the Torch

Carrying the torch is part of the healing process. It is a way to remember the child who died, pay tribute to that memory, acknowledge the child's life and the great loss, accept the alterations in life's plan, and re-invest in the lives of those who were left behind.

> During my daughter's battle and now for the last five years after her death, we pull together a group and sing Christmas carols in the hospital for all the children and families.—*Maurizia*

Responding to the needs of her own child, another mother created the Healing Heart Foundation to fund research in pain management for children with cancer. Among other fund-raising ideas, Healing Heart has a line of cards with illustrations by children.

> I knew the day my son died, something positive had to come out of it. He was very into giving back; he wanted to talk to other kids, he talked about all the people who gave to leukemia research before he was born. I wanted to do something in the area of pain management because it was such a gaping hole. Anything that helped him with pain, helped him to heal.

A mother maintained her involvement with the hospital where her son was treated but recognized that because her child died, some families with children undergoing treatment were uncomfortable turning to her as a resource.

> I brought my other children for child life therapy afterwards, and also went back when other kids relapsed, to help their families. There's something else that happens, when your child dies. You're not always that helpful to the people whose child is alive. Because they look at you and see the incarnation of their worst fear.—*Maureen*

If an avenue you've chosen is not as rewarding as you thought it would be, choose another. It may take you a few attempts to find the one that is right for you.

> To get out of the fog, we went on two trips. The first was a whale watch, without the kids. We thought, isn't this fantastic? I had a vision of Marco and my father (also deceased) swimming with the dolphins. I thought, he's doing better than we are. The second trip was to Europe. It was very healing for our relationship. We had such a wonderful time. It gave us a sense that there is still joy in life. A sense of hope.— *Vince*

Gentle Reminders for Carrying the Torch

- Focus on positives for yourself and your surviving children.
- Pick up your life where you left off, or head off in a new and exciting direction with your career, home, school, or social life.
- Rebuild relationships that were strained or neglected, with the siblings, your spouse, family members, and friends. Reach out to them, and be forgiving of yourself and them.
- Pack away the cancer literature and medical paperwork in a safe place.
- Help other families and children in some meaningful way.
- Write your grief story; write it, tape record it, or just keep it mentally in your head. Telling the story brings you peace and a sense of power over death and makes sense out of it. You "own" it. In sharing, you're sharing and releasing your child, your grief, and your experience. Writing or recording the story is a helpful act in itself; you do not have to make it public.
- Look at pictures and remember the good as well as the bad. Make photo albums, including some of your child when he or she was sick. Remind yourself of the time before the illness, of the relationship, joys, and pains.
- Write a letter to the deceased child, or talk to an empty chair or your child's doll. Tell it what you would want to say to the child.

CHAPTER 13

Surviving and Carrying the Torch

The storm had rolled away to faintness
like a wagon crossing a bridge.
—Eudora Welty, A Curtain of Green (1941)

Finding "normal" is difficult for many families in which a child has been treated for cancer. You feel changed. Your circumstances, priorities, and expectations are altered. At this transition, you really are forging a new life for yourself and your family. You have dedicated every moment during treatment to caring for your child, and now that focus is changing. You have to help your child make the adjustments to life after cancer. You have to find your way into new roles and resume past ones from a different perspective, whether those roles involve school, work, running a household, or other choices.

The hallmark of this phase is the gradual reintegration process. Life is changed by the cancer experience, but cancer is no longer the center. Parents report with surprise and delight that they have forgotten how to calculate an absolute neutrophil count (ANC) and other medical facts they used to rattle off in their sleep. However, parents tell us they have more reminders than they would like. Cancer parents may worry more about pesticides and drinking water or eating healthily. Survivors tend to like order and structure rather than spontaneity or surprises. Despite the changes, family members find their own personal ways to adapt and move forward in life.

> Recently while talking to an old friend that I had not seen in years, I did not tell him, "My son has cancer." Afterwards I reflected that it felt good not to say it, and that it was nice to reminisce over old times without my friend having to wonder what to say. The whole conversation was just like old times.—*Jenny*

* * *

We do go on, and it is okay. I know we have given Janie the best chance of survival: cutting-edge treatment, the latest protocol, total support for her during her illness. If anything happens, I know we did the best we could for Janie.—*Cecilia, grandmother*

* * *

My neighbor got into an accident. This time I was the one bringing over a roast chicken. It felt so good to have a turn on the giving side—when so many people had helped us. —*Neva*

Parents, survivors, and siblings may incorporate their experiences into a career.

I went back to college. Life had changed, and I needed to do something to reflect that change. I went to work in hospital-based social work. I found I had a knack for working with the other families as a peer. Social workers at the hospital encouraged me to pursue this.—*Val*

* * *

I hope to work in oncology. I am also interested in working in a school district on a child study team. I chose social work because I believe social work is a field that you go into not for the money but for the personal rewards and the way you can really help and touch someone's life. If I can make a difference in one person's life, than I am doing what I was meant to do.—*Hayley, long-term survivor*

Survivors and their families work to come to grips with the limitations and alterations brought about by the late effects of treatment. The more drastic the effects, the more difficult the task will be. A combination of medical and educational resources can help pinpoint your child's abilities and weaknesses and recommend ways to widen your child's horizons.

It is hard for me to hear about his delays. On a purely conceited level, I'm a professor and have some academic distinction. His dad is a computer analyst. We had pretty big dreams for this boy, and he was born with all the possibilities in the world. Then cancer came along like a speeding train. He's so happy, though, that I try not to think about it. I don't have any idea what he will end up able to do some 15 or 20 years from now. Who knows what talent or interest he'll have discovered that he can be productive with. Most of the time I focus on being thankful for what we have and positive about the future, but when I have to sit down and focus on his deficits, it brings up a lot of loss.—*Caroline*

* * *

There ought to be a "free pass" for life's battles after you fight cancer. Since that's not gonna happen, we just deal with it.—*Pat*

One way to move forward which may be a source of mixed emotions is the decision whether to have another child.

> He greets his new sister with such love. We couldn't have dreamed he would be so taken with her. She smiles at him more than anyone else, and I know we did the right thing in expanding our family.—*Rhonda*
>
> * * *
>
> I see an inherent danger in the need to have another child. It implies that the one who had cancer is damaged goods, or that we have to have another one in case she dies. I don't want to go there. We'll play the hand we've been dealt and enjoy the children we have for as long as we have them.—*Morgan*

A new pregnancy that occurred during a child's cancer treatment triggers anxieties also. Parents worry they will not be able to care for a new baby while a child is on treatment or if the child relapses. They worry that exposure to the drugs and radiation might harm the unborn baby. Whether or not their child's cancer is inherited, parents worry that the new baby might develop cancer or some other disease.

> The main worry was that I couldn't be in two places at once. It happened. Joseph was 3 weeks old. Aaron had the flu and spiked a high fever and had to be admitted. The hospital let me bring Joseph with me. But we were in a room with another child who also had the flu, so I couldn't take the baby in the room. I was sleeping in the family resource room. I would feed the baby and walk him up and down the hall. Then Mitch and I would meet in the hallway, and he'd take the baby and I'd go in with Aaron. Every time we went in or out of the room we had to put on gowns, gloves and masks or take it off. It was like keystone cops. After that, I didn't worry about it anymore. The worst happened. We did it.—*Debra*
>
> * * *
>
> The same day Andy was diagnosed with the kidney cancer, I found out I was pregnant. Talk about an emotional day! T. J. was born two weeks after Andy finished treatment. I was terrified that I couldn't "handle" the pregnancy. But I was so caught up and focused on Andy that I don't recall much morning sickness, and the pregnancy flew by. I was terrified of potential harm to the fetus that Andy's treatment might cause. Andy will be going for follow-up regularly and so will T. J., since this is a familial cancer. He's already been scanned and will continue to be watched closely. There are no guarantees. There is no contract to sign when children are born that promises they'll make it to adulthood or that they won't feel pain. Although cancer has me scared, worried, anxious, tired, and crazy, I guess, part of me refuses to let it completely rule everything I do.—*Diane*

Passing Management of the Disease to Your Grown Child

As the child who had cancer becomes an adult, many parents struggle with passing to him or her the management of the disease. When the child takes responsibility for his or her own health care and follow-up, the parent may feel out of the loop, left without a job. The parent reluctantly becomes an observer, as the child makes his or her own decisions and adjusts to accommodate any changes wrought by effects. Yet a parent's worry doesn't stop just because the child grows up. Luckily, the process is often a gradual one, which the child also feels more comfortable easing into slowly.

> You may give them your love
> but not your thoughts,
> For they have their own
> thoughts.
> You may house their bodies but
> not their souls.
> For their souls dwell in the
> house of tomorrow, which you
> cannot visit, not even in your
> dreams.
> You may strive to be like them,
> but seek not to make them like
> you.
> For life goes not backward nor
> tarries with yesterday.
> You are the bows from which
> your children as living arrows
> are sent forth.
> Kahlil Gibran, *The Prophet*
> (1923)

> I found it very disconcerting to be at home, knowing that Julian was at a checkup at the hospital and I had no idea what was going on. Even though he is all grown up I still find that I need to know the details of his health for my own peace of mind. He didn't tell me much. He did tell me that the nurses were great, and he was well cared for. That's all I got out of him before he headed back to school. Darn! I wanted to know every detail!—*Lorraine*

* * *

> Alicia (age 12) is pretty open with letting me see her body. She is also very good about coming to me with anything she notices. I think she passes it on to me, so she doesn't have to worry about it. That is a reassurance to me too. Since Alicia has passed her five-year mark, I really try to remind myself that a recurrence is unlikely and that if she developed a secondary cancer, she'd have the same chance as anyone else of beating it.—*Margaret*

If an adolescent is still on treatment, passing management of the disease can be a source of contention. Normal issues of control, care-taking, protection, and "empty-nest" syndrome take on added anxiety. The best ammunition a parent can give a survivor is information about the disease and follow-up care requirements. A good resource is *Childhood Cancer*

Survivors by Nancy Keene, Wendy Hobbie, and Kathy Ruccione (see Resources), which discusses possible effects of various treatments and includes a medical history form that parents can fill out and give to the child.

> It was hard at first just to trust that Cal was taking his meds on his own. When he was 18, I'd put his pills in a little cup by his computer and make sure they were taken. A few weeks before he moved to the dorm, I had to force him to take out his own pills. This was a big breakthrough for us. Now, he has made his first visit to his doctor on his own, and I have the doctor call him at his condo if they need to adjust his meds because of his ANC. He has yet to phone the doctor on his own to ask if he needs to come in because he has a fever, or the time he cut his finger badly.—*Jenny*

* * *

> Up until the end of treatment, my mother was at every visit. The follow-up visits were every six months, then once a year. By that time, I was pregnant. My oncologist was okay with my annual medical checkup being with the ob/gyn, who was aware of my history. As soon as I started seeing my doctor for my pregnancy, my mother was out of the picture. We still talk all the time, so she usually knows what little ailments I have. She didn't have a problem letting go of it because I had responded so well. I hadn't had any type of relapse. This was five years after I was diagnosed. At that point, she was ready to let go. I was 20.—*Gloria, long-term survivor*

Carrying the Torch

Some people cannot imagine leaving the entire cancer experience behind them without using their hard-earned knowledge or "giving something back" in some way. Many people find satisfaction in donating time, money, or gifts; volunteering at hospitals or camps; lobbying for improved health care and research; lecturing; fund-raising; writing; creating Web sites; forming support groups; or founding organizations devoted to helping other cancer parents and children. Using their unique skills, abilities, and networks, "torchbearers" may jump into existing programs or branch out with their own ideas.

> Camp Sunshine is a very special place for our family. Geoff has often said if he got one week of vacation a year, he would spend it volunteering there. Anne has a very special role there as a survivor—parents look at her and say, "My child can do this, too." We want to raise our girls to realize that in this world we all take care of each other. Camp Sunshine gives us that opportunity. I find my role to be that of a listener. People are very open—I think perhaps because we've been on similar journeys and also because they'll never see me again (there's a freedom in that!). It's also tremendously difficult to leave your child in

> someone else's care after you've been joined at the hip. Knowing my daughter was in treatment and had a Broviac and ng tube helps give them a feeling of safety, I think. It feels great to be on the other side, but I believe with it comes a responsibility and opportunity to give back.—*Pam*

A survivor and his family organized One Voice Foundation, Inc., to raise awareness and funds for cancer research. The young man, his family, and volunteers bicycle across the country, soliciting corporate and private pledges, visiting treatment centers, and speaking about childhood cancer issues.

Some people have a clear idea of a service that is needed but do not know how to go about forming an organization to provide it. Call your state's office of the Secretary of State and request the forms for starting a nonprofit charitable organization. Contact the Internal Revenue Service to apply for 501(c)(3) nonprofit status. The Children's Cancer Association was founded by the parents of a young girl who died of cancer. In Oregon and southwestern Washington state, the organization provides musical programs, wish fulfillment, visits from a "chemo pal," and information and support services to families. Nationally, it provides print and Web-based listings of resources for families via the Kids' Cancer Help Pages. Cofounder Regina Ellis discusses how she began:

> My background was in marketing, and my husband is an owner of a small manufacturing company, but we did not have nonprofit experience. We had lots of vision and knew others would join that vision with funding in time. We had enormous family, friend, and community support. We wanted to provide answers to the questions we had, to provide the fun and music that was missing, to offer the resources that were hard to access. I checked out books from the library and sought out professionals in business, foundations, and marketing for advice on how to start the organization. Our board was the pinnacle of compassion and willingness to make a difference and continues to be a driving force of our success. Today, CCA serves over 10,000 children annually. Our annual operating budget is close to $600,000. In addition to 9 staff members, we get help from 200 volunteers, corporate sponsors, and foundation partners.

Carrying the torch is not something everyone feels comfortable with; it can be an uncomfortable public role that keeps painful memories at the surface, seen as hanging on instead of moving on. It may become a bone of contention between family members. The founder of one informational support organization, the friend of a cancer parent, was dismayed when her friend wanted nothing to do with it and subsequently drifted out of the relationship. Another parent talks about her husband's discomfort with her project to raise research funds:

> When I wanted to start a foundation my husband wasn't sure he could be involved. Although I told him he didn't have to, I was kidding myself; I knew I would expect him to be part

of it, and others would, too. My friends were more into it than he was. He has helped, but it's so incredibly difficult for him. I've stopped expecting it.—*Simone*

Carrying the torch is a part of the healing process for families of children who survive, as well as for those whose children die. It is in the day-to-day living that cancer families transform their losses into an affirmation of life and renewal.

Gentle Reminders for Survivorship

- Focus on the positives for yourself and your growing children.
- Pick up your life where you left off, or head off in a new and exciting direction with your career, home, school, and social life.
- Rebuild relationships that were strained or neglected (with siblings, a spouse, family members, or friends). Reach out to them, and be forgiving of yourself and them.
- Get copies of medical records, then put the cancer literature and medical paperwork in a safe place so that your child will have it later.
- Educate your child on an ongoing basis about the illness, treatment, effects, and ramifications.
- Teach your child the importance and methods of self-exams, healthy living, cancer prevention, yearly physicals, screening exams, and so forth.
- Continue to advocate for your child's changing needs.
- Maintain valuable connections in the cancer world.
- Help other families and children in some meaningful way.
- Build your child's physical and emotional strength back up with activities such as karate, horseback riding, swimming, fencing, dance, gymnastics, pottery, painting, or musical instruments.

For the most part, adapting to survivorship will develop naturally and gradually. Your family will go at its own pace. As one parent put it, "I didn't realize how far we had moved on until I looked back."

Bibliography

Adams, C., and E. Fruge. 1996. *Why children misbehave: And what to do about it.* Oakland, CA: New Harbinger.

Adams, D. W., and E. J. Deveau. 1993. *Coping with childhood cancer: Where do we go from here?* New rev. ed. Hamilton, Ontario, Canada: Kinbridge.

______. 1986. "Helping dying adolescents: Needs and responses." In *Adolescence and death,* edited by C. A. Corr and J. N. McNeil, 79–85. New York: Springer.

American Psychiatric Association. 1994. *Diagnostic and Statistical Manual of Mental Disorders,* 4th ed. Washington, DC: American Psychiatric Association.

Benson, H. 1975. *The relaxation response.* New York: Morrow.

Berk, L. E. 2000. *Child development,* 5th ed. Boston: Allyn & Bacon.

Boyd, J. R., and M. Hunsberger. 1998. Chronically ill children coping with repeated hospitalizations: Their perceptions and suggested interventions. *Journal of Pediatric Nursing* 13(6):330–342.

Bronfenbrenner, U. 1981. *The ecology of human development.* Cambridge, MA: Harvard University Press.

______. 1986. Ecology of the family as a context for human development: Research perspectives. *Developmental Psychology* 22:723–742.

Bronfebrenner, U., and P. A. Morris. 1998. "The ecology of developmental processes." In *Handbook of child psychology. Vol. 1: Theoretical models of human development,* edited by R. M. Lerner, 5th ed., 535–584. New York: Wiley.

Buschman, P. 1988. "Pediatric orthopedics: Dealing with loss and chronic sorrow." In *Dying and disabled children: Dealing with loss and grief,* edited by H. M. Dick, D. P. Roye, Jr., P. R. Buschman, A. H. Kutscher, B. Rubinstein, and F. K. Forstenzer, 39–52. New York: Haworth Press.

CancerNet Web site: http://cancernet.nci.nih.gov (coping with cancer, supportive care, health professionals, depression).

Carpenter, P. J., and C. S. Levant. 1994. Sibling adaptation to the family crisis of childhood cancer. In *Pediatric psychooncology: Psychological perspectives on children with cancer,* edited by D. J. Bearison and R. K. Mulhern, 122–142. New York: Oxford University Press.

Chen, E., M. G. Craske, E. R. Katz, E. Schwartz, and L. K. Zeltzer. 2000. Pain-sensitive temperament: Does it predict procedural distress and response to psychological treatment among children with cancer? *Journal of Pediatric Psychology* 25(4):269–278.

Chen, E., L. K. Zeltzer, M. G. Craske, and E. Katz. 1999. Alteration of memory in the reduction of children's distress during repeated aversive medical procedures. *Journal of Consulting and Clinical Psychology* 67(4):481–490.

Chen, E., L. K. Zeltzer, M. G. Craske, and E. R. Katz. 2000. Children's memories for painful cancer treatment procedures: Implications for distress. *Child Development* 71(4): 933–947.

Chesler, M. A., J. Allswede, and O. A. Barbarin. 1991. Voices from the margin of the family: Siblings of children with cancer. *Journal of Psychosocial Oncology* 9(4):757–768.

Chesler, M. A., and O. A. Barbarin. 1987. *Childhood cancer and the family: Meeting the challenge of stress and support.* New York: Brunner/Mazel.

Chesler, M. A., and C. Parry. 1999. *Gender roles/styles in crisis: The experiences of fathers of children with cancer,* Monograph 577. Ann Arbor, MI: University of Michigan, Center for Research on Social Organization.

Chesler, M. A., S. P. Heiney, R. Perrin, G. P. Monaco, M. I. Kupst, N. F. Cincotta, E. R. Katz, P. Deasy-Spinetta, E. H. Whittam, and G. V. Foley. 1993. Principles of Psychosocial Programming for Children and Cancer. *Cancer Supplement* 71(10):3210–3212.

Cook, S. S. 1988. "The impact of the disabled child on the family." In *Dying and disabled children: Dealing with loss and grief,* edited by H. M. Dick, D. P. Roye Jr., P. R. Buschman, A. H. Kutscher, B. Rubinstein, and F. K. Forstenzer, 45–52. New York: Haworth Press.

Craig, K. D. 1984. Developmental changes in infant pain expression during immunization injections. *Social Science and Medicine* 19(12):1331–1337.

Davis, M., E. R. Eshelman, and M. McKay. 1995. *The relaxation and stress reduction workbook,* 4th ed. Oakland, CA: New Harbinger.

Drell, M. J., C. H. Siegel, and T. J. Gaensbauer. 1993. "Post-traumatic stress disorder." In *Handbook of infant mental health,* edited by C. Zeanah, 291–304. New York: Guilford Press.

Erdman, L. 1997. "Humor." In *Oncology nursing secrets,* edited by R. A. Gates and R. M. Fink, 446–449. Philadelphia: Hanley & Belfus.

Finkbeiner, A. K. 1996. *After the death of a child: Living with loss through the years.* Baltimore: Johns Hopkins University Press.

Fischer, K. W., and T. R. Bidell. 1998. "Dynamic development of psychological structures in action and thought." In *Handbook of child psychology. Vol. 1: Theoretical models of human development,* edited by R. M. Lerner, 5th ed., 467–561. New York: Wiley.

Fry, V. L. 1995. *Part of me died, too: Stories of creative survival among bereaved children and teenagers.* New York: Dutton Children's Books.

Gardner, H. 1999. *Intelligence reframed: Multiple intelligences for the 21st century.* New York: Basicbooks.

Gates, R. A., and P. W. Nishimoto. 1997. "Communicating, caring, and coping." In *Oncology nursing secrets,* edited by R. A. Gates and R. M. Fink, 428–436. Philadelphia: Hanley & Belfus.

Genius, M. 1995. The use of hypnosis in helping cancer patients control anxiety, pain, and emesis: A review of recent empirical studies. *American Journal of Clinical Hypnosis* 37(4): 316–325.

Golden, T. R. 1997. *Swallowed by a snake: The gift of the masculine side of healing.* Gaithersburg, MD: Golden Healing.

Goodheart, C. D., and M. H. Lansing. 1997. *Treating people with chronic disease: A psychological guide.* Washington, DC: American Psychological Association.

Greenberg, H. S., A. E. Kazak, and A. T. Meadows. 1989. Psychological functioning in 8- to 16-year-old cancer survivors and their parents. *Journal of Pediatrics* 114(3):488–493.

Grollman, E. 1990. *Talking about death: A dialogue between parent and child.* Boston: Beacon Press.

Haber, S., Ed. 1993. *Breast cancer: A psychological treatment manual.* New York: Springer.

Harter, S. 1998. "The development of self representations." In *Handbook of child psychology. Vol 3: Social, emotional, and personality development,* edited by N. Eisenberg, 5th ed., 553–618. New York: Wiley.

Heiney, S. P., L. M. Wells, B. Coleman, and E. Swygert. 1991. Lasting impressions: Adolescents with cancer share how to cope, a videotape program. *Journal of Pediatric Oncology Nursing* 8(1):18–23.

Heiney, S. P., L. M. Wells, B. Coleman, E. Swygert, and J. Ruffin. 1990. Lasting impressions: A psychosocial support program for adolescents with cancer and their parents. *Cancer Nursing* 13(1):13–20.

Ingebrigtsen, P., and M. W. Smith. 1997. "Family issues." In *Oncology nursing secrets,* edited by R. A. Gates and R. M. Fink, 459–462. Philadelphia: Hanley & Belfus.

Jay, S. M., E. Katz, C. H. Elliott, and S. E. Siegel. 1987. Cognitive–behavioral and pharmacological interventions for children's distress during painful medical procedures. *Journal of Consulting and Clinical Psychology* 55(6):860–865.

Jay, S., M. Ozolins, C. Elliott, and S. Caldwell. 1983. Assessment of children's distress during painful medical procedures. *Health Psychology* 2(2):133–147.

Johansen, B. B. 1988. "Care of the dying adolescent and the bereaved family." In *Dying and disabled children: Dealing with loss and grief,* edited by H. M. Dick, D. P. Roye, P. R. Buschman, A. H. Kutscher, B. Rubinstein, and F. K. Forstenzer, 59–67. New York: Haworth Press.

Johnson, S. E. 1987. *After a child dies.* New York: Springer.

Katz, F. R., J. Kellerman, and S. E. Siegel. 1980. Behavioral distress in children with cancer undergoing medical procedures: Developmental considerations. *Journal of Consulting and Clinical Psychology* 48(3):356–365.

Kazak, A. 1994. "Implications of survival: Pediatric oncology patients and their families." In *Pediatric psychooncology: Psychological perspectives on children with cancer,* edited by D. J. Bearison and R. K. Mulhern, 171–192. New York: Oxford University Press.

Kazak, A., M. Stuber, L. Barakat, K. Meeske, D. Guthrie, and A. Meadows. 1998. Predicting posttraumatic stress symptoms in mothers and fathers of survivors of childhood cancers. *Journal of the American Academy of Child Psychiatry* 37(8):823–831.

Keene, N. 1997. *Childhood leukemia.* Sebastopol, CA: O'Reilly & Associates.

Keene, N., W. Hobbie, and K. Ruccione. 2000. *Childhood cancer survivors: A practical guide to your future.* Sebastopol, CA: O'Reilly & Associates.

Kellerman, J. 1981. *Helping the fearful child: A guide to everyday problems and anxieties.* New York: Norton.

Koocher, G. P., and J. E. O'Malley, Eds. 1981. *The Damocles syndrome: Psychological consequences of surviving childhood cancer.* New York: McGraw-Hill.

Kupst, M. J. 1986. "Death of a child from a serious illness." In *Parental loss of a child,* edited by T. A. Rando, 191–199. Champaign, IL: Research Press.

Kupst, M. J. 1994. "Coping with pediatric cancer: Theoretical and research perspectives." In *Pediatric psychooncology: Psychological perspectives on children with cancer,* edited by D. J. Bearison and R. K. Mulhern, 35–60. New York: Oxford University Press.

Kupst, M. J., and J. L. Schulman. 1988. Long-term coping with pediatric leukemia: A six-year follow-up study. *Journal of Pediatric Psychology* 13:7–22.

Kushner, H. 1994. *When bad things happen to good people.* New York: Harper Collins.

Kuttner, L. 1996. *A child in pain: How to help, what to do.* Point Roberts, WA: Hartley & Marks.

Lange, A. J., and P. Jakubowski. 1980. *Responsible assertive behavior: Cognitive/behavioral procedures for trainers.* Champaign, IL: Research Press.

Lazarus, R. S. 1966. *Psychological stress and the coping process.* New York: McGraw Hill.

———. 1991. *Emotion and adaptation.* New York: Oxford University Press.

Lobato, D. J. 1990. *Brothers, sisters, and special needs: Information and activities for helping young siblings of children with chronic illnesses and developmental disabilities.* Baltimore: Brookes.

Mason, S., M. Johnson, and C. Woolley. 1999. A comparison of distractors for controlling distress in young children during medical procedures. *Journal of Clinical Psychology in Medical Settings* 6(3):239–248.

Masten, A., and J. D. Coatsworth. 1998. The development of competence in favorable and unfavorable environments: Lessons from research on successful children. *American Psychologist* 53(2):205–220.

Maurer, A. M., J. B. Burgess, S. S. Donaldson, K. A. Rickard, V. A. Stallings, J. Van Eyes, and M. Winick. 1990. Special nutritional needs of children with malignancies. *Journal of Parenteral and Enteral Nutrition* 14(1):315–324.

McCubbin, M. A., and H. I. McCubbin. 1991. Family stress theory and assessment: The T-double ABCX model of family adjustment and adaptation. In *Family assessment interventions for research and practice,* edited by H. I. McCubbin and A. I. Thompson, 3–34. Madison: University of Wisconsin Press.

National Institutes of Health, National Cancer Institute. 1995. *Understanding gene testing.* Washington, DC: U.S. Department of Health and Human Services.

Nelson, C. A., and F. E. Bloom. 1997. Child development and neuroscience. *Child Development* 68:970–987.

New Jersey Department of Education. 2000. *Parental rights in special education.* Trenton: Author, Office of Special Education Programs.

O'Malley, J. E., G. Koocher, D. Foster, and L. Slavin. 1979. Psychiatric sequelae of surviving childhood cancer. *American Journal of Orthopsychiatry* 49(4):608–616.

Orr, D., M. Hoffmans, and G. Bennetts. 1984. Adolescents with cancer report their psychosocial needs. *Journal of Psychosocial Oncology* 2(2):47–59.

Osterweis, M., F. Solomon, and M. Green. 1984. *Bereavement: Reactions, consequences, and care.* Washington, DC: National Academy Press.

Perrin, J. M., and W. E. McLean, Jr. 1988. Children with chronic illness: The prevention of dysfunction. *Pediatric Clinics of North America* 35:1325–1337.

Pynoos, R. S. 1990. "Post-traumatic stress disorder in children and adolescents." In *Psychiatric disorders in children and adolescents,* edited by B. Garfinkel, G. Carlson, and E. Weller, 48–53. Philadelphia: Saunders.

Ramey, C., and S. L. Ramey. 1998. Early intervention and early experience. *American Psychologist* 53(2):109–120.

Rando, T. A. 1986. "Unique issues and impact of the death of a child." In *Parental loss of a child,* edited by T. A. Rando, 5–43. Champaign, IL: Research Press.

Redd, W. 1994. "Behavioral interventions to reduce child distress." In *Handbook of psychooncology,* edited by J. C. Holland and J. H. Rowland, 573–581. New York: Oxford University Press.

Ricker, K. A., A. Lopez, B. J. Godshall, R. Weetman, and J. Grosfeld. 1991. Nutrition strategies for children with cancer. *Nutrition Focus* 6(5):1–9.

Ries, L. A. G., M. A. Smith, J. C. Gurney, M. Linet, T. Tamra, J. L. Young, and G. R. Bunin, Eds. 1999. *Cancer incidence and survival among children and adolescents: United States SEER Program 1975–1995,* NIH Publication No. 99-4649. Bethesda, MD: National Cancer Institute, SEER Program.

Rivers, D. 2000. *The seven challenges cooperative communication skills workbook and reader.* Santa Barbara, CA: Cooperative Communication Skills Internet Resource Center (Web site: www.coopcomm.org).

Rolland, J. S. 1994. Working with illness: Clinicians' personal and interface issues. *Family Systems Medicine* 12(2):149–169.

Rosen, M. 2000, April 9. "I feel like I have a secret key to every door." *Parade Magazine,* p. 14.

Sacks, N., and F. D. Ottery. 1996. Nutrition for the child with cancer. *Candlelighters Childhood Cancer Foundation Newsletter* 11(2):1–5.

Sanger, S., and M. Petrillo. 1980. *Emotional care of hospitalized children.* Philadelphia: Lippincott.

Screening for Mental Health Web site: http://www.nmisp.org (National Screening Day project).

Sommer, D. 1994. Exploring the spirituality of children in the midst of illness and suffering. *The ACCH Advocate* (Association for the Care of Children's Health, Bethesda, MD) 1(2): 7–12.

Sourkes, B. 1982. *The deepening shade: Psychological aspects of life-threatening illness.* Pittsburgh, PA: University of Pittsburgh Press.

Spinetta, J. J. 1977. Adjustment in children with cancer. *Journal of Pediatric Psychology* 2: 49–51.

Stevens, B. 1989. "Nursing management of pain in children." In *Family-centered nursing care of children,* edited by R. L. Foster, M. M. Hunsberger, and J. J. Tackett-Anderson, 882–914. Philadelphia: Saunders.

Stuber, M. L. 1995. Stress responses to pediatric cancer: A family phenomenon. *Family Systems Medicine* 13(2):163–172.

Stuber, M., D. Christakis, B. Houskamp, and A. Kazak. 1996. Posttrauma symptoms in childhood leukemia survivors and their parents. *Psychosomatics* 37:254–261.

Swaney, J. R. 1997. "Religion and spirituality." In *Oncology nursing secrets,* edited by R. A. Gates and R. M. Fink, 437–445. Philadelphia: Hanley & Belfus.

Taylor, S. 1983. Adjustment to threatening events: A theory of cognitive adaptation. *American Psychologist* 38(11):1161–1173.

Taylor, S. E., L. C. Klein, B. P. Lewis, T. L. Gruenewald, R. A. R. Gurung, and J. A. Updegraff. 2000. Biobehavioral responses to stress in females: Tend-and-befriend, not fight-or-flight. *Psychological Review* 107(3):411–429.

Thelen, E., and L. B. Smith. 1994. *A dynamic systems approach to the development of cognition and action.* Cambridge, MA: MIT Press.

Thompson, R. H. 1985. *Psychosocial research on pediatric hospitalization and health care: A review of the literature.* Springfield, IL: Charles C Thomas.

Thompson, R. J., and Gustafson, K. E. 1998. "Psychological interventions in childhood chronic illness." In *Psychologists desk reference,* edited by G. P. Koocher, J. C. Norcross, and S. S. Hill, 261–265. New York: Oxford University Press.

Tyc, V., R. Mulhern, D. Barclay, B. Smith, and A. Bieberich. 1997. Variables associated with anticipatory nausea and vomiting in pediatric cancer patients receiving ondansetron antiemetic therapy. *Journal of Pediatric Psychology* 22(1):45–58.

Tyson, R. 1986. The roots of psychopathology and our theories of development. *Journal of the American Academy of Child Psychiatry* 25:12–22.

Weeks, D. 1992. *The eight essential steps to conflict resolution.* Los Angeles, CA: Jeremy P. Tarcher (Web site: www.qvctc.commnet.edu/classes/conflict).

Winnicott, D. W. 1965. *The maturational processes and the facilitating environment.* New York: International University Press.

Wong, D. L., M. Hockenberry-Eaton, D. Wilson, M. L. Winkelstein, and P. Schwartz. 2001. *Wong's essentials of pediatric nursing,* 6th ed. St. Louis, MO: Mosby.

Wong, D., and L. Whaley. 1990. *Clinical manual of pediatric nursing.* St. Louis: C. V. Mosby.

Worchel, F., B. Nolan, V. Willson, J. Purser, D. Copeland, and B. Pfefferbaum. 1988. Assessment of depression in children with cancer. *Journal of Pediatric Psychology* 13:101–112.

Youngs, B. 1995. *Stress and your child.* Columbine, NY: Fawcett.

Zeltzer, L. 1994. "Pain and symptom management." In *Pediatric psychooncology: Psychological perspectives on children with cancer,* edited by D. J. Bearison and R. K. Mulhern, 61–83. New York: Oxford University Press.

Resources

Because we cannot possibly list all of the available resources here, we have chosen those that can link you to other resources and those with national or regional access. Find local organizations through national ones or by contacting your social worker, networking with other parents, searching the Internet, or looking in the *Encyclopedia of Associations* in the reference section of your local library.

The amount of information and support on the Internet is staggering, making it one of the most valuable resources. However, please be careful. Personal or commercial (for-profit) Web sites may not have information that is entirely objective or accurate. Talk with your doctors before trying anything you find on the Internet. Remember, not all chat rooms or discussion sites are moderated, private, or secure. Read privacy statements carefully. Web addresses can change more quickly than books are published—with a little searching on your own, you can find new links.

The resources are separated into two general categories: organizations and websites; and books and videos. Within organizations and websites, resources are grouped by general topics or types of information or service. Many of the organizations' services overlap, so check multiple categories. The books are separated into sections for adults and children, then further organized by topic; the videos are separated into sections for parents, children, and older children and mature teenagers.

Information provided here was accurate at the time this book went to press, June 2001.

ORGANIZATIONS & WEB SITES

CANCER

National Cancer Institute
9000 Rockville Pike, Building 31, Room 10A16
Bethesda, MD 20892
800-4-CANCER, Fax: 301-231-6941, CancerFax: 800-624-2511
http://www.nci.nih.gov
Offers free booklets on eating, nutrition, clinical trials, teenagers, transplants, pain, finishing treatment, relapse, and caregiver support. CancerNet offers a dictionary, genetics services directory, kids' page, Physician Data Query (information on cancers, treatments), clinical trials, list of treatment centers, statistics, and CancerLit (medical literature database). CancerFax accesses PDQ information from a fax machine: Follow prompts.

National Childhood Cancer Foundation/Children's Oncology Group
440 East Huntington Drive
P.O. Box 60012
Arcadia, CA 91066-6012
626-447-1674 or 800-458-6223
http://www.nccf.org/
COG is a research organization, has patient advocacy committee, and lists member hospitals. NCCF supports research for COG. Newsletter provides information on new treatment and psychosocial support. Advocacy.

Oncolink
http://www.oncolink.com/
Offers information, news, tips, support, clinical trials, hospitals, financial assistance, pharmaceutical assistance programs, articles, patients' stories, jokes, and art. Links.

Specific Cancers

Brain Tumors

American Brain Tumor Association
2720 River Road
Des Plains, IL 60018
800-886-2282 or 847-827-9910
http://www.abta.org
Offers publications, listings of support groups, physicians involved in clinical trials; pen pal program, social services consultations.

Brain Tumor Foundation of Canada
650 Waterloo Street, Suite 100
London, Ontario, Canada N6B 2R4
800-265-5106 or 519-642-7755
http://www.btfc.org
Supports research, local programs, one-on-one telephone link with trained volunteers. Handbooks, pamphlets, medical journal articles.

Brain Tumor Society
124 Watertown Street, Suite 3H
Watertown, MA 02472
800-770-8287 or 617-924-9997
http://www.tbts.com
Support, education, research. Telephone network, access to support groups. *Color Me Hope Resource Guide:* brief overview, associated problems, and resources. *Brain Tumors: A Guide for the Primary Care Physician.* Support lines.

Children's Brain Tumor Foundation
274 Madison Avenue, Suite 1301
New York, NY 10016
212-448-9494
http://www.childrensneuronet.org
Information on school issues, special education.

National Brain Tumor Foundation
414 13th Street, Suite 700
Oakland, CA 94612-2603
800-934-2873 or 510-389-9777
http://www.braintumor.org
Information on clinical trials, treatments. Support groups. Medical advice nurse on staff for questions. On-line chatrooms.

Pediatric Brain Tumor Foundation of the US
302 Ridgefield Court
Asheville, NC 28806
800-253-6530 or 828-665-6891
http://www.pbtfus.org
On-line conferences, family support programs.

Histiocytosis

Histiocytosis Association of America
302 North Broadway
Pittman, NJ 08071
800-548-2758 (United States and Canada) or 856-589-6606 (other countries)
http://www.histio.org/us

Leukemia

Leukemia & Lymphoma Society
1311 Mamaroneck Avenue, 3rd Floor
White Plains, NY 10605
800-955-4LSA (4572) or 914-949-5213
http://www.leukemia-lymphoma.org
50+ local chapters in the United States. Information, financial assistance, free booklets. Support groups, telephone links to other families. On-line discussion. Newsletter. *I'm Having a Bone Marrow Transplant:* coloring book. *What It Is That I Have, Don't Want, Didn't Ask for, Can't Give Back and How I Feel About It:* diary for children and teenagers, with comments from others.

Neuroblastoma

Neuroblastoma Children's Cancer Society
P.O. Box 957672
Hoffman Estates, IL 60195-7672
800-532-5162 or 847-490-4240
http://www.granitewebworks.com/nccs.htm
Information, support, chat, public awareness.

Neuroblastoma Home Page
Center for Medical Genetics
University Hospital, Gent, Belgium
http://allserv.rug.ac.be/fspelema/neubla/nb.htm
Explanation of NB, images of cells, genetics, staging, research, links.

A Starting Point: Pediatric Neurooncology Resources on the Internet
http://www.med.miami.edu/neurosurgery/startintro.htm

Pituitary Tumors

Pituitary Tumor Network Association
P.O. Box 1958
Thousand Oaks, CA 91358
800-642-9211 or 805-499-2262
http://www.pituitary.com
Information, resource guide.

Rare Disorders

National Organization for Rare Disorders
100 Route 37, P.O. Box 8923
New Fairfield, CT 06812-8923
800-999-6673 or 203-746-6518
http://www.rarediseases.org
Databases on rare diseases, organizations, orphan drugs. Local chapters.

Canadian Order for Rare Disorders
2740 4th Avenue South
Lethbridge, AB CAN T1J 0N9
403-345-3948 or 403-345-4544

Retinoblastoma

National Retinoblastoma Parent Group
P.O. Box 317
Watertown, MA 02471
800-562-6265
Family networking, publications, newsletter, workshops/conferences for families. Consultation for development of support groups. Advocacy.

Retinoblastoma International
Children's Hospital of Los Angeles
4650 Sunset Boulevard
Los Angeles, CA 90027
888-353-0080 or 323-669-2299
http://www.kidseyecancer.org/rbi/index_rbi.htm
Research funding, parent support.

The Retinoblastoma Society
c/o St. Bartholomew's Hospital
West Smithfield, London, UK EC1A 7BE
0171 600 3309, Fax: 0171 600 8579
Support and information.

FINANCIAL ASSISTANCE

Cancer Fund of America
2901 Breezewood Lane
Knoxville, TN 37921
800-578-5284 or 423-938-5281
http://www.cfoa.org
Help with expenses not covered by insurance (food, crutches, medical supplies, liquid dietary supplements). Average grant: $50.00.

The National Transplant Assistance Fund
3475 West Chester Pike, Suite 230
Newtown Square, PA 19073
800-642-8399 or 610-353-9684
http://www.transplantfund.org
Fundraising assistance and donor awareness material to transplant and catastrophic illness patients nationwide. Lists of transplant centers, information on insurance, finances, lodging, statistics.

Social Resource Homepage
University of Maryland Baltimore County, Social Work Department
http://www.gl.umbc.edu/~ddixon1/charitie/national/independ/
List of independent charities maintained for social workers and other caretaking professionals.

The Sparrow Foundation
4192 NW 61st Street
Redmond WA 97756
541-549-1144 x 8307 (Jeff Leeland)
http://www.sparrowfdn.org
Helps families set up fundraising for medical or related family maintenance costs. Call or download application off website. Foundation's non-profit status fund designates $2560 grant for child. Child is matched up with local school, where students/peers earn that grant doing community service, or raising money (foundation will match in addition). Template for fundraising.

Air Travel

Air Care Alliance
6202 S. Lewis Avenue, Suite F2
Tulsa, OK 74136-1014
800-260-9707 or 918-745-0384
http://aircareall.org/
Nationwide association of humanitarian flying organizations.

AirLifeLine
50 Fullerton Court, Suite 200
Sacramento, CA 95825
977-AIRLIFE or 916-641-7800
http://www.airlifeline.org

Corporate Angel Network, Inc.
Westchester County Airport, Building 1
White Plains, NY 10604
914-328-1313, Fax: 800-328-4226
Nationwide nonprofit program gives child (up to age 20) and two adults available seats on corporate private aircraft (will fly donor, too). Patient must be able to walk and travel without life-support system or medical attention.

DreamLine, Inc.
c/o Bob Iverson
117 North Merrill Street
Park Ridge IL 60068
847-910-3940
http://www.bobiverson.com/dreamline
Free airline travel for emergency medical treatment or vacation.

Mission Air Transportation Network
Proctor & Gamble Building
4711 Young Street
North York, Ontario, Canada M2N 6K8
416-222-6335
Free air transport to Canadians in financial need who must travel for medical care.

National Patient Travel Center
Mercy Medical Airlift
800-296-1217 (United States) or 757-318-9145 (other countries)
http://www.PatientTravel.org
Twenty-four-hour hotline referrals to inexpensive or free air service, volunteer pilot organizations, and special airline transport programs.

College Scholarships

Gullikson Foundation College Scholarship Program
8000 Sears Tower
Chicago IL 60606
888-GULLIKSON
Scholarships for brain tumor survivors.

Jay's World Childhood Cancer Foundation College Scholarship Program
5 Knoll Lane
Glen Head NY 11545
516-671-7410
http://www.jaysworld.org
Children cured, in remission, or able to attend college while on treatment can apply.

Credit Counseling

A Consumer Credit Counseling Foundation/National Credit Counseling Agency
877-426-6363
http://www.4-creditcounseling.com
Free, 24-hour counseling. Reduce payments, rates; consolidate debt; stop collection calls. Budgeting, debt management, deferred or excused interest, lower payments, some portion of debt excused. On-line application service.

Genus Credit Management
800-210-4455
http://www.nccs.org
Nonprofit organization. Free debt management and educational programs.

National Foundation for Credit Counseling
8611 Second Avenue, Suite 100
Silver Spring, MD 20910
800-388-2227
http://www.cccs.org
Local financial care centers offer counseling, debt solver, on-line counseling. Free or low-cost.

Drug Reimbursement/Assistance

Pharmaceutical Research and Manufacturers of America
1100 15th Street NW
Washington, DC 20005
202-835-3400
Hotline for physicians: 1-800-PMA-INFO
http://www.phrma.org/search/cures/dpdpap
Directory of patient assistance programs.

Needy Meds
http://www.needymeds.com
Information on patient assistance programs at pharmaceutical companies; oncology drugs, antibiotics, etc.

Government Assistance

Try state and local programs, as well as federal.

Department of Health and Human Services
http://www.hhs.gov/
Oversees agencies that focus on health care issues, insurance, assistance, etc.

Health Care Financing Administration
7500 Security Boulevard
Baltimore, MD 21244
410-786-3000
http://www.hcfa.gov/
Information on Medicaid, Medicare, SCHIP, HIPAA. Publications. Directory of local help.

Health Resources & Services Administration
Hill-Burton Funds: 800-638-0742.
http://www.hrsa.dhhs.gov/osp/dfcr/obtain/consfaq.htm
Hospitals receiving these funds must serve a certain number of uninsured or underinsured patients.

State Children's Health Insurance Program
877-KIDS-NOW
http://www.insurekidsnow.gov
Referral to state program offering low-cost or free health insurance coverage to uninsured children of low-wage, working parents.

Internal Revenue Service
800-TAX-FORM
http://www.irs.ustreas.gov
Publication 502 from library or IRS office will tell you which medical expenses are deductible.

Revenue Canada
800-959-8281
Ask for IT-519R—Medical Expense and Disability Tax Credits.

Social Security Administration
6401 Security Boulevard
Baltimore, MD 21235
800-772-1213 or 800-325-0778 (TTY)
http://www.ssa.gov

FUN STUFF

National Childhood Cancer Awareness Quilt Project
Quilts honor survivors and children who have died as well as raise awareness.
http://www.kidscancerprojects.com

Project Linus
P.O. Box 5621
Bloomington, IL 61702-5621
http://www.projectlinus.org
Hand-made blankets for sick kids.

SpeciaLove
117 Youth Development Court
Winchester, VA 22602
540-667-3774
http://www.speciallove.org/
Local programs, downloadable oncology camp songs (some with Christian slant). Links.

Starbright Foundation
11835 W. Olympic Boulevard, Suite 500
Los Angeles, CA 90064
800-315-2580 or 310-479-1212
http://www.starbright.org
Free products and programs for kids/teenagers. CD-ROM, videos, on-line network. "Videos With Attitude" for teenagers (e.g., *What Am I, Chopped Liver? Communicating With Your Doctor*) teaches how to speak up, ask questions, and feel more in control.

Sunshine Kids Foundation
2814 Virginia Street
Houston, TX 77098
713-524-1264
Free group activities to children with cancer.

Camps

Candlelighters and Association of Cancer Online Resource's Ped-Onc Resource Center both have extensive camp listings. See "Support."

Camp Simcha
151 West 30th Street
New York, NY 10001
877-CHAI-LIFE
http://www.chailifeline.org
National nonprofit Jewish organization Kosher camp.

Children's Oncology Camping Association, International
c/o The Children's Memorial Hospital
2300 Children's Plaza
Chicago, IL 60614
800-737-2667 or 312-880-4564
http://www.coca-intl.org/
Umbrella organization with newsletter, directory. Assists in establishment of new camps.

The Silver Lining Foundation
1490 Ute Avenue
Aspen, CO 81611
970-925-9540
http://www.kidstuff.org
Tennis player Andrea Jaeger's camp. Hope chest, newsletter, gift packs.

Expressive Arts

Changing Images Art Foundation, Inc.
30 Forest Place
Towaco, NJ 07082
973-334-2547, Fax: 973-263-0329
http://www.changingimages.org
Artists bring color and beauty to institutions geared to children. Involve patients, staff, and family in creation of murals.

Children's Art Project
MD Anderson Cancer Center
Houston, TX
800-231-1580
http://www.childrensartproject.org
Books, cards, and art by kids with cancer.

National Storytelling Network
116½ West Main Street
Jonesborough, TN 37659
800-525-4514 or 423-913-8201
http://www.storynet.org
Teacher's guide, links to local storytellers.

Humor

Anatomical Chart Company
8221 North Kimball
Skokie, IL 60076
800-621-7500
Funny props and novelties.

Bearable Times: The Kids' Hospital Network
P.O. Box 533
Harwich, MA 02645
508-430-7122
http://www.harwich.edu/bear/

Humor and Health Letter
P.O. Box 16814
Jackson, MS 39236
601-957-0075
Bimonthly newsletter. Interviews with humor experts, reviews of latest research and books on humor and laughter. $22.00/year.

Humor Project
110 Spring Street
Saratoga Springs, NY 12866
518-587-8770
"Laughing Matters" (quarterly), free catalog of humor and creativity books.

Johns Hopkins University
http://ww2.med.jhu.edu/peds/neonatology/fun.html

Parents Against Cancer
http://www.parentsagainstcancer.com/funny_pages.htm
Funny pages, encouragement. Captain Chemo Comic by teen survivor.

Whole Mirth Catalog
1034 Page Street
San Francisco, CA 94117
415-431-1913
Humorous items, toys, gags, books.

Music

Celebration Shop, Inc.
P.O. Box 355
Bedford, TX 76095
817-268-0020, Fax: 817-285-9548
http://www.celebrationshop.org
Nonprofit organization provides healing experiences for the special needs of children of all ages through performing arts and media.

Peter Alsop's Uplifting Children's Music
Moose School Productions
P.O. Box 960
Topanga, CA 90290
800-676-5480
http://www.peteralsop.com
Audiotape with songs about kids in hospitals.

Songs of Love Foundation
P.O. Box 750809, Dept. P
Forest Hills, NY 11375
800-960-7664 or 718-997-7548
http://www.songsoflove.org
Nonprofit organization produces personalized musical portraits for children and teenagers with chronic or life-threatening diseases.

Pen Pals/Newsletters

Children's Hopes and Dreams Foundation
280 Route 46
Dover, NJ 07801
973-361-7348
http://www.childrenswishes.org
Nonprofit group. Free, worldwide pen-pal program for children ages 5–17 with disabilities, chronic illnesses, or life-threatening illnesses. Retreat weekend program for parents (in NJ, NY, PA, CT) of kids with life-threatening illnesses.

Famous Phone Friends
9109 Sawyer Street
Los Angeles, CA 90035
310-204-5683
Links children confined to a hospital or home due to injury or illness with entertainers and athletes by telephone. Obtain referral from physician, nurse, hospital volunteer, or social worker.

Funletter
Friends Network
P.O. Box 4545
Santa Barbara, CA 93140
805-693-1017
http://www.kidscancernetwork.org
Activities newsletter for children with cancer. $10.00/year for a bimonthly issue. On-line resources.

The Laughter Prescription
Karen Silver
P.O. Box 7985
Northridge, CA 91327
Fun newsletter for parents and professionals.

Love Letters, Inc.
P.O. Box 41675
Chicago IL 60641
630-620-1970
Free service by volunteers who send letters, cards, and gifts to catastrophically ill children. Not pen pals. Confidentiality guaranteed.

Make a Child Smile
http://www.makeachildsmile
Solicits cards/letters for your child.

Products

Beautiful Bald Buddies
888-828-6978
http://www.baldbuddies.com/
Vermont artist Leni Lavin makes dolls for children.

ChemoCare Headwear
420 Hillcrest
Grosse Pointe Farms, MI 48236
http://www.chemocareheadwear.com
Hats, scarves, sleep caps, teddy bears, mouth care, cookbooks, relaxation tapes, other products for adults and children.

The Close Friends Story
Kendal & Co., Ltd.
P.O. Box 1935
Dayton, OH 45401-1935
937-279-0795
http://www.getclosefriends.com
Catheter covers for central lines; links to free games for kids.

Dolls With Disabilities
5959 Triumph Street
Commerce, CA 90840
800-227-3800
Soft-sculptured dolls (19 in.) help children with disabilities develop a positive self-image. $40.00 to $45.00 each.

Funtastic Learning
http://www.funtasticlearng.com
Developmental and fun toys, both challenging and classic.

GloGerm
P.O. Box 189
Moab, UT 84532

800-842-6622
http://www.glogerm.com
Product shows you what you missed when you washed your hands.

Gold Ribbons for Childhood Cancer Awareness
c/o Gigi Thorsen
8814 Oak Valley Drive
Sandy, UT 84093
801-944-2464, Fax: 801-944-0209
http://www.goldribbons.org
$2.50 each; $2.00 shipping for 1-10.

"Hair by Chemo"
P.O. Box 216
Wauzeka, WI 53826
800-729-9713
T-shirts and hats. "not by choice" on back.

Hip Hat
108 West Adalee St.
Tampa, FL 33603
813-447-4287 or 813-229-2377
http://www.hip-hat.com
Hats with hair free to children with cancer.

Illusions in Art Cards
Y&B Associates, Inc.
33 Primrose Lane
Hempstead, NY 11550
518-481-0256
http://www.illusionworks.com/html//_b_associates.html

Kidz With Leukemia
The Degge Group, Ltd.
703-276-0067, Fax: 703-276-0069
http://www.kidzwithleukemia.com
CD-ROM teaches children about leukemia.

Kimo Bear Project, Inc.
http://www.kimobear.org/
Educational and therapeutic play aid bear has central line that can be attached to IV tubing; loses its hair.

Nines
c/o Patty Robison
1814 Larrabee Avenue
Bellingham, WA 98225
360-671-0399
Hats for women and girls. Order a brochure.

S&S Worldwide
800-243-9232
Indoor and outdoor toys and games.

tlc catalog
800-850-9445 FAX 800-757-9997
Helpful products and clothes for cancer patients (mostly for adults, but some helpful things for children).

Wish Fulfillment

Many local organizations grant wishes, too. Get a comprehensive list from Candlelighters or on O'Reilly's Patient-Centered Guides Web site.

Aladdin Children's Charity: Wish Programs
http://www.aladdincharity.org
Provides simple, practical wishes to children in Canada ages 3–16 diagnosed with serious illness or life-threatening medical condition.

Brass Ring Society
551 E. Semoran Boulevard, Suite E-5
Fern Park, FL 32730
800-666-WISH or 407-339-6188
http://www.worldramp.net/brassring

Children's Wish Foundation International
7840 Roswell Road, Suite 301
Atlanta, GA 30350
770-393-WISH or 800-323-WISH
Wishes for terminally ill children in the United States and Europe.

The Children's Wish Foundation of Canada
95 Bayly Street, Suite 404
Ajax, Ontario, Canada L1S 7K8
905-426-5656, 800-267-WISH, or 800-700-4437, Fax: 905-426-4111
http://www.childrenswish.ca/
Provide once-in-a-lifetime experience for children ages 3–18 with life-threatening disease.

Dial-a-Dream
7 Addison Road
Wanstead London England E11 2RG
http://www.dial-a-dream.co.uk/index2.html
Wishes to children in U.K. suffering from life-threatening or debilitating illness.

The Dream Factory, Inc.
1218 S. Third Street
Louisville, KY 40203
800-456-7556 or 502-637-8700
http://www.dreamfactoryinc.com
Grants wishes of seriously or chronically ill children ages 3–13.

Give Kids the World
407-239-2308
Wish granting trips to Walt Disney World.

Grant a Wish Foundation
P.O. Box 21243
Baltimore, MD 21228
800-933-5470 or 410-744-1032
http://www.grant-a-wish.org
Wish granting, in-hospital entertainment, tickets, and several retreat/respite facilities.

Kids, Inc.
9300-D Old Keene Mill Road
Burke, VA 22015
703-455-KIDS
Grants wishes to gravely ill children ages 16 and younger, anywhere in the United States.

The Lisa Madonia Memorial Fund
409 Veloit
Forest Park, IL 60130
708-366-2057, Fax: 708-366-2065
Grants wishes and provides support to 18- to 25-year-olds with cancer. No geographic boundaries, but limited to $300.00.

Make-a-Wish Foundation of America
100 West Clarendon, Suite 2200
Phoenix, AZ 85013
800-722-WISH or 602-279-WISH
http://www.wish.org
Grants wishes to children younger than 18 with life-threatening illnesses. International chapters and affiliates.

A Special Wish Foundation, Inc.
2244 S. Hamilton Road, Suite 202
Columbus, OH 43232
800-486-WISH or 614-575-WISH
http://www.spwish.org
Grants wishes to children younger than 20. Chapters throughout the United States and in Moscow, Russia.

Starlight Children's Foundation
5900 Wilshire Boulevard, Suite 2530
Los Angeles, CA 90036
800-274-7827 or 323-634-0080
http://www.starlight.org
Wishes for seriously ill children ages 4–18. Chapters in United States, Canada, Australia, and UK.

Sunshine Foundation
1041 Mill Creek Drive
Feasterville, PA 19053
215-396-4770
http://www.sunshinefoundation.org
Wishes to chronically or terminally ill children ages 3–21.

A Wish With Wings
Arlington, TX
http://www.awishwithwings.org
Grants wishes to children with serious illnesses.

PSYCHOSOCIAL

American Association of Pastoral Counselors
9504-A Lee Highway
Fairfax, VA 22031-2303
703-385-6967
http://www.aapc.org

American Association of Sex Educators, Counselors, and Therapists
P.O. Box 5488
Richmond, VA 23220-0488
http://www.aasect.org

American Family Therapy Academy
2020 Pennsylvania Avenue NW, Suite 273
Washington, DC 20006
202-944-2776

American Psychological Association
750 First Street NE
Washington, DC 20002-4242
202-336-5500
http://www.apa.org
Finding Help: How to Choose a Psychologist free brochure.

American Psychiatric Association
1400 K Street NW
Washington, DC 20005
888-357-7924
http://www.psych.org

Anxiety Disorders Association of America
11900 Parklawn Drive, Suite 100
Rockville, MD 20852
301-231-9350
http://www.adaa.org

Canadian Mental Health Association
2160 Yonge Street, 3rd Floor
Toronto, Ontario, Canada M4S 2Z3
416-484-7750
http://www.cmha.ca

Federation of Families for Children's Mental Health
1101 King Street, Suite 420
Alexandria, VA 22314
703-684-7710
http://www.ffcmh.org

Find-a-Therapist, Inc.
5150 North 16th Street, Suite A-116
Phoenix, AZ 85016
800-865-0686 or 602-294-6677
http://www.find-a-therapist.com
Referrals at no charge to client.

International Association of Marriage and Family Counselors
225 Yale Avenue
Claremont, CA 91711
http://www.iamfc.org

National Association of School Psychologists
4340 East-West Highway, Suite 402
Bethesda, MD 20814
301-657-0270
http://www.naspwebonline.org/index2.html

National Association of Social Workers
750 First Street NE, Suite 700
Washington, DC 20020
800-638-8799 or 202-408-8600
http://www.socialworkers.org

National Institute of Marriage and Family Relations
6116 Rolling Road, Suite 306
Springfield, VA 22152
703-569-2400

National Institutes of Mental Health
Public Inquiries Branch
6001Executive Boulevard, Room 8184 MSC 9663
Bethesda, MD 20892-9663
301-443-4513
http://www.nimh.nih.gov

National Mental Health Association
1021 Prince Street
Alexandria, VA 22314-2971
800-969-6642 or 703-684-5968
http://www.nmha.org

Behavioral Techniques

The Academy for Guided Imagery
P.O. Box 2070
Mill Valley, CA 94942

800-726-2070
http://www.healthy.net/agi/index_ie.html
Referral to practitioner skilled in teaching children visualization techniques.

American Art Therapy Association, Inc.
1202 Allanson Road
Mundelein, IL 60060-3808
888-290-0878 or 874-949-6064
http://www.arttherapy.org

American Massage Therapy Association
820 Davis Street
Evanston, IL 60201
847-864-0123
http://www.aamtamassage.org

American Music Therapy Association
8455 Colesville Road, Suite 1000
Silver Spring, MD 20910
301-589-3300
http://www.musictherapy.org

American Psychotherapy & Medical Hypnosis Association
280 Island Avenue, #404
Reno, NV 89501
775-786-5650
http://www.APMHA.com

The American Society of Clinical Hypnosis
130 E. Elm Court, Suite 201
Roselle, IL 60172-2000
630-980-4740
http://www.asch.net
Professional organization will refer you to local hypnotherapists on request. Videos/books.

Association for Applied Psychophysiology & Biofeedback
10200 West 44th Avenue, Suite 304
Wheat Ridge, CO 80033
303-422-8436

Association for Therapeutic Humor
4534 West Butler Drive
Glendale, AZ 85302
623-934-6068
http://www.aath.org/home_1.html
Networking source for practical applications of humor in all therapeutic modalities. Newsletter.

The Children's Legacy
P.O. Box 300305
Denver, CO 80203
303-830-7595
http://members.aol.com/Tclphoto
Books and resource materials for children. Photography, writing, drawing to document feelings and thoughts associated with illness. Workshops. Journals created by children available to purchase, including *My Stupid Illness; Let Me Show You My World*, ages 5–18; *An Alphabet About Kids With Cancer.*

Childswork/Childsplay Center for Applied Psychology
135 Dupont Street
Plainview, NY 11803-0760
800-962-1141
http://www.childswork.com
Addresses social and emotional needs of children and adolescents. Books/tapes/games/posters to help with conflict resolution, anger control, self-esteem, positive thinking, anxiety. For therapists, teachers, parents.

Spinoza, the Bear Who Speaks From the Heart
1876 Minnehaha Avenue West
St. Paul, MN 55104-1029
800-CUB-BEAR or 651-644-7251
http://www.spinozabear.com
Therapeutic stuffed bear with tape player inside. Nine cassette tapes, including relaxation, self-esteem, imagination, grief and loss. Ask your social worker, psychologist, or special needs state agency to refer you.

Child Development

Child Life Council
11820 Parklawn Drive, #202
Rockville, MD 20852
301-881-7090
http://www.childlife.org
Professional organization. Use play, recreation, education, self-expression, and theories of child development to promote well-being of children and families in health care settings. Publications: *For Teenagers: Visiting the Hospital* ($2.00); *Repeated or Extended Hospitalizations* ($2.00); *Pain, Pain, Go Away: Helping Children with Pain* ($2.00).

Child Development Institute
17853 Santiago Boulevard, Suite 107-328
Villa Park, CA 92861
714-998-8617
http://www.cdipage.com/stress.shtml
Resources, articles on teenagers, stress, learning disabilities, sibling rivalry, ADHD, behavior, disorders.

Institute for Child Development
http://www.kiddsmart.com
Educational resources for social and emotional development. For teachers, parents, and counselors. Research summaries, educational games.

National Academy for Child Development
P.O. Box 380
Huntsville, UT 84317
801-621-8606, Fax: 801-621-8389
http://www.nacd.org
Home programs, referrals to services and evaluations, information on learning disabilities, home schooling, deafness.

National Institutes of Child Health and Human Development
Building 31, Room 2A-32
9000 Rockville Pike

Bethesda, MD 20892
301-496-5133
http://www.nichd.nih.gov

National Network for Child Care
http://www.nncc.org/Child.Dev/stage.page.html
Developmental stages.

New York University Child Study Center
http://www.aboutourkids.org
Information about special education and law, ADA, IEPs, gifted children, dealing with bullies, ADHD, choosing a mental health professional, eating disorders, anxiety disorders, selective mutism. Warning signs of mental illness, questions to ask the pediatrician and other tips.

Depression

National Depressive and Manic Depressive Association
730 North Franklin, Suite 501
Chicago, IL 60610-7204
800-82-NDMDA (800-826-3632)
http://www.ndmda.org
Educational brochures, referrals to support groups. Information on adolescent depression; bipolar disorder screening tool; bookstore.

Drug Abuse

Alcoholics Anonymous World Services
475 Riverside Drive, 11th Floor
New York, NY 10115
http://www.alcoholics-anonymous.org
Referrals, information for families and professionals. Questions to ask yourself. You can also look in a phone book for a local chapter.

Narcotics Anonymous
P.O. Box 999
Van Nuys, CA 91409
818-773-9999
http://www.wsoinc.com

Psychosocial Oncology

Association of Pediatric Oncology Social Workers
http://www.aposw.org

Journal of Psychosocial Oncology
The Haworth Press, Inc.
10 Alice Street
Binghamton, NY 13904-1580
800-342-9678

Psych Central
http://www.psychcentral.com
Web sites, newsgroups, mailing lists, and support for mental health.

Vital Options
"The Group Room" Cancer Radio Talk Show
800-GRP-ROOM or 818-508-5657
http://www.vitaloptions.org
Weekly syndicated call-in cancer radio talk show for patients, survivors, families, physicians, therapists. Sunday, 4–6 p.m. EST. Live Web simulcast.

SUPPORT

American Cancer Society
1599 Clifton Road, NE
Atlanta, GA 30329-4251
800-ACS-2345
http://www.cancer.org
Information, books and pamphlets (many free), videos, support, financial assistance. Look Good, Feel Better has teenager program. Local chapters.

American Self-Help Clearinghouse
Northwest Covenant Medical Center
100 Hanover Avenue, 2nd Floor, Suite 202
Cedar Knolls, NJ 07927
973-326-6789
http://www.njgroups.org
Referrals to self-help and support groups.

Association of Cancer Online Resources, Inc.
http://www.acor.org
Dozens of e-mail support groups (listservs), general and specific topics, including ALL, pediatric oncology, retinoblastoma, hospice, long-term survivors. Messages archived. Hosts Web sites, including Pediatric Oncology Resource Center, Childhood Leukemia, and Neuroblastoma. Ped-Onc Resource Center gives medical and practical information, stories from families, help with school issues, getting kids to take pills, giving GCSF shots, finances, lists of resources, camps, links to numerous organizations, Web sites.

Cancer Care, Inc.
275 7th Avenue
New York, NY 10001
800-813-HOPE (4673) or 212-302-2400
http://www.cancercare.org
Professional counseling over the telephone. Referrals, support groups, educational programs, financial assistance for nonmedical expenses.

Canadian Cancer Society
10 Alcorn Avenue, Suite 200
Toronto, Ontario, Canada M4V3B1
888-939-3333
http://www.cancer.ca
Peer support, camps, lodges, financial aid, volunteer drivers.

Candlelighters Childhood Cancer Foundation
3910 Warner Street
Kensington, MD 20895
800-366-CCCF or 301-962-3520
http://www.candlelighters.org
Information clearinghouse, support groups, newsletters. Ombudsman referral (second medical opinions, insurance, employment, legal, school issues). Camp and wish foundation lists. Booklets, books, reprints of medical journal articles. On-line message board. Extensive

suggested reading list, many publications available free or low cost. The best resource for families.

Candlelighters Childhood Cancer Foundation Canada
55 Eglinton Avenue East, Suite 401
Toronto, Ontario, Canada M4P 1G8
800-363-1062 (in Canada) or 416-489-6440
http://www.candlelighters.ca
Books, resource guide, computer searches for protocols, match with families.

Center for Attitudinal Healing
19 Main Street
Tiburon, CA 94920
415-435-5022
http://www.healingcenter.org
Supportive programs and activities to ease stress and tension of illness. Telephone and pen-pal programs. Siblings. Art and music activities. Parent groups. Educational programs.

Chai Lifeline
151 West 30th Street
New York, NY 10001
212-465-1300 or 877-CHAI-LIFE
http://www.chailifeline.org/
Programs for Jewish families. Medical referrals, support groups, visits to hospitalized and housebound children, financial aid, processing insurance claims, toy distribution, transportation, crisis intervention, kosher camp, wish fulfillment, sibling program, publications, children's magazines, big brother/sister. Homebound Educational Learning Program in Jewish studies.

Children's Cancer Association
7524 SW Macadam, B
Portland, OR 97219 or
P.O. Box 19734
Portland, OR 97219
503-244-3141, Fax: 503-423-7466
http://www.KidsCancerHelp.org
Web site/book offer resource list; local programs

Children's Cancer Resources on the Internet
http://childrenscancer.20m.com

Coping Magazine
P.O. Box 682268
2019 North Carothers
Franklin, TN 37068
615-790-2400, Fax: 615-794-0179
Bimonthly publication for people whose lives have been touched by cancer. Separate magazine: *Coping —Living With Cancer.*

National Center for Grandparent Support
PACER Center
8161 Normandale Boulevard
Minneapolis, MN 55437
952-838-9000
http://www.PACER.org/parent/grand.htm
Support and information for grandparents of children with special needs.

National Children's Cancer Society
1015 Locust Street, Suite 600
St. Louis, MO 63101
314-241-1600 or 800-5-FAMILY
http://www.children-cancer.org
Financial assistance, education, information, emotional support. Advocacy program to help with insurance, home care, supplies, respite care, donor registries.

National Parent-to-Parent Support & Information System
4118 East First Street
Blue Ridge, GA 30513
800-651-1151 or 706-632-8822
http://www.iser.com/NPPSIS-GA.html
Nonprofit organization links families, information on managed care, parent and disability programs.

National Self-Help Clearinghouse
25 West 43rd Street, Room 620
New York, NY 10036
212-642-2944

R. A. Bloch Cancer Foundation
4435 Main Street, Suite 500
Kansas City, MO 64111
800-433-0464 or 816-932-8453
http://www.blochcancer.org
Informational materials, list of institutions that offer second opinions. Free hotline connects newly diagnosed with survivors. *Guide for Cancer Supporters: Step-by-Step Ways to Help a Relative or Friend Fight Cancer.* Groups in Missouri and Kansas.

SKIP (Sick Kids Need Involved People)
545 Madison Avenue, 13th Floor
New York, NY 10022
212-421-9161
Local chapters.

Sickkids Mailing List
E-mail: listserv@maelstrom.stjohns.edu
Moderated with adult supervision e-mail support group for children younger than 18 who have serious illnesses. Team of children who serve as discussion managers. To subscribe, leave e-mail subject line blank, in the message body type: subscribe SICKKIDS <your first and last name>. Adults can e-mail questions or concerns to advisor: Sickkids-request@maelstrom.stjohns.edu.

Squirrel Tales
http://www.squirreltales.com/
Practical tips and encouragement, stories from families.

Advocacy, Legal, and Insurance Help

American Bar Association
http://www.abanet.org
Directory by state, referral service, lawyer locator. Commission on Mental and Physical Disability Law.

American Council on Life Insurance
1001 Pennsylvania Avenue NW
Washington, DC 20004
http://www.acli.com
Information on brokers who specialize in high-risk life insurance.

Center for Patient Advocacy
1350 Beverly Road, Suite 108
McLean, VA 22101
800-846-7444 or 703-748-0400
http://www.patientadvocacy.org

Childhood Cancer Ombudsman Program
P.O. Box 595
Burgess, VA 22432
Fax: 804-580-2502 or 2304
E-mail: gpmonaco@rivnet.net
Free service assists families and survivors with insurance, second medical opinion, disability rights, employment, discrimination, education, medical care, health care cost coverage. Medical library searches, analysis of employment contracts, legal appeals, filing complaints, job interviews, outside review. Citations to medical and legal literature.

Children's Health Environmental Coalition
P.O. Box 1540
Princeton, NJ 08542
609-252-1915

Children's Health Matters
http://www.childrenshealthmatters.org
Helps uninsured children apply for Medicaid, state health insurance.

The Disability Rights Education and Defense Fund
2212 Sixth Street
Berkeley, CA 94710
800-466-4232 or 510-644-2555
http://www.dredf.org
National law and policy center answers questions about ADA, explains how to file complaints. Dispute resolution.

Equal Employment Opportunity Commission
800-669-4000
http://www.eeoc.gov/
Enforces Title 1 of the ADA (employment). Call for enforcement publications.

Families USA
1334 G Street NW, Suite 300
Washington, DC 20005
202-628-3030
http://www.familiesusa.org
List of state agencies regulating health care and information on state managed care laws. Publications list, listserv. Fights for insurance reform.

Foundation for Accountability
503-223-2228
http://www.facct.org
Information about health care.

Institute for Child Health Policy
http://www.ichp.edu/managed/materials/purchaser/Default.htm
Evaluating managed care plans for children with special health needs: a purchaser's tool.

Institute of Health Care Research & Policy
Georgetown University
http://www.georgetown.edu/research/ihcrp
Insurance help. Consumer guides by state. *Health Care Research & Policy, Kennedy-Kassenbaum Insurance Guides. A Consumer Guide for Getting & Keeping Health Insurance* for each state, available to read on-line or to print out (http://www.healthinsuranceinfo.net).

Job Accommodation Network
West Virginia University
918 Chestnut Ridge Road, Suite 1
P.O. Box 6080
Morgantown, WV 26506-6080
800-526-7234 (United States) or 800-526-2262 (Canada)
http://janweb.icdi.wvu.edu
International consulting service that provides free information about how employers can accommodate people with disabilities. Not a placement service.

My Health Score
http://www.mecqa.com
Prices on procedures and hospital stays to fight the "reasonable and customary" claim by insurance company. Provider rating reports.

National Association of Insurance Commissioners
http://www.naic.org/consumer.htm
State-designated contacts for resolving insurance complaints.

National Association of Protection and Advocacy Systems, Inc.
900 Second Street NE, Suite 211
Washington, DC 20002
202-408-9514
http://www.protectionandadvocacy.com
Help with social security, disability rights, special education law.

National Insurance Consumer Organization
121 North Payne Street
Alexandria, VA 22314
703-549-8050
Consumer advocacy organization independent of insurance industry. Provides books, newsletters, information for high-risk insurance buyers. Annual membership fee.

National Legal Aid & Defender Association
202-452-0620

Patient Advocacy Coalition
3801 East Florida Avenue, Suite 400
Denver, CO 80210
303-512-0544

Patient Advocate Foundation
753 Thimble Shoals Boulevard, Suite B
Newport News, VA 23606
800-532-5274 or 757-873-6668
http://www.patientadvocate.org
Information on drug assistance programs; insurance commissioner information by state.

Privacy Rights Clearinghouse
1717 Kettner Avenue, Suite 105
San Diego, CA 92101
619-298-3395
http://www.privacyrights.org

Public Citizen Health Research Group
1600 20th Street NW
Washinton, DC 20009
202-588-1000
http://www.citizen.org/hrg
Books: *Medical Records; Getting Yours; Questionable Doctors.*

U.S. Department of Labor
http://www.dol.gov
Insurance help, information about the Family and Medical Leave Act, etc.

U.S. Department of Justice
Civil Rights Division, Public Access Section
800-841-0301
http://www.usdoj.gov/crt/ada.html

Bereavement

Alive Alone, Inc.
c/o Kay Bevington
11115 Dull Robinson Road
Van Wert, OH 45891
http://www.alivealone.org
Support for parents whose only child is deceased or who have lost all of their children. Newsletter.

Bereavement & Hospice Support Netline
http://www.ubalt.edu/bereavement
Directory of no-fee bereavement support groups and services by state/national.

Bereavement Publishing, Inc.
5125 North Union Boulevard
Colorado Springs, CO 80918
888-604-HOPE
http://www.bereavementmag.com
Bereavement: A Magazine of Hope and Healing. Also, cards, gifts, video, music.

Bereaved Parents of the USA
P.O. Box 95
Park Forest, IL 60466-0095
http://www.bereavedparentsusa.org
Local chapters, support, books/tapes, conferences. Also for siblings and grandparents.

Grief, Inc.
9016 Taylorsville Road, #181
Louisville, KY 40229
502-671-0535
http://www.griefinc.com
Darcie Sims, PhD, Grief Therapist Articles and publications. Guided-imagery tape. Publications include *Why Are The Casseroles Always Tuna? A Loving Look at the Lighter Side of Grief* and *Am I Still A Sister?* Inspirational messages and tapes.

The Centre for Living with Dying
554 Mansion Park Drive
Santa Clara, CA 95054
408-980-9801
http://www.thecentre.org
Educational program for students, teachers, staff, parents. Design assemblies for school population to acknowledge and deal with the loss.

The Compassionate Friends National Office
P.O. Box 3696
Oak Brook, IL 60522-3696
630-990-0010 or 877-969-0010
http://www.compassionatefriends.org
Support for bereaved families: local chapters, telephone support. Newsletters for parents and siblings. Books, audio, and video materials on adult and sibling grief. Audiocassettes: siblings, marriage, single parent, fathers, holidays, anger, recovery. Recordings of workshops: "Mourning," "Emotional Healing," "When Is Professional Help Needed?" "Understanding Sibling Grief," "Where Is God in All of This?" "Dreams and Unusual Happenings," "Anger, God and You," "Siblings 1–12 Years," "Writing When It Hurts."

Compassionate Friends of Canada/ Les Amis Compatissants du Canada
685 William Avenue
Winnipeg, Manitoba, Canada R3E OZ2

Day-by-Day
E-mail: gigi@lgcy.com
On-line parent support group about end of life, hospice, and bereavement. Also has list for teenage siblings.

The Dougy Center
National Center for Grieving Children and Families
P.O. Box 86852
Portland, OR 97286
503-775-5683
http://www.dougy.org
Referrals to local support services. Free bibliography. Publications.

Golden Healing Publishing
149 Little Quarry Mews
Gaithersburg, MD 20878
301-670-1027
http://www.webhealing.com
Psychotherapist Tom Golden's site for and about fathers/men grieving. Excerpts from his books.

The Good Grief Program
Peds @ Boston Medical Center
1 Boston Medical Center, Mat 5
Boston, MA 02118
617-414-4005

Local and national training in crisis intervention to schools and community groups to help children and adolescents when a friend is terminally ill or dies. Consultations to teachers, administrators, group leaders, parents: how to respond to needs of children. Books and videos. Assists school in enlisting support of local resources to assure continuation of program.

GriefNet
http://www.rivendell.org/
E-mail support groups. Kidsaid compassion site for kids. Library, bookstore, resources, memorials.

Growth House, Inc.
415-255-9045
http://www.growthhouse.org/
Information on end-of-life care, hospice and home care, pain management, grief, bereavement.

In Loving Memory
1416 Green Run Lake
Reston, VA 22090
703-435-0608
http://www.inlvmemory.org
Support for death of only child.

Last Acts
Robert Wood Johnson Foundation
P.O. Box 2316
Princeton, NJ 08543-2316
609-452-8701
http://www.lastacts.org
Call-to-action campaign designed to improve care at end of life. Bring issues out in open and help individuals and organizations pursue better ways to care for the dying.

Pen-Parents, Inc.
P.O. Box 8738
Reno, NV 89507-8738
702-826-7332
http://www.penparents.com
Support network for bereaved parents. Articles, chat, virtual postcards, newsletter.

Rainbows
1111 Tower Road
Shaumberg, IL 60173-4305
800-266-3206
Referrals to peer support groups for parent, child, adolescent, college-age suffering from loss of sibling, parent, spouse, and so forth.

Rothman–Cole Center for Sibling Loss
1456 W. Montrose Avenue
Chicago, IL 60613
773-274-4600
Sibling bereavement, help surviving children cope with loss and grow.

The Shiva Foundation
http://www.goodgrief.org
Non-profit, non-sectarian organization offers support in grieving process. Workshops, retreats, book.

The Sometimes Line
705 Noth Avenue
La Grande, OR 97850
541-962-7984
http://www.thesometimesline.com/sometimesline.html
Greeting cards with comforting verses.

TeenAge Grief, Inc. (TAG)
P.O. Box 220034
Newhall, CA 91322-0034
661-253-1932
http://www.smartlink.net/~tag/index.html
Nonprofit organization teaches professionals how to help teenagers with grief. Has links and products, including *No One Ever Told Us* video and *Teen Grief—Teens Tell Their Story* audiotape.

Teens and Therapy
http://www.teens-and-therapy.com
Reassurance and information for teenagers about therapy, crisis, depression, normal pressures, suicide.

TIGERS (Teens in Grief: Educate, Rebuild, Support)
521 Garden Court
Quincy, IL 62301
Support to educate teenagers in grieving process and comfort them.

Out of the Blu'
P.O. Box 12111
El Paso, TX 79912
800-398-5661
Grief cards designed by a certified professional grief counselor.

Bone Marrow Transplant

Blood and Marrow Transplant Information Network
2900 Skokie Valley Road, Suite B
Highland Park, IL 60035
888-597-7674 or 847-433-3313
http://www.bmtinfonet.org
Transplant centers, drug database, resources. Reference book: *Bone Marrow Transplants: A Book of Basics for Patients.* Newsletter published six times a year. Free.

BMT Family Support Network
P.O. Box 845
Avon, CT 06001
800-826-9376
Information, resources, telephone links to families, bereavement.

BMT Mailing List
http://www.ai.mit.edu/people/laurel/Bmt-talk/bmt-talk.html
To subscribe, leave subject line blank and in body of message type: subscribe. Monitored discussion group.

BMTInformation
http://www.bmtinfo.org
Information; ask the expert.

National Bone Marrow Transplant Link
29209 Northwestern Highway, #624
Southfield, MI 48034
800-LINK-BMT or 810-932-8483

Peer support, library, information, suggestions for financial assistance.

Brain Tumor

Virtual Trials
http://virtualtrials.com/
Brain tumor forums and mailing lists, special needs

Educating Classmates (see also Videos and Books)

CancerEd
http://hometown.aol.com
90-minute workshop presentations to educate students (grades 3–12) or healthcare professionals about childhood cancer. Good way to start dialogue. Video, classroom discussion, presentation of medical apparatus, and art exploration, plus survivor speakers available.

Bandaides and Blackboards
http://funrsc.fairfield.edu/~jfleitas/contents.html
Information for kids, teachers, parents.

Kids on the Block
9385C Gerwig Lane
Columbia MD 21046.
800-368-KIDS.
Video *Each & Every One,* 1992. Puppet program helps students be sensitive to issues faced by people with disabilities. Book I grades K–3 (blind, wheelchair, slow learner); Book II grades 4–6 (hearing, learning disability, cancer).

Necessary Pictures Film & Media
P.O. Box 107, Old Chelsea Station, New York NY 10011-0107
800-221-3170
http://hometown.aol.com/cancered
Workshop presentations for students in grades 3–12 or healthcare professionals. Video, workbook, teacher's guide.

Zink the Zebra Foundation, Inc.
5150 North Port Washington Road
Suite 151
Milwaukee WI 53217
414-963-4484
http://www.zinkthezebra.org
Nonprofit organization presents dynamic programs to schools to educate and encourage compassion and acceptance for children and adults with cancer or other illness or physical difference. Grades K-8. Also scouting programs and preschool programs. Book, videos, posters, other products. Web site has fun pages for children.

Facial Difference

AboutFace International
123 Edward Street, Suite 1003
Toronto, Ontario, Canada M5G 1E2
800-665-FACE
http://www.aboutfaceinternational.org
Support and information network concerned with facial difference. Educational programs.

AboutFace U.S.A.
P.O. Box 458
Crystal Lake IL 60014
888-486-1209
http://www.aboutface2000.org

Let's Face It
P.O. Box 29972
Bellingham, WA 98228
360-676-7325
http://www.faceit.org
U.S. branch of international mutual-help network for facial differences. Support, educational services, newsletter.

Genetics

Genetic Alliance, Inc.
4301 Connecticut Avenue NW, #404
Washington, DC 20008
800-336-GENE or 202-966-5557
http://www.geneticalliance.org/
Referrals to support and information organizations.

The National Society of Genetic Counselors
233 Canterbury Drive
Wallingford, PA 19086
610-872-7608 (Voicemail)
http://www.nsgc.org/resourcelink.asp
Referrals to local genetic counseling services.

Hospice

Children's Hospice International
2202 Mount Vernon Avenue, Suite 3C
Alexandria, VA 22301
800-2-4-CHILD or 703-684-0330
http://www.chionline.org
Clearinghouse for support groups and research programs, educational materials, pain management.

Christian Nursing Hospice, Inc.
http://christiannursing.org/index.htm
Tips to help those facing serious illness, dying person's bill of rights, hospice philosophy.

Hospice Foundation of America
2001 South Street NW, Suite 300
Washington, DC 20009
800-854-3402
http://www.hospicefoundation.org

Hospicelink
Hospice Education Institution
190 Westbrook Road
Essex, CT 06426-1510
800-331-1620
http://www.hospiceworld.org
Referrals to local support services, information about hospice and palliative care.

National Hospice Organization Help Line
1901 North Moore Street, Suite 901
Arlington, VA 22209
800-658-8898
http://www.nho.org

National Hospice & Palliative Care Organization
1700 Diagonal Road, Suite 300
Alexandria, VA 22314
800-658-8898 or 703-837-1500
http://www.nhpco.org
Bibliography of children's literature on death and dying, how to find hospice care. Conferences, books, pamphlets.

National Institute for Jewish Hospice
8723 Alden Drive, Suite 5107
Los Angeles, CA 90048
800-446-4448 or 323-467-7423

Medical Accreditation/ Certification (choosing a doctor/hospital)

American Academy of Pediatric Dentistry
http://www.aapd.org
Find a dentist.

American Board of Medical Specialties
http://www.abms.org
Find out whether doctor is board-certified.

Best Doctors Worldwide
800-675-1199
http://www.bestdoctors.com

Joint Commission on Accreditation of Healthcare Organizations
One Renaissance Boulvard
Oakbrook Terrace, IL 60181
630-792-5000
http://www.jcaho.org
Quality Chek: see if your hospital is accredited.

Health Grades
http://www.healthgrades.com
Results of patient satisfaction surveys on doctors, hospitals, hospice programs, etc.

Searchpointe
http://www.searchpointe.com
Verify credentials and get disciplinary information on doctors for $9.95.

Medical Information

American Society for Clinical Laboratory Science
http://www.ascls.org/labtesting/index.htm
Professionals answer questions about laboratory values.

Association of Pediatric Oncology Nurses
4700 West Lake Avenue
Glenview, IL 60025
847-375-4624
http://www.apon.org
Has handbooks on neuroblastoma, osteosarcoma, Ewing's, Wilm's, rhabdomyosarcoma, chemotherapy. Journal; legislative updates.

Children's Cancer Web
http://www.CancerIndex.org/ccw
Overview of Web pages with links (UK).

Center Watch
http://www.centerwatch.com
Clinical trials listing service.

Doctor's Doctor
http://www.thedoctorsdoctor.com
Pathologist's Web site helps you understand lab reports.

Healthfinder
http://www.healthfinder.gov
Directory of medical dictionaries, news sites, links to private information providers.

Lymphoma Information Network
http://www.lymphomainfo.net/lymphoma.html
Information about childhood Hodgkin's and no-Hodgkin's disease. Links, resources.

Med Help International
http://www.medhelp.org
Nonprofit consumer health information library. Medical glossary, articles, messages from the Medical Forums, articles from other Internet sites, and links to support groups.

Medical Matrix
http://www.medmatrix.org
Peer-reviewed, up-to-date clinical medical resources. Links to hundreds of sites ranked by medical experts.

Medscape
http://www.medscape.com/Home/Topics/oncology/oncology.html
Database of medical journal articles, dictionaries, drug information, medical images. Can search Medline (National Library of Medicine).

National Library of Medicine
http://www.nlm.nih.gov
Links to 24 biomedical journals, some free, some by subscription only.
Medline/PubMed: Database of medical information, medical journal citations, and abstracts.

National Network of Libraries of Medicine
800-338-7657

Online Medical Dictionary
http://www.graylab.ac.uk/omd/index.html

Quackwatch
http://www.quackwatch.com
Dr. Stephen Barrett's site combats health-related frauds, myths, and fads.

Rxlist
http://www.rxlist.com
Drug FAQs, patient monographs, medical encyclopedia, newsletter.

Clinical Trials Sites
http://ctep.info.nih.giv/relsites.htm
http://clinicaltrials.gov

Cord Blood Sites
http://www.cordblood.org

Parent's Guide to Choosing a Private Cord Blood Bank
http://www.parentsguide cordblood.com

Children's Hospital Oakland
Cord blood banking program
510-450-7605
http://www.siblingcordblood.org

Medical Support

HealthTouch
http://www.healthtouch.com
Information on drugs, vitamins, natural medicines; resource directory.

Medic Alert Foundation
2323 Colorado Avenue
Turlock, CA 95380
800-432-5378
http://www.medicalert.org
Bracelets, medallions for patients. Information on allergies, treatments, diagnosis, contact information, etc. Call 888-633-4298 or download Children's Emergency Information form for Children With Special Needs. Treatment information can be inputted.

National Neutropenia Network
6348 North Milwaukee Avenue
Box 205
Chicago, IL 60646
800-638-8768 or 312-792-8151
http://www.neutropenia.org

National Center for Complementary and Alternative Medicine
P.O. Box 8218
Silver Spring, MD 20907-8218
888-644-6226 or 301-402-2466
http://www.mccam.nih.gov/nccam
Information clearinghouse; medical journal articles.

Patient-Centered Guides
O'Reilly & Associates, Inc.
http://www.patientcenters.com
On-line excerpts from books in series, including Nancy Keene's excellent parent guides on childhood cancer. Information and tips. Links to onconurse.com.

Pediatrics Home Care Guide
http://www.hmc.psu.edu/pennstatechildrens/Hematologyoncology/homeguide/Homeguide.html
Practical information on caring for child with cancer at home, medical and social issues. For each topic: understanding the problem, when to get professional help, what you can do, possible obstacles.

Pediatric Services of America, Inc.
310 Technology Parkway
Norcross, GA 30092
800-950-1580, Referral center: 800-666-8865
http://www.psakids.com
Visiting nurses, pediatric home care.

Severe Chronic Neutropenia International Registry
Puget Sound Plaza
1325 4th Avenue, Suite 1365
Seattle, WA 98101-2509
800-726-4463 or 206-543-9749
http://depts.washington.edu/registry

Society of Critical Care Medicine
8101 East Kaiser Boulevard, 3rd Floor
Anaheim, CA 92808-2259
714-282-6000
http://www.sccm.org/consumer/consum_home_set.html
Information on critical care medicine (ICU) for professionals.

Visiting Nurse Associations of America
11 Beacon Street, Suite 910
Boston, MA 02108
617-523-4042
http://www.vnaa.org/Home.htm
More than 500 community associations in the United States provide community-based home care services, including skilled nurses, therapists, and home health care aides. Home care resources; VNA directory.

Nutrition

American Institute for Cancer Research
1759 R Street NW
Washington, DC 20069
800-843-8114 (hotline, 9-5 EST)
http://www.aicr.org/aicr
Registered dietician available to answer questions. Free materials on how to lower cancer risk. Eating hints.

The Oley Foundation
214 Hun Memorial
Albany Medical Center, A-28
Albany, NY 12208-3478
800-776-OLEY or 518-262-5079 (outside United States)
http://www.oley.org
Free information and support to patients requiring home nutritional support. Regional coordinators. Educational materials.

Society for Nutritional Oncology Adjuvant Therapy
3455 Salt Creek Lane
Arlington Heights, IL 60005
800-704-NOAT or 847-342-6484
http://www.noat.org

Pain

Agency for Health Care Research & Quality
800-358-9295

http://text.nlm.nih.gov/
Guidelines for management of postoperative and procedural pain in infants and children.

American Pain Society
4700 West Lake Avenue
Glenview, IL 60025
847-375-4715, Fax: 877-734-8758 (toll free)
http://www.ampainsoc.org/
Referrals to pain treatment centers; articles, news, links, journal.

American Society of Pain Management Nurses
7794 Grow Drive
Pensacola, FL 32514
888-34-ASPMN
http://www.aspmn.org

City of Hope Pain/Palliative Care Resource Center
1500 East Duarte Road
Duarte, CA 91010
818-301-8111 (ext. 3829)
http://mayday.coh.org
Publications, pain assessment scales, nondrug pain interventions.

International Pain Foundation
909 NE 43rd Street, Suite 306
Seattle, WA 98105-6020
206-547-2157
Publications about pain for general public. Fosters and encourages research.

National Foundation for the Treatment of Pain
1330 Skyline Drive, #21
Monterey, CA 93940
831-655-8812
http://www.paincare.org
Nonprofit organization offers support for patients suffering from intractable pain.

The Pediatric Pain Letter
Psychology Department
Dalhousie University
Halifax, Nova Scotia, Canada B3H 4J1
Fax: 902-494-6585
Quarterly publication, reviews scientific literature, reviews books. $25.00/year.

Wisconsin Cancer Pain Initiative
1300 University Avenue, Room 4720
Madison, WI 53706
608-265-4013
http://www.wisc.edu.molphorm/wcpi
Educational materials, regulatory updates, links to state initiatives. *Handbook of Cancer Pain Management.*

Talaria
http://www.talaria.org
Information on pain medications, clinical guidelines, library. For professionals.

Center for Control of Pain in Children and Adults
http://pedspain.nursing.uiowa.edu/
Helping children assess and describe pain, understand pain medications. Kids' drawings.

Practical Help

Angel Locks, Inc.
P.O. Box 7116
North Arlington, NJ 07031
877-93-LOCKS
http://www.angellocks.org
Free wigs for kids (up to age 18)

Hotels/Motels in Partnership, Inc.
602-264-0228
Safe home system for women and children who need emergency housing.

The Karing Book: A Patient's Pal
80601 Driver Road
Tygh Valley, OR 97063
Organizer/journal in neat binder: calendar, diary, charts, places for notes on meds, medical history, doctor's visits, chemo, visitors, gifts, financial information. $19.95 plus $4.00 shipping.

Locks of Love
1640 South Congress Avenue, Suite 104
Palm Springs, FL 33461
888-896-1588 or 561-963-1677
http://www.locksoflove.org/
Provides hairpieces to children younger than 18 who are financially disadvantaged.

Meals on Wheels Association of America
1414 Prince Street, Suite 202
Alexandria, VA 22314
800-677-1116 or 703-548-5558
http://www.mealsonwheelsassn.org
Information about meal programs in your community. May be run by private agencies.

National Association of Hospital Hospitality Houses, Inc.
P.O. Box 18087
Asheville, NC 28814-0087
800-542-9730 or 828-253-1188
http://www.nahhh.org

Ronald McDonald Houses
One Kroc Drive
Oak Brook, IL 60523
630-623-7048
http://www.rmhc.com/about/programs/education/rmh

Wheelchair Foundation
P.O. Box 2973
3700 Blackhawn Plaza Circle
Danville, CA 94526-7973
877-378-3839
http://www.wheelchairfoundation.org
Wheelchairs for people who can't afford them.

Wigs for Kids
Executive Club Building
21330 Center Ridge Road, Suite C
Rocky River, OH 44116
440-333-4433
http://www.wigsforkids.org
Need physician referral.

Siblings

Sibling Support Project—Sibshops
Children's Hospital and Medical Center
P.O. Box 5371 CL 09
Seattle, WA 98105-0371
206-368-4911
http://www.seattlechildrens.org/sibsupp/
Books, programs, newsletter, resources.

Sibling Information Network
Department of Educational Psychology
Box U-64
University of Connecticut
Storrs, CT 06288
Publishes newsletter for and about siblings of children with disabilities or chronic illnesses.

Survivors

American Cancer Society's Survivors' Network
http://www.acscsn.org/

Cancer Cured Kids
P.O. Box 189
Old Westbury, NY 11568
800-CCK-7525 or 516-484-8160
Information about educational and psychosocial needs of survivors.

Children's Hospital of Los Angeles
http://www.childrenshospitalLA.org/life.cfm
Survivorship and long-term effects, directory of long-term follow-up clinics, information about cognitive deficits, and links.

Cancervive
6500 Wilshire Boulevard, Suite 500
Los Angeles, CA 90048
310-203-9232
http://www.cancervive.org
Support for survivors. Publications. Articles, links. "Adventure Park" board game for kids. Teacher's guide, videos for back to school and siblings.

Cancer Survivors Gathering Place
http://www.teleport.com/~jimmc

Cancer Survivors Online
http://www.cancersurvivors.org
Lists of books and resources, financial assistance, glossary, talking to doctors, questions to ask.

Make Today Count
101½ South Union Street
Alexandria, VA 22314
703-548-9674
Two hundred chapters provide emotional help to survivors and families. Programs, group discussions, newsletters, social activities, workshops, seminars, education activities.

Medical Information Bureau, Inc.
P.O. Box 105, Essex Station
Boston, MA 02112
617-426-3660
http://www.mib.com/html/request_record.html
Medical data kept for insurance companies. To check accuracy, have medical information sent to your doctor and nonmedical information sent to you. Download "Request for Disclosure" form D-2. One report costs $8.50.

MEDISEND
214-386-4991
Collects medical surplus in the United States and sends to public and charity hospitals in developing countries. Donate unopened, leftover supplies.

National Cancer Institute's Office of Cancer Survivorship
http://dccps.nci.nih.gov/OCS/
Educates patients, physicians, and public.

National Coalition for Cancer Survivorship
1010 Wayne Avenue, Suite 770
Silver Spring, MD 20910-5600
877-NCCS-YES or 301-650-9127, Fax: 301-565-9670
http://www.cansearch.org
Information and advocacy addressing needs of long-term survivors. Extensive publications list (finishing treatment, working with doctor, health insurance). *Networker* (newsletter). Six audiotapes, *Cancer Survival Toolbox*, tell how to deal with doctors, employers and insurers. Resources.

Outlook—Life Beyond Childhood Cancer
800-322-1468
http://www.outlook-life.org/
Information on school, insurance, employment, health, long-term effects, hot topics. Excerpts from book *Kids With Courage* available.

***SURVIVING!* Newsletter**
Department of Radiation Oncology
Stanford University Medical Center
Division of Radiation Therapy, Room A035
Stanford, CA 94305-5304
650-723-7881
http://www-radonc.stanford.edu/surviving.html
For adult survivors (and adults who had cancer as children). Newsletter.

Webbugs
http://webbugs.wust.edu/patientsandfamilies/articles/late_effects1.htm
Information about late effects.

Teenagers

4YOUth
http://listserv.acor.org/archives/4Youth.html
On-line discussion group; medical and emotional experiences. Share

stories. Support. Talk with others who understand.

Ulman Cancer Fund for Young Adults
4725 Dorsey Hall Drive, Suite A
Ellicott City, MD 21042
888-393-FUND
http://www.ulmanfund.org
Support programs, scholarship information, survivors' issues, support groups, making treatment decisions.

CanTeen
CanTeen of Australia
http://www.canteen.com.au
CanTeen of Ireland
http://www.irishcancer.ie/support/canteen.html
CanTeen of New Zealand
http://www.canteen.org.nz
Peer support organizations for young people (12–24) with cancer and their siblings.

SPECIAL NEEDS

Ability Online Support Network
http://www.ablelink.org
Connects children and adolescents with disabilities to disabled or nondisabled peers and mentors for friendship and support.

Assistive Technology Loan Fund
804-662-7606 or 800-922-4684

Disabled Children's Relief Fund
50 Harrison Avenue
Freeport, NY 11520
516-377-1605
Funding for assistive technology for children with disabilities; priority given to those without insurance.

***Exceptional Parent* Magazine**
Subscriber Service
P.O. Box 3000, Dept. EP
Denville, NJ 07834
800-562-1973 (customer service)
http://www.eparent.com
Annual resource guide: *Directories of National Organizations, Associations, Products & Services.*

Family Village
http://www.familyvillage.wisc.edu
Information on disabilities, adaptive products, assistive technology, physical and occupational therapy and rehabilitation, dance, music, art, education, procedures.

Family Voices
3411 Candelria NE Suite M
Albuquerque, NM 87107
505-872-4744 or 888-835-5669
http://www.familyvoices.org
Network of volunteer coordinators, families, and professionals caring for children with special health care needs/chronic conditions. Information on social security, managed care, Medicaid, Katie Beckett waivers, other federal programs. English and Spanish. Advocacy and support.

Fathers' Network
http://www.fathersnetwork.org
National and Washington state fathers' network for fathers of children with special healthcare needs and/or developmental disabilities. Programs in United States, Canada, and New Zealand.

Federation for Children With Special Needs, Inc.
1135 Tremont Street, Suite 420
Boston, MA 02120
800-331-0688 (in MA) or 617-236-7210
http://www.fcsn.org

iCan
http://www.icanonline.net
Resources, issues, rights, relationships, recreation.

National Center for Youth With Disability
University of Minnesota
420 Delaware Street SE, Box 721
Minneapolis, MN 55455
800-333-6293 or 612-626-2825

National Information Center for Children and Youth With Disabilities
P.O. Box 1492
Washington, DC 20013-1492
800-695-0285 or 202-884-8200
http://www.nichy.org
Information for families. Publications: reading and resources, programs for infants, toddlers, preschoolers, medical bills, sibling issues.
Booklet: *Meeting the Medical Bills.*

National Lekotek Centers
708-328-0001
Network of early intervention programs for young children with disabilities, using adapted toys and computers at play centers or with toy lending libraries.

National Parent Network on Disabilities
1600 Prince Street, Suite 115
Alexandria, VA 22314
703-684-6763.
http://www.npnd.org
Lobbies for people with disabilities; legislative news. Parent training information centers. Links to agencies to help meet child's educational needs.

National Sports Center for the Disabled
303-726-5514
Year-round recreational activities.

Parent Pals
http://parentpals.com
General information, tips, games, links, newsletters about learning disabilities, traumatic brain injury, vision and hearing impairment, speech and language impairment, orthopedic impairments.

U.S. Organization for Disabled Athletes, Inc.
800-25-USODA

Amputation

Super Kids
Peter & Peggy McLoughlin
60 Clyde Street
Newton, MA 02160
Biannual newsletter for kids who wear prostheses. Information, support, personal experiences.

American Amputee Foundation, Inc.
P.O. Box 250218
Hillcrest Station
Little Rock, AR 72225
501-666-2523
http://www.arcat.com
Financial assistance, counseling groups, referrals, "give-a-limb" program, national resource directory.

Amputee Coalition of America
900 East Hill Avenue, Suite 285
Knoxville, TN 37915-2568
888-267-5669 or 423-524-8772
http://www.amputee-coalition.org/
Information, advocacy.

National Odd Shoe Exchange
Information request:
3200 North Delaware Street
Chandler, AZ 85225-1100
480-892-3484
International nonprofit shoe exchange for amputees and people with odd sizes.

Blindness

American Council of the Blind
1155 15th Street NW, Suite 1004
Washington, DC 20005
800-424-8666 or 202-467-5081
http://www.acb.org

American Foundation for the Blind
11 Penn Plaza, Suite 300
New York, NY 10001
1-800-AFB-LINE
http://www.afb.org

Blind Children's Fund
Resource Center
4740 Okemos Road
Okemos, MI 48864
517-347-1357
http://www.blindchildrensfund.org
Information, resources, articles, products, books.

The Institute for Families of Blind Children
P.O. Box 54700 MS# 111
Los Angeles, CA 90054-0700
323-669-4649
http://www.instituteforfamilies.org
Supports and provides information to families affected by retinoblastoma and visual impairment.

The Lighthouse National Center for Vision and Child Development
111 East 59th Street
New York, NY 10022
800-829-0500 or 212-821-9200
http://www.lighthouse.org

National Association for Parents of the Visually Impaired
P.O. Box 317
Watertown, MA 02272-0317
800-562-6265 or 617-972-7441
http://www.spedex.com/napvi
Information and resources. Emotional support, networking, outreach programs. Social and school issues; sibling and parent support.

National Library Service for the Blind and Physically Handicapped
Library of Congress
1291 Taylor Street NW
Washington, DC 20542
202-707-5100
http://www.loc.gov/nls

National Organization of Parents of Blind Children
Division of National Federation of the Blind
1800 Johnson Street
Baltimore, MD 21230
410-696-9314 (ext. 360)
http://www.nfb.org
Magazine, workshops, pen pals, camp, scholarships, handbooks for teachers.

Deafness

Alexander Graham Bell Association
3417 Volta Place NW
Washington, DC 20007
202-337-5220 or 202-337-5221 (TTY)
http://www.agbell.org
Financial aid, publications, advocacy. Local chapters.

The American Academy of Audiology
http://www.audiology.org
Consumer information about hearing loss and aids. Find an audiologist. Ask the expert. E-mail discussion list.

American Society for Deaf Children
P.O. Box 3355
Gettysburg, PA 17325
717-334-7922 (V/TTY)
800-942-ASDC (parent hotline)
http://www.deafchildren.org
National organization advocating for high-quality programs and services.

Go Hear
http://www.gohear.org
Parent- and kid-oriented Web site with resources for families of newly diagnosed hearing impaired children.

Handspeak
http://www.handspeak.com
Fun site demonstrates sign language

(from all over the world) dictionary.

HEAR NOW
9745 East Hampden Avenue, Suite 300
Denver, CO 80231-4923
800-648-HEAR

Miracle Ear Chidren's Foundation
800-234-5422
http://www.miracle-ear.com
Free hearing aids to children from low-income families

National Association of the Deaf
814 Thayer Avenue
Silver Spring, MD 20910-4500
301-587-1788 or 301-587-1789 (TTY)
http://www.nad.org

National Institute on Deafness and Other Communication Disorders
31 Center Drive, MSC 2320
Bethesda, MD 20892-2320
800-241-1044
http://www.nidcd.nih.gov

SHHH: Self Help for Hard of Hearing People
7910 Woodmont Avenue, Suite 1200
Bethesda, MD 20814
301-657-2248 or 301-657-2249 (TTY)
http://www.shhh.org
Advocacy, support.

Education

CanTeach
http://www.netwrxl.net/~canteach
Links children with long-term illness with teachers

Education Resources Information Center
621 Skytop Road, Suite 160
Syracuse University
Syracuse, NY 13244-5290
800-464-9107 or 315-443-3640
http://www.askERIC.org
National information system with 16 clearinghouses, abstracts of documents and journal articles, Q&A service, virtual library, database of education information for teachers, counselors, and parents.

Family Education
http://www.familyeducation.com
Education resources, learning network, tips on learning disabilities.

HEATH Resource Center of American Council on Education
One Dupont Circle NW
Washington, DC 20036
800-544-3284
http://www.heath-resource-center.org/
National clearinghouse on higher education for people with disabilities. Information on services available at American colleges and vo-tech schools. Scholarship information and referrals.

Internet Special Education Resources
http://iser.com/index/shtml
Directory of services, assessment, educational alternatives, therapy, rights, advocacy, search by state. Products, books, articles.

U.S. Department of Education
Office of Special Education and Rehabilitative Services
400 Maryland Avenue SW
Washington, DC 20202
800-USA-LEARN, 202-305-8134, or 202-205-4475 (TTY)
http://www.ed.gov/
Inquiries, referrals, publications. Information on ADA, rehabilitation, grants.

Wright Group, McGraw-Hill Publishing
19201 120th Avenue NE
Bothell, WA 98011
800-523-2371
http://www.wrightgroup.com/index.html
Publishes innovative children's educational materials (K-6); information for parents and teachers, workshops.

Learning Disabilities

Learning Disabilities Association of America
4156 Library Road
Pittsburgh, PA 15234-1349
412-341-1515, Fax: 412-344-0224
http://www.ldanatl.org/
Association of parents and professionals. Inquiries, pamphlets, books, local chapters.

Learning Disabilities Association of Canada
323 Chapel Street, Suite 200
Ottawa, Ontario, Canada K1N 7Z2
613-238-5721

Learning Disabilities Online
http://www.ldonline.org
Information for parents, teachers. News, technology.

National Center for Learning Disabilities
381 Park Avenue South, Suite 1401
New York, NY 10016
888-575-7373 or 212-545-7510
http://www.ncld.org

Neurological Disorder/ Stroke

National Institute of Neurological Disorders & Stroke
P.O. Box 5801
Bethesda, MD 20824
800-352-9424 or 301-496-5751
http://www.ninds.nih.gov

Products

Abilitations
One Sportime Way

Atlanta, GA 30340
800-850-8602
http://www.abilitations.com/products/shtml
Exercise products and physical therapy activity guides.

ABLEDATA
8630 Fenton Street, Suite 930
Silver Spring, MD 20910
800-227-0216 (voice) or 301-608-8912 (TTY)
http://www.abledata.com
Products and toys, assistive technology.

Crestwood Communication Aids, Inc.
6625 North Sidney Place
Milwaukee, WI 53209
414-352-5678
http://www.communicationaids.com
Communication aids for children and adults.

Flaghouse—Special Populations
601 Flaghouse Drive
Hasbrouck Heights, NJ 07604-3116
800-793-7900 or 201-288-7600
http://www.flaghouse.com/special.htm
Adaptive toys and therapy products.

Guide to Toys for Children Who Are Blind or Visually Impaired
Toy Manufacturers of America
200 Fifth Avenue, Suite 740
New York, NY 10010
212-675-1141
http://toy-tma.org/industry/publications/cover.html

Pediatric Projects
22711 Napa Street
West Hills, CA 91304
800-947-0947
Nonprofit information on 500 toys and books developed to explain medical conditions to children.

Plum Enterprises, Inc.
P.O. Box 85
500 Freedom View Lane
Valley Forge, PA 19481-0085
800-321-PLUM or 610-783-7377
http://www.plument.com
ProtectaCap and ProtectaHip. Protective gear (all sizes, children through adults) for postsurgery, kids with shunts, coordination issues, low counts, seizures, etc.

P.R.I.D.E. Foundation
391 Long Hill Road
Groton, CT 06340-1293
860-445-7320
National organization dedicated to solving dressing problems of people with disabilities. Resources include fact sheet on children's clothing modifications. Applicable to children in wheelchairs, amputees, or those who have trouble managing buttons.

Rehabilitation

Disabled Sports USA
451 Hungerford Drive, Suite 100
Rockville, MD 20850
310-217-9840 or 301-217-0963 (TDD)
http://www.dsusa.org/
Sports, recreation, educational programs, magazine, local chapters.

National Rehabilitation Information Center
8455 Colesville Road, Suite 935
Silver Spring, MD 20910-3319
800-346-2742 or 301-588-9284

North American Riding for the Handicapped Association
P.O. Box 33150
Denver, CO 80233
800-369-RIDE (7433)
http://www.narha.org
Referral to a local riding center.

Short Stature

Human Growth Foundation
997 Glen Cover Avenue
Glen Head, NY 11545
800-451-6434
http://www.hgfound.org

Little People of America
P.O. Box 745
Lubbock, TX 79408
888-LPA-2001
http://www.lpaonline.org
Resources, links, books, clothing, and product resources.

Speech Disorder

American Speech-Language-Hearing Association
10801 Rockville Pike
Rockville, MD 20852
800-638-8255 (v/TTY)
http://www.asha.org
Professional organization. Find an audiologist or speech-language pathologist. Speech, language, and swallowing issues.

National Aphasia Association (speech disorders)
156 Fifth Avenue, Suite 707
New York, NY 10010
800-922-4622
http://www.aphasia.org

BOOKS

PUBLISHERS/ DISTRIBUTORS

The following publishers have entire lines devoted to the kinds of issues cancer families face. Ask for a list of their publications or a catalog.

BOOKWORM Children's Books
1740 North Hermitage
Chicago, IL 60622
312-486-3586 or 312-486-8236
Children's storybooks on death, disabilities, sibling relationships. Annotated, grouped by age categories and topics. Referral information for families.

Centering Corporation
1531 N. Saddle Creek Road
P.O. Box 3367
Omaha, NE 68103-0367
402-553-1200
http://www.centering.org
More than 300 books and videos on coping with serious illness, loss, and grief.

Compassion Books
704-675-9670 (M–F, 9–5 EST)
Free catalogue. More than 400 books related to grief, death, and loss.

Center for Attitudinal Healing
33 Buchanan Drive
Sausalito, CA 94965
415-331-6161
http://www.healingcenter.org
Promotes use of the arts in a loving, supportive program to help children ages 6–16 share feelings.

Magination Press
http://www.maginationpress.com
Books written for parents and kids by mental health professionals, about fears, emotions, family issues, self-esteem, divorce, disabilities.

New Harbinger Publications, Inc.
5674 Shattuck Avenue
Oakland, CA 94609
800-748-6273
http://www.newharbinger.com
Quality self-help guides for consumers and professionals. Books, workbooks, videos, audiotapes. Most written for adults, but adaptable to children. Topics include chemo and radiation, trauma, relaxation/stress, anger, visualization, grief, couple skills, forgiveness, communication, conflict resolution, pain, getting to sleep, parenting.

O'Reilly & Associates, Inc.
101 Morris Street
Sebastopol, CA 95472
http://www.patientcenters.com
Patient-centered guides including books on leukemia, solid tumors, lymphoma, survivorship, visiting the hospital, and working with your doctor.

Gryphon House
P.O. Box 207
Beltsville, MD 20704-0207
888-GHBOOK1 or 800-638-0928
http://www.ghbooks.com
Activity and early childhood books for teachers and parents.

BOOKS FOR PARENTS

If a book is out of print, you might still find it at your library, or the library at a university. Your hospital social worker may have a copy, as well, to lend you.

Cancer

Bone Marrow Transplants: A Guide for Cancer Patients and their Families. Marianne Shaffer and George Santos. Philadelphia: Taylor. 1994.

Brain Tumor Resource Handbook: Pediatric Version. London, Ontario, Canada: Brain Tumor Foundation of Canada, 1994.

Childhood Cancer: A Handbook From St. Jude Children's Research Hospital. Grant Steen, PhD, and Joseph Mirro, MD, Eds. Memphis, TN: St. Jude Children's Research Hospital, 2000. What to expect, treatment options, clinical trials, pain, side effects, nutrition, educational concerns, finding medical information on the Web, financial issues. Ordering information: Available at book stores or order by calling 800-386-5656 ($30.00).

Childhood Cancer: A Parent's Guide to Solid Tumor Cancers. Hanna Jones-Hodder and Nancy Keene. Sebastopol, CA: O'Reilly & Associates, 1999.

Childhood Leukemia. Nancy Keene. Sebastopol, CA: O'Reilly & Associates, 1997.

Conquering Kids Cancer: Triumphs and Tragedies of a Children's Cancer Doctor. Kenneth Lazarus, MD. Houston, TX: Emerald Ink, 1999.

Gifts of Time. Fred Epstein, MD, and Elaine Fantle Smimberg. New York: William Morrow, 1993. Brain stem and spinal cord tumor cases. Description of neurosurgery. Out of print.

Know Before You Go: The Childhood Cancer Journey. Sheryl Lozowski-Sullivan. Kensington, MD:

Candlelighters Childhood Cancer Foundation, 1998. Free copy to families from Candlelighters.

Navigating Through a Strange Land: A Book for Brain Tumor Patients and Their Families. Patricia Ann Roloff. West Fork, AR: Indigo Press, 2001. Types of brain tumors, coping, treatment, dealing with medical system, resources, bibliography. Ordering information: Indigo Press, P.O. Box 968, West Fork, AR 72774-0968; 501-839-3944 ($16.95 + $3.50 shipping).

Non-Hodgkin's Lymphomas: Making Sense of Diagnosis, Treatment, and Options. Lorraine Johnston. Sebastapol, CA: O'Reilly. 1999.

One Day at a Time: Children Living With Cancer. Thomas Bergman. Wakeforest, NC: Gareth Stevens, 1989. Interviews with kids.

Surviving Childhood Cancer: A Guide for Families. Margot Fromer. Washington, DC: American Psychiatric Press, 1995.

They Never Want to Tell You: Children Talk About Cancer. David Bearison. Cambridge, MA: Harvard University Press, 1991. Children's own stories. Excellent discussion of how to inform children at diagnosis. Most of the children quoted are teenagers.

Coping

Armfuls of Time: The Psychological Experience of the Child With a Life-Threatening Illness. Barbara Sourkes, PhD. Pittsburgh, PA: University of Pittsburgh Press, 1995.

Cancer and Self-Help: Bridging the Troubled Waters of Childhood Illness. Mark A. Chesler and Barbara Chesney. Madison: University of Wisconsin Press, 1995. How self-help groups are formed, how they function and recruit, and why they are effective. Ordering information: 608-262-8782 (paperback, $19.95).

A Child in Pain: How to Help, What to Do. Leora Kuttner, PhD. Point Roberts, WA: Hartley & Marks, 1996. Understand, assess, and alleviate pain. Practical techniques for parents.

Childhood Cancer and the Family: Meeting the Challenge of Stress and Support. Mark Chesler and Oscar Barbarin. New York: Brunner/Mazel, 1987. Out of print.

Children With Cancer: Communication and Emotions. Anna M. Van Veldhuizen and Bob F. Last. Amsterdam, Holland: Swets & Zeitlinger, 1991. Emotional, coping and communicative aspects of childhood cancer. Technical, research methods. Also helps sort out feelings.

Coping With Childhood Cancer: Where Do We Go From Here? David Adams, MSW, and Eleanor Deveau, BScN. Reston, VA: Reston, 1984.

Emotional Aspects of Childhood Leukemia: A Handbook for Parents. J. P. Spinetta and F. H. Kung. New York: Leukemia Society of America, 1994.

Healing Visualizations: Creating Health through Imagery. Gerald Epstein. New York: Bantam, 1989. Imagery exercises for medical problems adaptable for children.

The Human Side of Cancer: Living With Hope, Coping With Uncertainty. Jimmie C. Holland and Sheldon Lewis. New York: HarperCollins, 2000. Emotional issues, coping strategies, psychological effects, emotional baggage of surviving.

Reaching Children Through Play Therapy: An Experiential Approach. Carol and Byron Norton. Denver, CO: Pendleton Clay, 1997. Explains model of play therapy used by Kid Power therapists. For parents and therapists.

The Relaxation Response. Herbert Benson, MD. New York: Avon Books, 1990. Relaxation method of pain relief.

Spinning Inwards. Maureen Murdock. Boston: Shambhala, 1987. Using imagery with children.

Therapeutic Play Activities for Hospitalized Children. Robyn Hart, CCLS, Patricia L. Mather, PhD, Jeanne F. Slack, RN, DNSc, and Marcia Powell, MA, CTRS. St. Louis, MO: Mosby Year Book, 1992.

When Life Becomes Precious: A Guide for Loved Ones and Friends of Cancer Patients. Elise Needell Babcock. New York: Bantam Books, 1997.

You Are Not Alone: A Sourcebook for Support Groups for Families of Children with Cancer. Mark Chesler and Sara Eldridge. Kensington, MD: Candelighters Childhood Cancer Foundation. 2000.

Death/Bereavement

After the Death of a Child: Living With Loss Through the Years. Ann Finkbeiner. New York: Harvest Books, 1996.

The Art of Condolence: What to Write, What to Say, What to Do at a Time of Loss. Leonard M. Zunin and Hilary Stanton Zunin. New York: Harperperennial Library, 1992.

Bereaved Children & Teens: A Support Guide for Parents and Professionals. Boston: Beacon Press, 1996.

Beyond Grief: A Guide for Recovering From the Death of a Loved One. Carol Staudacher. Oakland, CA: New Harbinger, 1995.

Books to Help Children Cope With Separation and Loss. J. E. Bernstein. New York: Bowker, 1983. Guide to bibliographical resources. Extensive indexes, summaries, assessments. Helpful organizations.

A Child Dies: A Portrait of Family Grief. Joan Hagen Arnold and Penelope Buschman Gemma. Philadelphia: Charles Press, 1994.

Children Grieve, Too: A Book for Families Who Have Experienced a Death. Joy Johnson and Marvin Johnson. Omaha, NE: Centering, 1998.

Children Mourning, Mourning Children. Kenneth Doka, PhD, Ed. Washington, DC: Hospice Foundation of America, 1995. Children's understanding of death, answering questions, role of schools.

The Dying Child: The Management of the Child or Adolescent Who Is Dying. William M. Easson. Springfield, IL: Charles C Thomas, 1981. Tasks facing the child and those who deal with him or her.

The Dying and the Bereaved Teenager. John D. Morgan, Ed. Philadelphia: Charles Press, 1998. For counselors and caregivers. Dying teenagers, bereaved teenagers, school protocols. Not all about cancer, but most applicable for dying teenagers or teenaged siblings. Coping mechanisms. Ordering information: 215-925-3995 ($16.95 plus $2.25 shipping).

Final Gifts: Understanding the Special Awareness, Needs, and Communications of the Dying. Maggie Callanan and Patricia Kelley. New York: Poseidon Press, 1992. Written by two hospice nurses with decades of experience. Helps families understand and communicate with terminally ill patients.

Goodbye My Child. Margaret M. Pike. Omaha, NE: Centering Corp., 1992.

Good Grief. Deborah Morris Coryell. Tucson, AZ: Shiva Foundation, 1997. Jewish perspective. The nature of loss, healing.

Grandma's Tears: Comfort for Grieving Grandparents. June Cerza Kolf. Grand Rapids, MI: Baker Book House, 1995. Ordering information: 800-877-2665 ($5.40 plus $3.00 shipping).

Grief: Climb Toward Understanding: Self-Help When You Are Struggling. Phyllis Davies. Sunnybank, 1998. Checklists of what you can do.

Grief Quest: Reflections for Men Coping With Loss. Robert J. Miller, with Stephen Hrycyniak, St. Meinrad, IN: Abbey Press, 1998. Christian perspective. Ordering information: 800-621-1588.

Grieving: How to Go on Living When Someone You Love Dies. Therese A. Rando, PhD. New York: Bantam Books, 1991.

The Grieving Child: A Parent's Guide. Helen Fitzgerald. New York: Fireside, 1992. Therapist with personal experience working with bereaved children. Practical solutions.

At Home With Terminal Illness: A Family Guide to Hospice in the Home. Michael Appleton and Todd Henschell. Upper Saddle River, NJ: Prentice Hall, 1995.

Hospice and Palliative Care: Questions and Answers. Virginia Sendor and Patrice O'Connor. Lanham, MD: Scarecrow Press, 1991.

Life and Loss. Linda Goldman. New York: Hemisphere, 2000. How children view losses, debunking myths, avoiding cliches. Ways to help child say goodbye to loved one and commemorate the loss.

Living With Grief: Children, Adolescents, and Loss. Kenneth Doka, Ed. Washington, DC: Hospice Foundation of America, 2000.

Men and Grief: A Guide for Men Surviving the Death of a Loved One. Carol Staudacher. Oakland, CA: New Harbinger, 1992. Out of print.

On Children and Death. Elizabeth Kubler-Ross, MD. New York: Collier Books, 1997. Practical help in living through terminal period of child's life with love and understanding.

150 Facts About Grieving Children. Erin Linn. Incline Village, NV: Publisher's Mark, 1990. Mother of bereaved sibs. Helpful guide for parents, teachers, peers to understand fears, anger, and grief. List of support groups.

Parental Loss of a Child. Therese Rando, PhD, Ed. Champaign, IL: Research Press, 1986. Death from a serious illness; guilt and grief; advice to physicians, clergy and funeral directors; professional help and support organizations.

The Private Worlds of Dying Children. Myra Bluebond-Langner. Princeton, NJ: Princeton University Press, 1980.

Recovering From the Loss of a Sibling: When a Brother or Sister Dies. Katherine Fair Donnelly. iUniverse.com, 2000.

Shadows in the Sun: The Experiences of Sibling Bereavement in Childhood. Betty Davies. New York: Brunner/Mazel, 1998.

Sibling Grief: How Parents Can Help the Child Whose Brother or Sister Has Died. M. Scherago. Redmond, WA: Medic, 1997. Ordering information: 402-553-1200 (12 pp.).

Stuck for Words: What to Say to Someone Who Is Grieving. Doris Zagdanski. Melbourn, Australia: Hill of Content, 1994.

Talking About Death: A Dialogue Between Parent and Child. Earl Grollman. Boston, MA: Beacon Press, 1990. How to explain death, how children react to specific types of death, and when to seek professional help.

35 Ways to Help a Grieving Child. Portland, OR: Dougy Center for Grieving Children, 1999.

A Time to Grieve: Meditations for Healing After the Death of a Loved One. Carol Staudacher. New York: HarperCollins, 1994.

When Your Friend's Child Dies: A Guide to Being a Thoughtful and Caring Friend. Julane Grant. Scappoose, OR: Angel Hugs, 1998. What to say and what not to say. Ordering information: P.O. Box 843, Scappoose, OR, 97056. 800-431-1579. $6.95,

Words to Comfort, Words to Heal: Poems and Meditations for Those Who Grieve. Juliet Mabey. Oxford, England: Oneworld, 1998.

The Worst Loss: How Families Heal From the Death of a Child. Barbara D. Rosof. New York: H. Holt, 1995.

Unspoken Grief: Coping With Childhood Sibling Loss. Helen Rosen. Lexington, MA: Lexington Books, 1986. Out of print.

Disabilities/Special Needs

Children With Visual Impairments: A Parents' Guide. M. Cay Holbrook, PhD, Ed. Bethesda, MD: Woodbine House, 1996.

Choices in Deafness: A Parent's Guide to Communication Options. Sue Schwartz. Bethesda, MD: Woodbine House, 2nd ed., 1996.

Kid Friendly Parenting With Deaf and Hard of Hearing Children: A Treasury of Fun Activities Toward Better Behavior. Daria Medwid and Denise Chapman Weston. Washington, DC: Clerc, 1995.

Making Sense of Sensory Integration (audiotape and booklet). Jane Koomer, et al., Curve Records, 1998.

The Out-of-Sync Child. Carol Stock Kranowitz. New York: Perigree, 1998. Sensory integration issues.

The Source for Non-Verbal Learning Disabilities. Sue Thompson. Linguisystems, 1997.

Uncommon Fathers Reflections on Raising a Child With a Disability. Donald Meyer. Bethesda, MD: Woodbine House, 1995. By fathers of children with disabilities; emotions are very similar to cancer parents.

The Silent Garden: Raising Your Deaf Child. Paul W. Ogden. Washington, DC: Gallaudet University Press, 1996.

Short and OK: A Guide for Parents of Short Children. Patricia Rieser and Heino F. L. Meyer-Bahlburg. Glenhead, New York: Human Growth Foundation, 1991. Schooling, medical, psychosocial issues, causal issues, resources. Ordering information: 800-451-6434.

Education (for parents and teachers)

Adaptive Education Strategies. Margaret C. Wang. Baltimore, MD: Paul H. Brookes, 1992. Ordering information: Paul H. Brookes, P.O. Box 10624, Baltimore, MD 21285-0624.

Adolescents With Chronic Illnesses—Issues for School Personnel. Minneapolis, MN: National Center for Youth with Disabilities, 1990. Bibliography.

Back to School: A Handbook for Parents of Children With Cancer. American Cancer Society (free; Pub. no. 88-20M-No. 2640-LE).

Back to School: A Handbook for Educators of Children With Life-threatening Diseases in the Yeshiva/Day School System. 1995. School re-entry, infection control, needs of high school students, special education, saying good-bye. Ordering information: Chai Lifeline, 212-465-1300 or 877-CHAI-LIFE.

Back to School: Teens Prepare for School Reentry. Ordering information: Starbright, 800-315-2580 (free).

Cancer in the Classroom. Immune-suppression, teasing, effects on learning, changes in medical status. Ordering information: Portland Oregon Candlelighters, 3145 NE 20th Street, Portland, OR 97212.

Cancervive Teacher's Guide for Kids With Cancer. Susan Nessim and Ernest R. Katz, PhD. 1995. Ordering information: Cancervive; 310-203-9232.

Children With Limb Loss: A Handbook for Teachers. Grand Rapids, MI: Area Child Amputee Center, 1993. Ordering information: Area Child Amputee Center, 235 Wealthy SE, Grand Rapids, MI 49503.

The Class in Room 44: When a Classmate Dies. Lynn Bennett Blackburn, PhD. Omaha, NE: Centering, 1991. K-3rd grade.

Death and the Adolescent. Grant Baxter and Wendy Stuart. 1999. Handbook to help teens deal with death. Ten-week school-based grief support group.

Death and the Classroom: A Teacher's Guide to Assist Grieving Students. Kathleen K. Cassini and Jacqueline L. Rogers. 1990. Ordering information. Griefwork of Cincinnati, 1445 Colonial Drive, Suite B, Cincinnati, OH 45238; 513-922-1202.

Death Education: An Annotated Resource Guide. H. Wass, C. A. Corr, R. A. Pacholski, and C. M. Sanders. Washington, DC: Hemisphere, 1980. Resources for educators.

Educating the Child With Cancer: School Reentry Resource Manual. Patricia Deasy-Spinetta and Elisabeth Irvin. Kensington, MD: Candlelighters Childhood Cancer foundation. Useful for teachers and parents. Ordering information: Single copy, free from Candlelighters.

Keyboarding For Kids. Chandler, AZ: Ellsworth. Teaches typing. Grades 1–6. Ordering information, Ellsworth Publishing, P.O. Box 6727, Chandler, AZ 85246; 602-963-4817.

Helping the Chronically Ill Child in School: A Handbook for Teachers, Counselors, and Administrators. Gertrude Morrow. Englewood Cliffs, NJ: Prentice-Hall, 1985.

Helping Schools Cope With Childhood Cancer: Current Facts and Creative Solutions. 1993. Ordering information: Pediatric Cancer School Support Program, Psychology Dept., Room 2192, Children's Hospital of Western Ontario, 800 Commissioner's Road, East, London, Ontario, Canada N6A 4G5.

Helping Your Child, A Manual for Parents of Children With Brain Tumors and *Teaching the Child With a Brain Tumor.* Booklets. Ordering information: Children's Health Care St. Paul, Dept. of Hematology/Oncology, 345 North Smith Avenue, St. Paul, MN 55102 ($1.00 each including shipping).

Including Your Child. Washington, DC: U.S. Dept. of Education. Ordering information: National Library of Education, 800-424-1616 or Fax: 202-219-1696 (single copy free for parents of children with special needs up to age 8).

Just Will. Cincinnati, OH: Children's Hospital School Liaison Program, 1993. Picture book for preschoolers about child with cancer. Ordering information: 513-559-8604.

Managing Chronic Illness in the Classroom. Dorothy B. Wishnietsky and Dan H. Wishnietsky. 1996.

Negotiating the Special Education Maze: A Guide for Parents and Teachers. Winifred Anderson, Stephen Chitwood, and Deidre Hayden. Bethesda, MD: Woodbine House, 1997. Step-by-step guide to obtaining help for child. Eligibility, evaluation, laws.

The Special Education Sourcebook. A Teacher's Guide to Programs, Materials, and Information Sources. Michael S. Rosenberg, PhD and Irene Edmond-Rosenberg, MPA. Bethesda, MD: Woodbine House, 1994.

Special Like You, Special Like Me. Beth Canarie. Cincinnati, OH: Children's Hospital Cincinnati School Liaison Program, 1992. Workbook for classmates. Basic facts, emphasizes child still same person. Spaces to draw. K–4.

Students With Cancer: A Resource for the Educator. Cancer, treatment, prognosis, ways teachers can help, resources for more info. Free copy from National Cancer Institute.

Suggestions for Teachers and School Counselors. The Compassionate Friends.

The Survival Guide for Kids With LD. Rhoda Cummings and Gary Fisher. Minneapolis, MN: Free Spirit, 1991. Ordering information: Free Spirit Publishing, 400 First Avenue North, #616, Minneapolis, MN 55401; 800-735-7323.

Understanding Learning Disabilities: A Parents' Guide and Workbook. Richmond, VA: Learning Disabilities Council and National Center for LD, 1991. Coping, evaluation, advocacy, resources. Ordering information: Learning Disabilities Council and National Center for LD, P.O. Box 8451, Richmond, VA 23226; 804-748-5012.

When Your Child Is Ready to Return to School. American Brain Tumor Association. Pamphlet.

With a Little Help From My Friends: Living With Leukemia and Lymphoma and *Making the Grade: Back to School After Cancer for Teens.* Ordering information: Leukemia and Lymphoma Society.

You Have a Student With Cancer. 1980. For school personnel, feelings, information, hints about contact while child absent, return, etc. Booklets about pain, coping, unproved methods, etc. Programs: transportation, equipment, and supplies (wigs, prostheses, wheelchairs, hospital beds), support groups, housing, educational, literature, camps.

You, Your Child, and Special Education: A Guide to Making the System Work. Barbara Coyne

Cutler. Baltimore, MD: Brookes, 1993. Ordering information: P.O. Box 10624, Baltimore, MD 21285-0624.

Finances

Beyond Profit: The Complete Guide to Managing the Nonprofit Organization. Fred Setterberg and Kary Sculman. New York: HarperCollins. Out of print.

Financial Aid for the Disabled and Their Families. Gail Ann Schlacter and R. David Weber, Eds. San Carlos, CA: Reference Service Press, 2000. Scholarships, fellowships, loans, grants, awards, internships. State-related benefits. Ordering information: 100 Industrial Road, #9, San Carlos, CA 94070; 415-594-0743.

Financial Resource Management for Nonprofit Organizations. Leon Haller. Englewood Cliffs, NJ: Prentice Hall, 1982. Out of print.

For Fun and Funds: Creative Fund Raising Ideas for Your Organizaton. Carole DeSoto. New York: Simon & Schuster. Out of print.

Fundraising: Hands-On Tactics for Nonprofit Groups. Peter L. Edles. New York: McGraw-Hill, 1993.

Grass Roots Fund Raising Book: How to Raise Money in Your Community. Joan Flanagan for The Youth Project. Chicago: Swallow Press, 1977.

How to Form a Nonprofit Corporation. Anthony Mancuso. Berkely, CA: Nolo Press, 1998.

The Insider's Guide to HMOs: How to Navigate the Managed-Care System and Get the Health Care You Deserve. Alan J. Steinberg, MD. New York: Plume, 1997.

One Small Sparrow: Michael's Story and Hope of Compassion in the Classroom. Jeff Leeland. Sisters, OR: Multnomah Books, 2000. Ideas for fundraising methods. Christian perspective.

Starting and Managing a Nonprofit Organization: A Legal Guide. Bruce Hopkins. New York: John Wiley & Sons, 2000.

Humor

Compassionate Laughter—Jest for Your Health. Patty Wooten, RN. Salt Lake City, UT: Commune-A-Key, 1996.

Healing Power of Humor. Allen Klein. Los Angeles: J. P. Tarcher, 1989.

I Want to Grow Hair, I Want to Grow Up, I Want to Go to Boise. Erma Bombeck. New York: Harper & Row, 1990.

A Life in the Balance. Scott Burton. www.sburton.com/inconnav.htm Stand-up comic tells about his battle with osteosarcoma.

Life and Depth: Very Funny Stories About Very Scary Things (audiotape). Joe Kogel. Survivor talks about the use of humor for recovery. Ordering information: 50 Summit Avenue, Providence, RI 02906; 401-351-0229.

Thank God It's Only Cancer. Steve Gould. Miami, FL: Mondays, 1995. And *A Lighter Look at the "C" Word: More Cartoons and Comments on Cancer.* Miami, FL: Mondays, 1997. Ordering information: Mondays, P.O. Box 162605, Miami FL 33116.

Illness/Care

Both Sides of the White Coat: An Insider's Perspectives on the Critically Ill Child. Scott E. Eveloff, MD. iUniverse.com, 2000. Applicable insights on critical care, physician hierarchy, ethical issues, good/bad encounters with medical profession. Ordering information: www.iUniverse.com.

Burnout—The Cost of Caring. Christina Maslach, PhD. Englewood Cliffs, NJ: Prentice-Hall, 1982. How to recognize, prevent, and cure the burnout syndrome for nurses, teachers, counselors, doctors, therapists, police, social workers, and caregivers.

Cancer Clinical Trials. Robert Finn. Sebastopol, CA: O'Reilly & Associates, 1999.

Cancer Pain Relief and Palliative Care in Children. Washington, DC: World Health Organization, 1998. Ordering information: 49 Sheridan Avenue, Albany, NY 12210; 518-436-9686 ($16.50).

Cancer Patient's Workbook. Joanie Willis. New York: Dorling Kindersley, 2001. Helps keep track of and organize treatment information.

Caring for Children With Chronic Illness: Issues and Strategies. Ruth E. K. Stein, Ed. New York: Springer, 1989.

The Chronically Ill Child: A Guide for Parents and Professionals. Audrey McCollum. New Haven, CT: Yale University Press, 1981. Out of print.

Cognitive Aspects of Chronic Illness in Children. Ronald T. Brown, Ed. New York: Guilford Press, 1999. Written for psychologists and pediatricians. Impact of diseases and treatments on learning and behavior.

The Complete Idiot's Guide to Managed Healthcare. Sophie Korczyk and Hazel A. White. New York: Alpha Books, 1998.

Coping with Prednisone and other Cortison-Related Medicines: It May Work Miracles, but How do You Handle the Side Effects? Eugenia Zukerman, Julie Ingelfinger, MD. New York: St. Martin's, 1998.

Fight Back and Win: How to Get HMOs and Health Insurance to Pay Up. William M. Shernoff. Boardroom Books, 1999.

Home Care for the Seriously Ill Child: A Manual for Parents. D. Gay Modlow and Ida M. Martinson. Alexandria, VA: Children's Hospice International, 1991. Ordering information: Children's Hospice International ($7.95).

Hospice Care for Children. Ann Armstrong-Dailey, Ed. New York: Oxford University Press, 1993.

The Intelligent Patient's Guide to the Doctor-Patient Relationship: Learning How to Talk So Your Doctor Will Listen. Barbara M. Korsch, MD and Caroline Harding. New York: Oxford University Press (trade), 1998. For adults.

Making Informed Medical Decisions. Nancy Oster, et al. Alexandria, VA: O'Reilly, 2000.

Medical Choices, Medical Chances: How Patients, Families and Physicians Can Cope With Uncertainty. Harold Bursztajin and Richard Feinbloom, et al. New York: Routledge, 1990.

Meeting the Challenge of Disability or Chronic Illness—A Family Guide. Lori Goldfarb. Baltimore, MD: Brookes, 1986.

Numb Toes and Aching Soles: Coping with Peripheral Neuropathy. John Senneff. Med Press. 1999.

Supportive Care of Children With Cancer: Current Therapy and Guidelines. Arthur Ablin, MD, Ed. Baltimore, MD: Johns Hopkins University Press, 1997. Handbook for clinicians. Ordering information: 800-537-5487 (paperback, $29.95 plus $4.00 shipping).

Surviving Modern Medicine: How to Get the Best From Doctors, Family and Friends. Peter Clarke and Susan H. Evans. New Brunswick, NJ: Rutgers University Press, 1998. Getting doctors to pay attention, making medical decisions, seeking support, protecting your choices in critical care. For adults.

Why Mine? A Book for Parents Whose Child Is Seriously Ill. Joy Johnson. Omaha, NE: Centering, 1981.

Working With Your Doctor: Getting the Healthcare You Deserve. Nancy Keene. Sebastopol, CA: O'Reilly & Associates, 1998.

The Yale University School of Medicine Patient's Guide to Medical Tests. Yale University School of Medicine. Boston, MA: Houghton-Mifflin, 1997.

Your Child in the Hospital: A Practical Guide for Parents. Nancy Keene and Rachel Prentice. Sebastopol, CA: O'Reilly & Associates, 1999.

Parenting

Ages and Stages. Karen Miller. Marshfield, MA: Telshare, 1985. Stages of physical, emotional, and intellectual development.

Common Sense Discipline Building Self-Esteem in Young Children: Stories From Life. Grace Mitchell and Lois Dewsnap. Marshfield, MA: Telshare, 1995. Story-oriented approach; real-life issues and conflicts; practical approaches to solutions.

Dribble Drabble Art Experiences for Young Children. Deya Brashears. Beltsville, MD: Gryphon House, 1985.

Games to Play With Babies; Games to Play With Toddlers; More Games to Play With Toddlers; Games to Play With Two Year Olds; 500 Five Minute Games; Quick and Easy Activities for 3 to 6 Year Olds. All by Jackie Silberg. Beltsville, MD: Gryphon House.

Growing a Girl: Seven Strategies for Raising a Strong, Spirited Daughter. Barbara Mackoff. New York: Bantam Doubleday Dell, 1996.

Helping Your Child Handle Stress: The Parent's Guide to Recognizing and Solving Childhood Problems. Katherine Kersey. Washington, DC: Acropolis Books, 1986. Normal stresses: toilet training, eating, sibling rivalry, school, divorce, stepfamilies, moving, depression, illness, physical disabilities, adoption, alcoholism, death in the family. Gives story examples.

Homemade Books to Help Kids Cope. Robert Ziegler. Washington, DC: Magination Press, 1992. For parents and their children ages 4–13.

How to Develop Self-Esteem in Your Child. Bettie B. Youngs, PhD, EdD. New York: Fawcett Columbine.

How to Say It to Your Kids: The Right Words to Solve Problems, Soothe Feelings, and Teach Values. Paul Coleman. Paramus, NJ: Prentice-Hall, 2000.

How to Talk So Kids Will Listen and Listen So Kids Will Talk. Adele Faber. New York: Avon, 1999.

Make-Believe: Games and Activities for Imaginative Play. Dorothy Singer and Jerome Singer. Washington, DC: Magination Press, 2000. Ages 2–5.

More Annie Stories: Therapeutic Storytelling Techniques. Doris Brett. Washington, DC: Magination Press, 1992.

A Parent's Guide to Early Childhood Education. Diane Trister Dodge and Joanna Phinney. In English, Chinese, or Spanish. Goals of developmentally appropriate program. What you can learn from activities, conversation, etc. How parents and teachers can work together to help children acquire skills, attitudes, and habits to excel in school and life.

Raising a Son: Parents and the Raising of a Healthy Man. Celestial Arts, 1996. And *Raising a Daughter,* Ten Speed Press, 1994. Both by Don Elium and Jeanne Elium.

Raising a Thinking Child: Help Your Young Child to Resolve Everyday Conflicts and Get Along With Others and *Raising a Thinking Pre-Teen.* Myrna Shure, PhD. New York: Holt, 2000. Clear examples of wrong way and right way to react and respond. Good for adults, too.

Sticks and Stones: 7 Ways Your Child Can Deal With Teasing, Conflict and Other Hard Times. Scott Cooper. New York: Times Books, 2000.

Stress and Your Child: Helping Kids Cope With the Strains and Pressures of Life. Bettie B. Youngs, PhD, EdD. New York: Fawcett Columbine, 1995.

When Your Child Needs Help: A Parents' Guide to Therapy for Children. Norma Doft. New York: Crown, 1994.

When a Hug Won't Fix the Hurt. Karen Dockrey. Brooklyn, NY: New Hope, 2000. Advice on coming to grips with feelings, working with friends, child and school, expectations and choices of family. Christian theme.

Siblings

Remember that any book about cancer or feelings can be useful for the siblings as well.

Beyond Sibling Rivalry: How to Help Your Children Become Cooperative, Caring and Compassionate. Peter Goldenthal, PhD. Owl Books, 2000.

Brothers and Sisters: A Special Part of Exceptional Families. Thomas Powell and Peggy Gallagher. Baltimore, MD: Paul H. Brookes, 1993.

Brothers, Sisters and Special Needs: Information and Activities for Helping Young Siblings of Children With Chronic Illnesses and Developmental Disabilities. Debra J. Lobato. Baltimore, MD: Paul H. Brookes, 1990. Out of print.

In the Shadow of Illness: Parents and Siblings of the Chronically Ill. Myra Bluebond-Langner. Princeton, NJ: Princeton University Press, 2000. About the experiences of families of children with cystic fibrosis; but the emotional issues are similar.

It Isn't Fair: Siblings of Children With Disabilities. S. D. Klein and M. J. Schleifer, Eds. Westport, CT: Exceptional Parent Press, 1993.

Loving Each One Best: A Caring and Practical Approach to Raising Siblings. Nancy Samalin. New York: Bantam Books, 1997.

Mixed Feelings: Love, Hate, Rivalry, and Reconciliation Among Brothers and Sisters. Francine Klagsbrun. New York: Bantam Books, 1992.

Siblings Without Rivalry: How to Help Your Children Live Together So You Can Live Too. A. Faber and E. Mazlish. New York: Avon Books, 1998.

Sibshops: Workshops for Siblings of Children With Special Needs. Donald Meyer and Patricia Vadasy. Baltimore, MD: Brookes, 1994. How to implement an ongoing program like the one started at Children's Hospital in Seattle, WA. Ideas for games, discussion activities. For siblings of children with cancer, chronic illness, or disability. Ordering information: Brookes Publishing, P.O. Box 10624, Baltimore, MD 21285 ($32.00).

Spiritual

Chicken Soup for the Soul. Jack Canfield. Deerfield Beach, FL: Health Communications, 2001. Many in the series for: fathers, teenagers, survivors, pre-teens, kids, couples, etc.

Head First: The Biology of Hope and the Healing Power of the Human Spirit. Norman Cousins. New York: Penguin Books, 1990.

Kitchen Table Wisdom: Stories That Heal. Rachel Remen, NY: Riverhead Books, 1996.

Naming the Silence: God, Medicine, and the Problem of Suffering. Stanley Hauerwas. Grand Rapids, MI: Eerdmans, 2000.

The Spiritual Life of Children. Robert Coles. Boston, MA: Houghton-Mifflin, 1991. Ideas about God from children of various religions.

When Bad Things Happen to Good People. Harold Kushner. New York: Avon, 1994.

When God Doesn't Make Sense. James Dobson. Carol Stream, IL: Tyndale House, 1993. Christian psychologist worked in cancer units in California. Childrearing, human relationships.

Survivorship

Some of these books will be appropriate for a mature teenager.

After Cancer: A Guide to Your New Life. Wendy Harpham. New York: Norton, 1994. Q&A format, written by doctor/survivor, addresses medical, psychological, and practical issues of recovery.

Cancervive: The Challenge of Life After Cancer. Susan Nessim and Judith Ellis. Boston, MA: Houghton-Mifflin, 1991. Emotions, employment, insurance, effects, family, fertility issues.

Childhood Cancer: A Practical Guide to Your Future. Nancy Keene, Wendy Hobbie, and Kathy Ruccione. Sebastopol, CA: O'Reilly & Associates, 2000.

Dancing in Limbo: Making Sense of Life After Cancer. Glenna Halvoson-Boyd and Lisa Hunter. San Francisco: Jossey-Bass, 1995.

The Damocles Syndrome: Psychosocial Consequences of Surviving Childhood Cancer. Gerald Koocher and John O'Malley. New York: McGraw-Hill, 1981. Out of print.

Testimonials

(Books by cancer families or survivors)

Anatomy of an Illness. Norman Cousins. New York: Bantam Doubleday Dell, 1991.

Against the Odds: The True Story of Michele, a Cancer Survivor. Patrick and Patricia Nolan. Clinton, WA: Alchemy, 1995. Ordering information: Alchemy Publishing Co., P.O. Box 285, Clinton, WA 98236; 360-321-7705.

Amanda's Gift. Scott MacLellan. Roswell, GA: Health Awareness Communications, 1998. Father's story of daughter's battle with histiocytosis, cancer, and liver transplant. Ordering information: 215 Spearfield Trace Roswell GA 30075. ($15.95; GA residents add 7% sales tax).

Autobiography of a Face. Lucy Grealy. New York: Houghton-Mifflin, 1994.

Being Brett: Chronicle of a Daughter's Death. Douglas Hobbie. New York: Henry Holt, 1998. Father recalls his daughter's struggle with Hodgkin's.

Blood of the Lamb. Peter DeVries. Boston, MA: Little Brown, 1961. Out of print.

Cancer Ward. Aleksandr Solzhenitsyn. New York: Noonday Press, 1991. Fiction based on his own treatment. Survival, hope, growth of spirit in horrible conditions in the USSR.

Choices: A Journey of Faith—Torrey's Miracle. Margaret Berger Morse. New York: Vantage Press, 1999. Alternate treatments. Short book, profits go to fund for parents seeking alternative therapies.

Count It All Joy. Sheila Ethier, RN. Edmonton, Alberta, Canada: Speedfast Color Press, 1999. Nurse and single mom; son has leukemia. Sixteen-month journal dealing with her depression, emotional pain, begun 10 years after diagnosis, talks about treatment and effects, including ADHD and her volunteer work.

Death Be Not Proud. John Gunther. New York: Harper & Row, 1949. Teenage son's terminal illness.

Eric. Doris Lund. New York: Harperperennial, 2000. By mother about teenage son's terminal illness. Acute leukemia.

Finding Strength: A Mother and Daughter's Story of Childhood Cancer. Juanne N. Clarke and Lauren N. Clarke. New York: Oxford University Press, 1999.

Fireflies. David Morrell. New York: Warner Books, 1999. Father's love and struggle to accept 15-year-old son's illness and death. Ewing's sarcoma, BMT. Faith, doubt, suffering, peace.

For the Love of Mike: A Mother's Story of Her Son's Lifetime Journey With Childhood Cancer. Linda Gillick. Waco, TX: WRS, 1994. Out of print. Neuroblastoma.

It's Not About the Bike: My Journey Back to Life. Lance Armstrong and Sally Jenkins. New York: Putnam, 2000. Inspiring story of athlete's experience. Medical details, long training to recovery.

Kids With Courage: Thoughts and Stories About Growing up With Cancer. Maury Cotter Kelly. Madison: Wisconsin Clearinghouse, 1998. Ordering information: University of Wisconsin Comprehensive Cancer Center, K4/666 Clinical Science Center, 600 Highland Avenue, Madison, WI 53792.

Making Miracles Happen. Gregory White Smith and Steven Naifeh. Boston: Little, Brown & Co., 1992. Anecdotes of medical miracles, doctors' insights, issue of control. Keep searching. Keep asking questions. Glosses over decision to stop looking.

Perfect Vision: A Mother's Experience With Childhood Cancer. Sharon Higgins Brunner. Fuquay-Varina, NC: Research Triangle, 1996. Mother of baby with retinoblastoma. Ordering information: Research Triangle Publishing, P.O. Box 1130, Fuquay-Varina, NC 27526; 800-941-0020 ($10.00 plus $2.50 shipping).

Six Months to Live: Learning From a Young Man With Cancer. Daniel Hallock. Farmington, PA: Plough, 2000. Terminal illness.

Victoria, My Daughter: A True Story of Courage. Elizabeth Hart. Sydney, Australia: Bodley Head. Mother's story of her daughter's battle with osteosarcoma and death.

BOOKS FOR KIDS

Children's Book Council
12 West 37th Street, 2nd Floor
New York, NY 10018-7480
800-999-2160 or 212-966-1990
http://www.cbcbooks.org
Look at the showcase archives.

American Library Association
http://www.ala.org/parents

Amputees

Adolescents With Limb Loss: A Handbook for Adolescents and Their Families and *Children With Limb Loss: A Handbook for Families.* Kirsten W. Lundeen, compiler. Grand Rapids, MI: Area Child Amputee Center, 1987. Booklets for birth–5 years and 6–12 years. Limb loss, physical aspects, medical care, prosthesis, self-image, independence, activities, sexuality and dating, rights and needs of teenagers and parents, resources. Ordering information: Area Child Amputee Center, 235 Wealthy, SE, Grand Rapids, MI 49503; 616-454-7988.

Annie Loses Her Leg but Finds Her Way. Sandra J. Philipson. Aurora, OH: Greenleaf Book Group, 1999. Annie, a springer spaniel, loses her leg to cancer. She is sad, her brother Max is in denial. They meet Samantha, a three-legged dog, and through her they both begin to heal. Optimistic. Friendship, love, loss. Ages 4–8.

To Walk on Two Feet. Marjorie Cook. Philadelphia, PA: Westminster Press, 1978. Out of print. Disablement, anger, and depression a teenage amputee feels vividly portrayed in this book.

You're Not Alone. John Sabolich. Oklahoma City, OK: Sabolich Prosthetic & Research Center, 1991. Out of print. Personal stories of 38 amputees. Ordering information: Sabolich Prosthetic & Research Center, P.O. Box 60509, Oklahoma City, OK 73146; 800-223-2336.

Bone Marrow Transplants

The Gift: For Children Who Are Bone Marrow Donors. Columbia, SC: Center for Cancer Research and Treatment. Help understand and deal with stress, express feelings, open-ended activities, explains harvesting, real photos, coping with anxiety and pain. Instructions for caregivers. Through metaphor of garden and special gift of seeds. Ordering information: Sue Heiney, Center for Cancer Treatment and Research Richland Memorial Hospital, Seven Richland Medical Park Drive, Columbia, SC 29203; 803-434-3460, Fax: 803-434-3095. (Make checks payable to Psychosocial Oncology/CCTR; one copy, $9.00.) http://www.rmh.edu

Stevie's New Blood. Kathryn Ulberg Lilleby. Pittsburgh, PA: Oncology Nursing Press, 1999. BMT explanation. Two books in one: One for 6–10, adjacent page is more detailed text for older children and adults.

There's a Little Bit of Me in Jamey. Diana Amadeo. Niles, IL: Albert Whitman, 1989. Ages 8–13.

Cancer

Afraid to Ask: A Book for Families to Share about Cancer. Judylaine Fine. New York: William Morrow, 1986. Ages 9–12.

George's Button. Columbia, SC: Children's Center for Cancer and Blood Disorders. Educational booklet about subcutaneous ports. Colorfully illustrated. Preschool/primary school level. Ordering information: Children's Center for Cancer and Blood Disorders, Children's Hospital of Richland Memorial, Suite 203, Seven Richland Medical Park, Columbia, SC 29203; 803-434-3533 ($11.00).

A Day With Dr. Waddle: An Introduction to Cancer Written for Children. Center for Basic Cancer Research staff. Manhattan, KS: Kansas State University Center for Basic Research, 1988. Coloring book. Ages 4–8.

Dear Bruno. Alice Trillin. New York: New Press, 1996. Woman who survived cancer writes this to a 12-year-old boy with cancer. Great cartoons. Simple but not simplistic.

Draw Me a Picture. Susan Nessim and Barbara Wyman. Los Angeles, CA: Cancervive, 1993. Coloring book for children with cancer. Marty Bunny talks about how it was when he was in hospital for cancer and invites readers to draw about their experiences. Ages 3–6. Ordering information: Cancervive, 310-203-9232.

Draw Me a Picture II: A Friend for Life. Susan Nessim and Barbara Wyman. Los Angeles, CA: Cancervive, 1994. Story and activity book for children with cancer. Ages 7–11. Ordering information: Cancervive, 310-203-9232.

I'm Still Me: Coping With Leukemia. Tim Peters. Peapack, NJ: Dr. Wellbook Collection, 1997. Picture book. Herbie the chick has leukemia. Friends make Herbie feel included. Good for classmates, friends, siblings. Ordering information: Tim Peters and Co. Publishing, 87 Main Street, Peapack NJ 07977; 908-234-2050 or 800-543-2230. http://www.captainbio.com (also books about diabetes, epilepsy, hearing loss, asthma, human anatomy board books)

Let's Talk About When Kids Have Cancer. Melanie Apel Gordon. Center City, MN: Hazelden, 1999. Ages 4–8. Other subjects of Let's Talk Library books: allergies, asthma, living in a blended family, alcohol abuse, being afraid, being shy, deafness, drug abuse, feeling sad, going to a funeral, going to the hospital.

Life Isn't Always a Day at the Beach. Pam Ganz, MS, ped-onc counselor. Lincoln, NE: High Five, 1996. For school-age children with cancer and siblings. Facilitates discussion. Ordering information: High Five Publishing, 4030 South 31st Street, Lincoln, NE 68502; 402-489-6060 ($9.95 plus $2.75 shipping).

Living With Cancer. Simon Smail. New York: F. Watts, 1990. Life for children with cancer, treatments, and prospects for the future. Ages 9–12.

My ABC Book of Cancer. Shannin Chamberlain. San Francisco, Synergistic Press, 1991. Ten-year-old survivor uses alphabet to discuss hospital experiences. Ordering information: Synergistic Press, 3965 Sacramento Street, San Francisco, CA 94118; 415-387-8180 ($6.95). Or through bookstores.

My Book for Kids With Cansur: A Child's Autobiography of Hope. Jason Gaes. Aberdeen, SD: Melius & Peterson, 1987.

My Fake Eye: The Story of My Prosthesis and *My New Glasses: A Book for Parents and Children.* Nancy Chernus-Mansfield, MA, and Marilyn Horn, LCSW. Los Angeles, CA: Institute for Families of Blind Children, 1991 and 1993. Ordering information: Institute for Families of Blind Children, 213-669-4649 (free).

One Day at a Time: Children Living With Leukemia. Thomas Bergman. Milwaukee, WI: Gareth Stevens, 1989. Out of print. Stories, photos. Ordering information: 800-433-0942.

The Problem With Hair: A Story for Children Who Are Learning About Cancer. Karen Sue Foss. Omaha, NE: Centering, 1996.

Sammy's Syringe (ages 2–5); *Marvin's Marvelous Medicine* (ages 6–9); *Your Body and G-CSF* (ages 12 and up). Intro books on g-csf therapy. Available in Spanish. Distributed by Amgen. Ordering information: Physician may call 800-232-9997.

Some Things Change and Some Things Stay the Same. Fred Rogers. Atlanta, GA: American Cancer Society, 1989. Comforting book for preschool-age children with cancer and their siblings.

The Talking Lady Presents: Having a Brain Tumor. Doris Rosenberg, MSW, CSW. North York, Ontario, Canada: Talking Lady Press, 1996. Describes procedures. Space to draw and express feelings. Not much about radiation and chemo. Ages 4–12. Ordering information: Talking Lady Press, 4949 Bathurst Street, #201, North York, Ontario, Canada M2R 1Y1; 888-512-TALK ($19.95 plus $3.75 shipping). http://www.canadamalls.com/talkinglady

What Happened to You, Happened to Me. Mary Kjosness and Laura Rudolph, Eds. Atlanta, GA: American Cancer Society, 1984. Ages 6–19.

What Is Cancer Anyway? Explaining Cancer to Children of All Ages. Karen L. Carney, RN, LCSW. Montclair, NJ: Dragonfly, 1998. Picture book with definitions: cancer, radiation, chemotherapy; emphasizes everyone's cancer is different. Hopeful. Ages 4–8.

You and Leukemia: A Day at a Time. Lynn Baker, MD. Philadelphia, PA: WB Saunders, 1988. Guide to leukemia. Explanation of diagnostic tests, treatment, emotional response to chronic disease process. Ages 10 and up.

Death

Annie and the Old One. Miska Miles. Boston: Little, Brown, 1971. Navajo reservation. Annie's grandmother says she will "return to the earth" when Annie's mother finishes rug she's weaving. Annie doesn't understand why mother keeps weaving and tries to stop her. Grandmother talks about natural cycles of life and death. Magical beliefs about death. Ages 4–8.

Anne and the Sand Dobbies. J. B. Coburn. New York: Seabury, 1967. Dan experiences death of little sister, Anne, and of dog. Questions answered by father and neighbor. Unusual: includes complete funeral service. Ages 9–12.

Beat the Turtle Drum. Constance Greene. New York: Viking, 1976. Girl's sister dies in accident falling from a tree. She has feelings of jealousy and being left out by her parents.

Belle Pruitt. Vera Cleaver. New York: J. B. Lippincott, 1988. Eleven-year-old helps family deal with the loss of her baby brother when her mother retreats into mourning. Ages 9–12.

A Birthday Present for Daniel: A Child's Story of Loss. Juliet Rothman. Amherst, NY: Prometheus, 1996. Sister's grief, acknowledgment of birthday of brother who died. Memories, remembering. Ages 9–12. Ordering information: order from bookstores or Prometheus Books, 59 John Glenn Drive, Amherst, NY 14228; 716-691-0133 ($14.95).

Bridge to Terabithia. Katharine Paterson. New York: Thomas Crowell, 1977. Boy and girl are friends, have special place; girl dies in storm. Inspires boy to assert himself. Ages 9–12.

Children Are Not Paperdolls. Erin Linn. Greely, CO: Harvest Printing, 1982. Drawing and comments by bereaved children, can be used to strengthen communication.

Children Facing Grief: Letters From Bereaved Brothers and Sisters. Janis Loomis Romand, Ed. St. Meinrad, IN: Abbey Press, 1989.

The Dead Bird. Margaret Wise Brown. Reading, MA: Addison-Wesley, 1965. Children find a dead bird and bury it, without input from adults. Ages 4–8.

Dying Is Different. P. R. Hughes. Mahomet, IL: Mech Mentor Educational Publishers, 1978. Children's pages use drawings, colors, poems about living and dead flowers, ants, fish, cat, grandmother. Depictions of inevitability of death, justification, remembering, acceptance, grief, funerals, cemetaries. Remarks for parents and teachers suggest questions and guidelines for discussion. Preschool to age 8.

The Empty Place: A Child's Guide Through Grief. Roberta Temes, PhD. Far Hills, NJ: New Horizon Press, 1992. Feelings after death of a sibling, empty place in the house, at the table, in brother's heart. Ordering information: 402-553-1200.

The Empty Window. Eve Bunting. New York: F. Warne, 1980. Out of print. 5th and 6th grade.

The Fall of Freddie the Leaf. Leo Buscaglia. New York: Holt, Rinehart & Winston, 1982. Allegory about balance between life and death. Ages 4–8.

Fire in My Heart, Ice in My Veins: A Journal for Teenagers Experiencing a Loss. Enid Samuel Traisman. Omaha, NE: Centering, 1992.

For Those Who Live: Helping Children Cope With the Death of a Brother or Sister. Kathy LaTour. Omaha, NE: Centering, 1983. Ages 13–18.

Gentle Willow. Joyce Mills. Washington, DC: Magination Press, 1993. Story for children about dying. Ages 4–8.

The Golden Bird. Hans Stolp. New York: Dial, 1990. Eleven-year-old boy dying from cancer. Visited by speaking bird from God and boy's father, who prepare him for his transformation into a new form.

The Grieving Teen: A Guide for Teenagers and Their Friends. Helen Fitzgerald. New York: Simon & Schuster, 2000.

Hang Tough, Paul Mather. Alfred Slote. New York: HarperTrophy, 1993. Sixth grader, baseball pitcher, has leukemia. In 3rd remission. Parents move around to find hospitals. He joins new team. New doc is very helpful: becomes personally invovled. Struggle of boy, protectiveness of parents. Ages 9–12.

Help Me Say Goodbye: Activities for Helping Kids Cope When a Special Person Dies. Janis Silverman. Minneapolis, MN: Fairview Press, 1999. Art therapy and activity book.

I Had a Friend Named Peter: Talking to Children About the Death of a Friend. Janice Cohn. New York: William Morrow, 1987. Out of print.

If Nathan Were Here. Mary Bahr Fritts. Grand Rapids, MI: Eardmans, 2000. Boy grieves loss of his friend. Ages 4–8.

The Kids' Book About Death and Dying. Eric Rofes, Ed. Boston: Little, Brown, 1985. Child-to-child perspective, 11–14 year olds share experiences.

Koko's Kitten. Francine Patterson. New York: Scholastic, 1985. Love and loss. Picture book. Ages 4–8.

Life and Death. H. Zim and S. Bleeker. New York: William Morrow, 1970. Out of print. Plain language, biology and chemistry of death. Natural life cycle. Attitudes toward death, funeral customs. Ages 9 and up.

Life and Death in the Third Grade. Maureen Burns and Cara Burns. Greenville, MI: Empey Enterprises, 1988. Sudden accident of close friend. Ages 9–12.

Lifetimes: The Beautiful Way to Explain Death to Children. Bryan Mellonie and Robert Ingpen. New York: Bantam Books, 1983. Paintings and simple text explain death is part of life. Ages 4–8.

Life Without Alice. Elizabeth Benning. Out of print. Lily's twin sister Alice is diagnosed with a brain tumor. Lily withdraws from school and friends to spend every waking moment with her sister, certain she can't live without her. For teenagers. Ages 12 and up.

A Little Bit of Rob. Barbara J. Turner. Morton Grove, IL: Albert Whitman, 1996. Parents and sister finally take boat out again, to get lives back to normal. Ages 4–8.

Losing Someone You Love. Elizabeth Richter. New York: Putnam, 1986. Young people share experiences of death of sibling.

Loss and How to Cope With It. J. E. Bernstein. New York: Seabury Press, 1977. Discusses responses of people to death of a loved one, normalizes "bizarre" reactions. Personal stories. Practical advice. Ages 12 and up.

Lost and Found. Rabbi Marc Gellman and Monsignor Thomas Hartman (the God Squad). New York: Seabury Press, 1999. Heartening guide for kids coping with loss. Ages 9–12.

The Magic Moth. Virginia Lee. New York: Houghton-Mifflin, 1972. 5th–6th grade.

Meeting Death. Margaret O. Hyde and Lawrence E. Hyde. New York: Walker, 1989. Myths, realities, feelings; technical and philosophical explanations. Reading suggestions, information sources. Ages 12 and up.

Mustard. C. Graeber. New York: Macmillan, 1982. Mustard, a cat with heart ailment. Owner Alex is 8. Increasing infirmities, can't shield Mustard from harsh realities of life. Cope with death. "If only" questions after death. Ages 4–8.

My Brother's Ghost. Allan Ahlberg. New York: Viking Children's Books, 2001. Mystery story with a twist. Ages 9–12.

My Twin Sister, Erika. Ilse-Margaret Vogel. New York: Harper & Row, 1986. Out of print. Young girl tells of loss, relief in sharing feelings with mother.

On the Wings of a Butterfly: The Story About Life and Death. Marilyn Maple. Seattle, WA: Parenting Press, 1992. Little girl comes to understand the concept of death as a transformation, like the metamorphosis of a butterfly. Ages 4–8.

Remembering You. Rose Resler. Workbook for children who have lost a sibling. Space to write feelings. Ages 6–teens. Ordering information: Rainbow Babies & Children's Hospital, Child Life Dept., Room 838, 11100 Euclid Avenue, Cleveland, OH 44106 ($2.25 plus $3.00 shipping).

Remember the Secret. Elisabeth Kubler-Ross. Berkeley, CA: Celestial Arts, 1998. Heaven. Ages 4–8.

Rudi's Pond. Eve Bunting. New York: Houghton-Mifflin, 1999. When Rudi dies, his friends and classmates build a schoolyard pond as a memorial. Ages 4–8.

Run, Run as Fast as You Can. Mary Pope Osborne. New York: Dial, 1982. 5th–6th grade.

Sad Isn't Bad: A Good-Grief Guidebook for Kids Dealing With Loss. Michaelene Mundy. St. Meinard, IN: Abbey Press, 1998. Ages 4–8.

The Saddest Time. Norma Simon. Morton Grove, IL: Albert Whitman, 1992. Death as inevitable end of life, anticipated death of adult, accidental death of a child (reaction of classmates), feelings. Ages 4–8.

Saying Goodbye. Jim Boulden and Joan Boulden. Santa Rose, CA: Boulden, 1991. Activity book. Ordering information: Boulden Publishing, P.O. Box 1186, Weaverville, CA 96093; 800-238-8433.

Straight Talk About Death for Teenagers: How to Cope With Losing Someone You Love. Earl Grollman. Boston, MA: Beacon Press, 1993. Denial, pain, anger, sadness, physical symptoms, depression.

A Summer to Die. Lois Lowry. New York: Laurel Leaf, 1984. Family life and friendships. Older sister dies. Young adult.

Teenagers Face to Face With Bereavement. Karen Gravelle and Charles Haskins. Englewood Cliffs, NJ: J. Messner, 1989. Perspectives and experience of 17 teens coping with grief.

There Is a Rainbow Behind Every Dark Cloud. Center for Attitudinal Healing. Berkeley, CA: Celestial Arts, 1979. Pictures and words; children come to terms with terminal illness.

Two Weeks With the Queen. Morris Gleitzman. New York: HarperTrophy. Out of print. Colin is sent from Australia to stay with relatives in England when his younger brother is diagnosed. Friendship with a young gay man whose companion is dying of AIDS helps Colin come to terms with his brother's death.

When I Die, Will I Get Better? Joeri and Piet Breebart. New York: Peter Bedrick Books, 1993. Six-year-old boy coming to terms with little brother's sudden death from meningitis. Father and son make up story about Joe and Fred Rabbit (boys' alter egos). Funeral, loss, healing process.

When People Die. J. E. Bernstein and S. V. Gullo. New York: E. P. Dutton, 1977. Explains reactions to death of loved one, grieving process, biological and physiological aspects of death. Answers children's questions. Beautiful photographs. Ages 6–10.

When Someone Very Special Dies: Children Can Learn to Cope With Grief. Marge Heegaard. Minneapolis, MN: Woodland Press, 1991. Workbook. Ages 6–12. Ordering information: Woodland Press, 99 Woodland Circle, Minneapolis, MN 55424; 612-926-2665 ($6.95 plus tax plus $2.50 shipping).

When Dinosaurs Die: A Guide to Understanding Death. Laurie Krasny Brown. Boston, MA: Little Brown, 1996. Ages 4–8.

When I Was Older. Garret Freymann-Weyr. New York: Houghton-Mifflin, 2000. Girl tries to understand life, death, and the time in between after her brother dies of leukemia. Ages 9–12.

Where's Jess? Joy and Marv Johnson. Omaha, NE: Centering, 1982. Ages 4–8.

Feelings/Coping

Aarvy Aardvark Finds Hope: A Read Aloud Story for People of All Ages About Loving and Losing, Friendship and Hope. Donna O'Toole. Burnsville, NC: Compassion Books, 1988. Aarvy Aardvark and his friend Ralphie Rabbit show how a family member or friend can help one another in distress.

Alexander and the Terrible, Horrible, No Good, Very Bad Day. Judith Viorst. New York: Simon & Schuster. Ages up to 3 years.

Amazing Grace. Mary Hoffman. New York: Scholastic, 1991. You can do whatever you set your mind to do.

Bad Case of Stripes. David Shannon. New York: Scholastic, 1998. Okay to be "you."

Bloomability. Sharon Creech. New York: HarperTrophy, 1999. Domenica Santolina Doone discovers beauty of nature, her place in the world, value of friendship, and that life is full of "bloomabilities." Ages 8–12.

The Carrot Seed. Ruth Krauss. New York: Harper & Row, 1945. Pics by Crockett Johnson. Very simple. Hope. Perseverance.

Dark Day, Light Night. Jan Carr. New York: Hyperion, 1995. 'Manda's Aunt Ruby helps her deal with angry feelings by making lists of all the things they like in the world. Ages 4–8.

Dealing With Feelings. I'm Frustrated; I'm Mad; I'm Sad; I'm Scared; I'm Proud; I'm Excited. Series. Elizabeth Crary. Seattle: Parenting Press, 1992 Fun, gamelike books to teach children how to handle feelings and solve problems. Ages 4–8.

Don't Pop Your Cork on Monday (anti-stress); *Don't Feed the Monster on Tuesday* (self-esteem); *Don't Rant and Rave on Wednesday* (anger control); *Don't Despair on Thursdays* (grief management); *Don't Tell a Whopper on Fridays* (truth-control); *Don't Fall Apart on Saturdays* (divorce survival). Adolph Moser, EdD. Kansas City, MO: Landmark Editions, 1991. Ages 4–12.

Double-dip Feelings: Stories to Help Children Understand Emotions. Barbara S. Cain. Milwaukee, WI: Gareth Stevens, 1993. Natural to feel contradictory emotions.

Emotional Ups and Downs. Enid Fisher. Milwaukee, WI: Gareth Stevens, 1998. Feelings of shyness, embarrassment, anger. Relationships. Death of a loved one. Fighting with family members. Ages 9–12.

Everybody Has Feelings. Charles E. Avery. Beltsville, MD: Gryphon House, 1998. Photographs. In English and Spanish. Ages 3–6.

Fears, Doubts, Blues and Pouts: Stories About Handling Fear, Worry, Sadness and Anger. H. Norman Wright and Gary Oliver. Colorado Springs, CO: Chariot Victor, 1999. Ages 4–8.

The Feelings Book. Todd Parr. Boston: Little Brown, 2000.

Fortunately. Remy Charlip. New York: Aladdin, 1993. Every event has a fortunately and an unfortunately side.

Friska, The Sheep That Was Too Small. Rob Lewis.New York: Farrar Straus Giroux, 1987. Being small.

Hooway for Wodney Wat. Helen Lester. New York: Houghton-Mifflin, 1999. The kids make fun of Rodney's lisp, until it helps rid the class of a bully. Ages 4–8.

Hope for the Flowers. Trina Paulus. New York: Paulist Press, 1972.

People. Peter Spier. New York: Doubleday, 1980. People are all different. Ages 4–8.

I Am So Angry I Could Scream. Laura Fox. Far Hills, NJ: Small Horizons, 2000.

Ignatius Finds Help: A Story About Psychotherapy for Children. Matthew Galvin. Washington, DC: Magination Press, 1987. Ages 4–8.

I Know I Made It Happen: A Gentle Book About Feeling Guilt. Lynn Blackburn. Omaha, NE: Centering, 1990.

It's Hard to Tell You How I Feel: Helping Children Express and Understand Their Feelings. Richard Krebs. Minneapolis, MN: Augsburg, 1981.

I Want Your Moo! A Story for Children About Self-Esteem. Marcella Baku Weiner and Jill Neimark. Washington, DC: Magination Press, 1994. Ages 4–8.

Jessica and the Wolf: A Story for Children Who Have Bad Dreams. Ted Lobby. Washington, DC: Magination Press, 1990. Ages 3–8.

The Jester Has Lost His Jingle. David Saltzman. Jester, 1995. Fable about value of laughter. Ordering information: The Jester Company, 800-9-JESTER (book, $20.00; doll, $32.00; set, $45.00). Also in bookstores.

Kate's Giants. Valiska Gregory. Cambridge, MA: Candlewick Press, 1995. Mother helps turn fears of night into friends. Calming techniques. Ages 4–8.

Leo the Lop. Stephen Cosgrove. New York: Price Stern Sloan, 1995. Normal is whatever you are.

Livingstone Mouse. Pamela Duncan Edwards. New York: HarperCollins, 1996. Mouse wants to make his nest in the "best" place in the world, searches all over for "China," only to find that the best place is the one that makes him happy and comfortable (in an old piece of china). Ages 3–7.

My Best Friend Is Me. Beth Ann Marcozzi. Plainview, NY: Child's Work, Child's Play. Social rejection. Ages 4–8.

The Missing Piece. Shel Silverstein. New York: HarperCollins, 1976. Being different. Ages 4–8.

The Moon Balloon: A Journey of Hope and Discovery for Children and Families. Joan Drescher. Bethesda, MD: Association for the Care of Children's Health, 1996

My Feelings Are Like Wild Animals! How Do I Tame Them? A Practical Guide to Help Teens (and Former Teens) Feel and Deal With Painful Emotions. Gary Egeberg. New York: Paulist Press, 1998. Christian perspective dealing with teenage anger, fear, hate.

Sometimes I Like to Cry. Elizabeth and Harry Stanton.Morton Grove, IL: Albert Whitman. Out of print. Ages 3–6.

Sometimes I Like to Fight, But I Don't Do It Much Anymore: A Self-Esteem Book for Children With Difficulty in Controlling Their Anger. Laurence Shapiro. Plainview, NY: Child Works, Childs Play, 1995. Ages 4–8.

Songs of Myself: An Anthology of Poems and Art. Georgia Heard, Ed. New York: Mondo, 2000. Poetry to celebrate your uniqueness. Ages 7–10.

The Soul Bird. Michal Snunit. New York: Hyperion, 1999. Inside each of us is a soul bird that expresses our feelings and should be listened to and appreciated.

Taming Monster Moments: Tips for Turning on Soul Lights to Help Children Handle Fear and Anger (Creative Meditations for Children). Daniel J. Porter, et al. New York: Paulist Press, 1999. Cartoons. Christian perspective. Ages 4–8.

Tanya and the Tobo Man: A Story for Children Entering Therapy. Lesley Koplow. Washington, DC: Magination Press, 1991. Available in English and Spanish. Ages 4–8.

The Temper Tantrum Book. Edna Preston Mitchell. New York: Viking, 1996. Ages 4–7.

Thank You, Mr. Falker. Patricia Polacco. New York: Philomel Books, 1998. Teacher helps girl who has trouble learning to read.

That's Good! That's Bad! Margery Cuyler. New York: Owlet, 1993. Each turn of events has an up side and a down side.

Tough Boris. Mem Fox. New York: Harcourt Brace, 1994. Even tough old pirates cry when they're sad.

The Very Angry Day That Amy Didn't Have. Laurence Shapiro. Plainview, NY: Child Works, Childs Play, 1994. About handling anger. Prekindergarten–elementary.

Weslandia. Paul Fleischman. New York: Scholastic, 1999. Boy who's "different" uses his imagination and creativity to make his own "country."

When the Wind Stops. Charlotte Zolotow. New York: HarperCollins, 1995. Every ending is a beginning. Ages 4–8.

When They Fight. Kathryn White. New York: Winslow Press. Picture book about family discord. Ages 3–6.

Wilfrid Gordon McDonald Partridge. Mem Fox. Kane Miller, 1989. Boy discovers the meaning of memories. Ages 4–8.

The Woman in the Wall. Patrice Kindl. New York: Houghton-Mifflin, 1997. Anna, extremely shy, retreats into herself and her secret rooms to hide from the outside world. Ages 10–14.

The Worry Stone. Marianna Dengler. Flagstaff, AZ: Northland, 1996.

Zink the Zebra: A Special Tale. Kelly Weil. Milwaukee, WI: Gareth Stevens, 1996. Zebra with spots instead of stripes: being different makes you special. Ages 4–8. Ordering information: Zink the Zebra Foundation, 414-963-4488.

Zink. Cherie Bennett. New York: Dell Yearling, 1999. Inspired by the author of Zink the Zebra, author intertwines 10-year-old Becky's life with leukemia and a rich fantasy/imagery which helps her cope. Ages 9–12.

Humor/Fun Stuff

Try Jack Prelutsky's poetry, the Captain Underpants series by Dav Pilkey, Amelia Bedelia series by Peggy Parrish, or the dark humor of Lemony Snicket's Series of Unfortunate Events.

Adventures in Art: Arts & Crafts Experiences for 8 to 13-year-olds. Susan Milord. Charlotte, VA: Williamson, 1997.

Brainstorm! The Stories of Twenty American Kid Inventors. Tom Tucker. New York: Farrar, Straus & Giroux. Ages 9–12.

Button, Button, Who's Got the Button? 101 Button Games. Hajo Bucken. Herndon, VA: Anthroposophic Press, 1995.

Cat's Cradle. Camilla Gryski. Econo-Clad Books, 1999. Also, *Many Stars* and *Super String Games.* Minneapolis, MN: Econo-Clad Books, 1999. Ages 9–12.

Curses, Inc., and Other Stories. Vivian Van Velde. New York: Harcourt, Brace. Magic always has consequences. Ages 12 and up.

Frindle. Andrew Clements. New York: Aladdin, 1998. Boy makes up his own word and sets about getting everyone else to use it. Ages 10–12.

How to Write Poetry. Paul Janeczko. New York: Scholastic, 1999. Ages 9–14. Also, *Favorite Poetry.* Lessons for grades 4–8.

Instant Activities for Poetry (Grades 3–6). Merrily Hansen. New York: Scholastic Trade, 1999.

Kids Create Art and Craft Experiences for 3 to 9 Year Olds. Laurie Carlson. Charlotte, VA: Williamson Press, 1999.

Laugh-eteria: Poems and Drawings. Douglas Florian. New York: Puffin, 2000. Ages 6 and up.

Mrs. McNosh Hangs Up Her Wash. Sarah Weeks. New York: HarperCollins, 1998. Also, *Mrs. McNosh and a Great Big Squash,* 2000.

One Potato, Two Potato, Three Potato, Four! 165 Chants for Children. Mary Lou Colgin, compiler. Beltsville, MD: Gryphon House, 1990.

Roald Dahl's Revolting Rhymes. Roald Dahl. Puffin Books, 1995. Ages 9–12. Also, *Dirty Beasts.* New York: Viking, 1996.

The Secret Knowledge of Grown-Ups. David Wisniewski. New York: Lothrop, Lee & Shepard Books, 1998. The real reasons grown-ups tell you to do things. Ages 4–8.

Silly Sally. Audrey Wood. San Diego, CA: Harcourt Brace Jovanovich, 1992.

Sit on a Potato Pan, Otis! Jon Agee. New York: Farrar, Straus & Giroux, 1999. Palindromes illustrated with silly cartoons. Ages 6 and up. Also *So Many Dynamos! and Other Palindromes,* 1997; *Go Hang a Salami! I'm a Lasagna Hog,* 1992; and *Who Ordered the Jumbo Shrimp? and Other Oxymorons.* New York: Harpercollins Juvenile, 1998.

Signing for Kids. Mickey Flodin. New York: Berkley, 1991. Introduction to American Sign Language, including words for thoughts and feelings.

The Sixth Grade Nickname Game. Gordon Korman. New York: Hyperion, 2000. Ages 8–12.

String Games. Anne Akers Johnson. Ages 9–12. Also, *Cat's Cradle.* Palo Alto, CA: Klutz, 1993.

Things That Make You Feel Good, Things That Make You Feel Bad. Todd Parr. Boston: Little, Brown, 1999. Age 3–6.

Underwear Do's and Don'ts. Todd Parr. Boston: Little, Brown, 2000. Ages 4–8.

Illness/Hospital Experience

Advice to Doctors and Other Big People From Kids. Gerald Jampolsky. Berkeley, CA: Celestial Arts, 1991. Share this one with all grown-ups!

The Coping Library: Coping With a Learning Disability. Jaydene Morrison and Lawrence Clayton. Center City, MN: Hazelden Information Education, 1999. Grades 7–12.

The Girl in the Opposite Bed. Honor Arundel. New York: T. Nelson, 1971. Fourteen-year-old girl, shy and snobbish, struggles with mixed feelings about the "lower class" girl in the opposite hospital bed.

Going Home. Margaret Wild. New York: Scholastic, 1994. While waiting to leave the hospital, Hugo takes imaginary excursions with exotic animals in faraway lands.

Henry and the White Wolf. Tim Karu and Tyler Karu. New York: Workman, 2000. Allegory of sick hedgehog undergoing treatments offered up by the White Wolf, a feared figure. Comes with a "talisman stone."

Little Tree: A Story for Children With Serious Medical Problems. Joyce Mills. Washington, DC: Magination Press, 1992. Overcome fear, sadness, serious medical changes; Magic Happy Breath Exercise.

My Round Rainbow: Helping Children Manage Illness. Maxine Walker. Greenville, SC: Children's Hospital. Story and coloring book activity. Therapeutic activities to help children articulate their feelings. Ordering information: Chaplain Maxine Walker, c/o The Children's Hospital, 701 Grove Road, Greenville, SC 29605-5601; 864-455-3195 ($12.50 each). Also available in computer-based program.

My Worst Friend. P. J. Peterson and Meredith Johnson. New York: Dutton Books, 1998. Humorous story of two girls who dislike each other. When one gets a brain tumor, the other feels obliged to be nice, but it turns out that's not what either needs, as they come to terms with an unusual friendship. Ages 9–12.

A Night Without Stars. James Howe. New York: Atheneum, 1983. Eleven-year-old Maria goes to the hospital for open heart surgery, finds strength in friendship with a badly scarred burn victim.

No Dragons to Slay. Jan Greenberg. Farrar, Straus, & Giroux, 1983. High school senior has cancer, learns new perceptions from friendship with beautiful young archaeologist.

The Only Way Out. Deborah Kent. Pittsburgh, PA: Apple Books, 1997. Fourteen-year-old Shannon makes decisions about how to deal with her disease. Goes on trip to see a healer in New Orleans.

The Revenge of the Incredible Dr. Rancid and His Youthful Assistant, Jeffrey. Ellen Confort. Boston: Little, Brown, 1980. Short, skinny Jeffrey, always picked on by bully, finds solace in writing a fantasy story in which he, with the help of Dr. Rancid, emerges as a hero.

Secret Magic. Zeno Zeplin. Nel Mar, 1991. Lauren's hair loss due to chemo, her classmates' teasing, and Uncle David's plan to win her friends.

This Is a Hospital, Not a Zoo! Roberta Karim. New York: Clarion Books, 1998. Magical animal crackers turn Filbert MacFee into a rhino, giraffe, etc. Ages 4–8.

Those Mean Nasty, Dirty Downright Disgusting but . . . Invisible Germs. Judith Rice. St. Paul, MN: Redleaf Press, 1989.

When Someone Has a Very Serious Illness: Children Learn to Cope With Loss and Change (The Drawing Out Feelings Series). Marge Heegard. Minneapolis, MN: Woodland Press, 1992. Workbook, draw about feelings and experiences. Elementary and junior high. Ages 9–12.

Why Me? Harnessing the Healing Power of the Human Spirit. Garrett Porter and Patricia Norris Pelad. New York: E.P. Dutton, 1985. Nine-year-old and therapist. Visualization and imagery.

Siblings

And to Think That We Thought That We'd Never Be Friends. Mary Ann Hoberman. New York: Crown, 1999. Siblings fight, make up, unite the world to make music. In Seuss-like verse.

The Barefoot Book of Brother and Sister Tales. Mary Hoffman. New York: Barefoot Books, 2000. Fairy tales of devoted siblings. Ages 9–12.

Brothers and Sisters Are Like That! Stories to Read to Yourself. Child Study Association of America. New York: Thomas Y. Cromell, 1971. Out of print.

Busy Days: For Boys and Girls Whose Brother or Sister Is Very Sick. Omaha, NE: Centering, 1985. Ages 3–8.

The Fear Place. Phyllis Reynolds Naylor. New York: Atheneum, 1994. Boy faces fears and feelings about brother on camping trip alone together.

Good as Goldie. Margie Palatini. Location: Disney Press, 2000. Ages 4–8.

Happy Birthday to You. Su Chen Fang. 1997. Boy meets girl who is undergoing treatment, comes up with a way to make her birthday special.

The Kite Flyers. Linda Sue Park. New York: Houghton-Mifflin, 2000. Set in 15th-century Korea, intense sibling rivalry, but teamwork, between brothers. Ages 9–12.

Koala Lou. Mem Fox. New York: Harcourt Brace, 1994. Sibling rivalry, parent loves child for who she is, not what she can or can't do.

Living With a Brother or Sister With Special Needs: A Book for Sibs. Donald J. Meyer, Patricia F. Vadasy, and Rebecca R. Fewell. Seattle: University of Washington Press, 1985. About feelings of siblings of children with disabilities, disabilities.

The One in the Middle Is the Green Kangaroo. Judy Blume. New York: Yearling Books, 1982. Middle child feeling left out. Ages 4–8.

Straight From the Siblings: Another Look at the Rainbow. Gerald Jamplosky and Gloria Murray. Berkeley, CA: Celestial Arts, 1983. Ordering information: Center for Attitudinal Healing, 415-435-5022. Ages 8–18.

The Two Princesses of Bamarre. Gail Carson Levine. New York: HarperCollins. Two very different sisters work together. Ages 9–12.

The Trolls. Polly Horvath. New York: Farrar Straus & Giroux, 1999. Ages 9–12.

The Tunnel. Anthony Browne. London: Walker Books, 1989. Modern fable about brother and sister who discover a tunnel and what they mean to each other. Ages 4–8.

When Sophie Gets Angry—Really, Really Angry. Molly Bang. New York: Scholastic Trade, 1999.

Simple story about handling anger and sibling rivalry. Ages 2–7.

What about Me? When Brothers and Sisters Get Sick. Alan Peterkin. Washington, DC: Magination Press, 1992.

Teenagers

The Adventures of Blue Avenger. Norma Howe. New York: Henry Holt, 2000. Humor, philosophy, romance. Boy explores concept of free will after the death of his father. Also *Blue Avenger Cracks the Code.* Ages 12 and up.

Angela Ambrosia. Ray Errol Fox. New York: Alfred A. Knopf, 1979. Story of girl's winning fight with leukemia.

Beauty and Cancer: Looking and Feeling Your Best. Diane Doan Noyes and Peggy Mellody. Dallas, TX: Taylor, 1992. Wigs, headwraps, skin care, clothing, manicures and pedicures, nutrition, exercise. Illustrations, resources.

Cancer in the Young: A Sense of Hope. Margaret O. Hyde and Lawrence E. Hyde. Philadelphia, PA: Westminster, 1985. Case histories, fears, myths, list of camps and other resources. Ages 12–15.

Chemo Girl: Saving the World One Tx at a Time. Christina Richmond. Sudbury, MA: Jones & Bartlett, 1996. Written by a 12-year-old with rhabdomyosarcoma, this book describes a superhero who shares hope and encouragement.

Chemo Kid. Robert Lipsyte. New York: HarperTrophy, 1992.

The C-word: Teenagers and Their Families Living With Cancer. Elena Dorfman (rhabdo survivor). Troutdale, OR: New Sage Press, 1998. Interviews with five patients, their parents, sibs, photos, treatment, positive and negative effects, changes in relationships, etc.

Easy for You to Say: Questions and Answers for Teens Living With Chronic Illness or Disability. Miriam Kaufman. Toronto, Ontario, Canada: Key Porter Books, 1995. Medical issues, sexuality. Grades 9–12.

Hunter in the Dark. Monica Hughes. Stoddart Kids, 1997. Seventeen-year old Mike, suddenly ill with leukemia. Parents hide truth from him. In hospital, he dreams of hunting. Ages 12 and up.

Invincible Summer. Jean Ferris. New York: Farrar, Straus & Giroux, 1994. Fictional relationship of two adolescents with cancer. Love story. (Parental warning: sex between teenage characters.)

Jeff Asks About Cancer Pain: A Booklet for Teens About Cancer Pain. Madison: Wisconsin Cancer Pain Initiative, 1990. Questions of 16-year-old boy with cancer: pain, narcotics, side effects, school and peer concerns. Illustrations. Ordering information: Wisconsin Cancer Pain Initiative, 608-265-4013 (free).

Life Happens. Kathleen McCoy and Charles Wibbelsman. New York: Berkley, 1996. Advice for teenagers on coping with common feelings of sadness, anger, anxiety.

Miriam's Well. Lois Ruby. Out of print. Christian Miriam (bone cancer) loves Jewish Adam. Complicated issues of religion and beliefs in faith healing are given in alternating viewpoints of two teens trying to understand each other. Ages 12 and up.

My Journal: Reflections on Life. Omaha, NE: Centering. For teenagers coping with life-threatening or terminal illness.

No Way! It Can't Be: A Young Adult Faces Cancer. Doug and Diana Ulman. Ellicott City, MD: Ulman Cancer Fund. Booklet.

Princes in Exile. Mark Schreiber. Beaufort, SC: Beaufort Books, 1983. Out of print. Gifted, asocial teen with a brain tumor gets a shift in perspective when he spends a summer at a cancer camp.

The Specter. Joan Lowery Nixon. New York: Laurel Leaf, 1993. Mystery. Seventeen-year-old Dina has cancer. Roommate Julie was in a car accident, is convinced someone is trying to kill her. Dina gets involved in case, but afraid she has made herself a target.

The Teenage Hospital Experience: You Can Handle It. Elizabeth Richter. New York: Coward, McCann, & Geohegan, 1982. Out of print.

Teenagers Face to Face With Cancer. Karen Gravelle and Bertram A. John. New York: Julian Messner, 1986. Seventeen teenagers talk openly about their cancer.

Teens Face to Face With Chronic Illness. Susan LeVert. Parsippany, NJ: Silver Burdett Press, 1993.

A Time for Dancing. Davida Wills Hurwin. Boston: Little Brown, 1995. Two best friends, one with cancer, tell about their senior year of high school. Ages 12 and up.

Too Old to Cry, Too Young to Die. Edith Pendleton. Nashville, TN: Thomas Nelson, 1980. Records experiences of 35 teenagers and young adults with cancer.

When a Friend Dies: A Book for Teens About Grieving and Healing. Marilyn E. Gootman. Minneapolis, MN: Free Spirit, 1994. Quotes from teenagers, and brief explanations and advice from author. No feelings are wrong. Comforting. Validating (you are not alone).

Jessi's Wish (Babysitter's Club #48). Ann Martin. Milwaukee, WI: Gareth Stevens, 1996. Out of print. Jessi volunteers at Kids Can Do Anything Club, meets 9-year-old Danielle, who has cancer. Not wholly medically accurate.

Six Months to Live. Lurlene McDaniel. New York: Bantam Starfire, 1995. Teenage girl with leukemia. Five other books in the series: *Now I Lay Me Down to Sleep,* teenager with leukemia deals with divorce and death of a friend; *Don't Die, My Love,* story of sweethearts, boy has Hodgkins, community support, dealing with illness and death; *Somewhere Between Life and Death,* story of girl whose younger sister is in an accident, family decides to turn off life-support; *Time to Let Go,* sequel about sibling grief. These books are romance novels; they are not heavy duty on medical facts but appeal to some, especially younger teenage girls.

Testimonials/True Stories

Hang Tough. Matthew Lancaster. New York: Paulist Press, 1985. Out of print. Ewing's survivor and illustrator.

Having Leukemia Isn't So Bad; Of Course, It Wouldn't Be My First Choice. Cynthia Krumme. Winchester, MA: Sargasso Enterprises, 1993. Diary entries, photos. Girl diagnosed at 4 with leukemia; goes to age 16.

I'll Never Walk Alone: The Inspiring Story of a Teenager's Struggle Against Cancer. Carol Simonides. New York: Macmillan. Out of print.

Keep Your Finger on the Boat. Lisa Pugh and Virginia Y. Pugh. Kalamazoo, MI: Ana, 1990. Journals, poetry, tapes, essays, girl in mid-teens shares feelings and experiences during four-year journey thru myelocytic leukemia. Ordering information: Ana Publishing, P.O. Box 625, Kalamazoo, MI 49005.

Lance Armstrong: The Race of His Life. Kristin Armstrong and Ken Call. Concord, NH: Platt & Munk, 2000. Ages 9–12.

Leukemia and Me, a Fight for Survival. Lisa Nicole Shinault. Benton Harbor, MI: Community Centre Group, 1991. Journal recordings. BMT. CML. Ordering information: Community Centre Group, 1385 East Empire Avenue, Benton Harbor, MI 49022; 616-925-0033.

My Journey of Hope. Sarah Jean Kovar. Grand Rapids, MI: Zondervan, 1993. Out of print. Eleven-year-old with brain tumor. Treatment, feelings, family relationships, relapse, death. Ordering information: 800-727-8004.

My Stupid Illness. Katy Tartakoff. Denver, CO: Children's Legacy, 1994. Ordering information: The Children's Legacy, P.O. Box 300305, Denver, CO 80203; 303-830-7595

My Treatment. Joe Bannah. Brisbane, Australia: Children's Leukemia and Cancer Society, 1982. Non-Hodgkins lymphoma. Ordering information: Children's Leukemia and Cancer Society, P.O. Box 361, North Brisbane, Queensland 400 Australia.

On With My Life. Patti Trull. New York: Putnam, 1983. Long-term survivor of osteogenic sarcoma shares experiences with amputation, family life, school, sports, work as occupational therapist.

Seeing Things My Way. Alden Carter. Albert Whitman, 1998. Second grader Amanda had a tumor in her head, and now she has blind spots when she looks at things. Hope and determination. Ages 4–8. Ordering information: Blind Children's Fund, 517-347-1357.

Shira: A Legacy of Courage. Sharon Grollman. New York: Bantam Doubleday Dell, 1991. Biography of child's coming to terms with own dying. Reactions of family, community.

Sunshine. Norma Klein. New York: Avon, 1974. Based on real-life diaries and tapes of dying 19-year old mother, for her daughter.

Todd. Bonnie Dempewolf. South Colby, WA: Bonnie Dempewolf, 1991. Mother's account of son's three-year treatment for ALL, with son's version, and how well he is doing now. Ordering information: Bonnie Dempewolf, P.O. Box 4268, S. Colby, WA 98384 ($9.95).

VIDEOS

Most of these videos will be more accessible through your hospital social worker, family resource center, or library. Some of them are out of print, others are simply too expensive for a family to purchase on their own, or were designed by hospital staff to be educational tools.

CHILDREN

Cancer in the Classroom. Portland Oregon: Candlelighters. Immune-suppression, teasing, effects on learning, changes in medical status. Ordering information: 3145 NE 20th St., Portland, OR 97212.

Childhood Cancer: Patients Speak Out. 16 min. Children's Hospital of Denver, 1991. Also, *Childhood Cancer: Siblings Speak Out.* For children. Feelings about physical and other changes, demonstrate involvement in normal activities.

Fighting Back. Color, 90 min. New York: Documentary Films, 1981. Four children ages 9–16 with leukemia in Ontario. Treatment, reactions, remissions, relapses, reactions of parents. For caregiver education, prepared students, and patients.

Hairballs on My Pillow. 15 min. Upbeat look at world of children with cancer. Comes with newsletter with exercises and activities. Good for classmates. Includes a teacher's notebook. Ordering information: Central Arkansas Radiation Therapy Institute, Communication Division, Markham University, P.O. Box 5210? 55050, Little Rock, AR 72215; 800-482-8561 or 501-660-7630; http://www.carti.com.

The Healing Path. 35 mins. Compassionate Friends. 1993. Addresses concerns of surviving sibling. Ordering information from Compassionate Friends.

I'm Still Me. 18 mins. Leukemia Society of America, 1989. Video and handbook. Puppets. Hair loss, guilt, worry, teasing, physical changes and feelings. Classroom resource.

Making a Difference . . . Together. 22 mins. Maywood, IL: Loyola University Medical Center, 1990. Children and teens talk about going back to school. Classroom resource for primary and junior high. Suggestions for teachers and nurses. Ordering information: Loyola University Medical Center, Social Work Dept. 2160 South First Avenue, Maywood IL 60153; 708-216-5044. ($20).

Mr. Rogers Talks About Childhood Cancer. 45 min. 1990. Two videos, guidebook, storybook. Stresses importance of talking about feelings. Ordering information: American Cancer Society.

My Brother Is Sick. 13 min. Kids Corner Series, 1984. Puppets and music, emotional responses of well sibling. Ordering information: Kids Corner, 2027 North Tejon, Colorado Springs, CO 80907.

My Hair's Falling Out . . . Am I Still Pretty? A Childhood Cancer Education Video. 22 mins. New York: Necessary Pictures, 1992. One woman show tells the story of a child with leukemia. Classroom education video for grades 1–5. Ordering information from Necessary Pictures Film & Media (see Educating Classmates).

School: Obstacle or Opportunity? Coping with Chronic Illness in the Elementary [Secondary] Classroom. 25 mins. Cincinnati, OH: Children's Hospital Medical Center. Experiences of principals, teachers, counselors, school nurses, parents, patients. Teacher guide. Classroom resource. Ordering information: rental from Hematology-Oncology Division, Elland and Bethesda Aves., Cincinnati, OH. 513-559-8604.

Standing Together, Standing Strong. 30 mins. New York: Cancer Cured Kids. School reintegration. Informs educator about cancer, treatment, side effects, impact on child's function. Emphasizes communication with parents, hospital. Classroom resource elementary through high school. Ordering information: Cancer Cured Kids. 888-995-KIDS.

Stop and Go Ahead with Success. Social skills at the elementary school level. Non-verbal learning disability. Classroom resource. Ordering information: http://www.ldam.org

Understanding Grief: Kids Helping Kids. Earl Grollman. 14 min. Interviews with children who have lost pet or loved one talking about emotions. 4T's: talk, touch, tears, time. Ages 9–14. Ordering information: DD Batesville Management Services, 1069 SR 46E, Batesville, IN 47006-9169.

Welcome Back. 14 min. Baltimore, MD: Johns Hopkins Children's Center, 1994. School reentry. Teacher's guide. Order: Aquarius Productions 508-651-2963, fax 508-650-4216. Email: aqvideos@ix.netcom.com $140 to purchase, $50 to preview.

Why Charlie Brown Why? Video version of book; 1990. Friend of Linus has leukemia. Explains in simple terms and also shows the feelings the friends and siblings may have.

You Don't Have to Die: Jason's Story. Jason Gaes. Video version of book. Ordering information: Ambrose Video Publishing, 381 Park Avenue South, Suite 1601, New York, NY 10016; 800-526-4663.

OLDER CHILDREN AND TEENAGERS

An Adolescent Copes With Death: Debbie. Color, 27 min. 1979. In interview, Debbie explains her disease, Ewing's sarcoma, reactions to treatment, attitude to prognosis. Ordering information: St. Louis University Medical Center, Audiovisual Dept., 1402 South Grand Boulevard., St. Louis, MO 63104.

Back to School. Washington, DC: Universal Health Associates, 1987. Interviews with students, different ages and illnesses, most cancer, treated at MD Anderson. Feelings and experiences returning to school. Ordering information: 1701 K St. NW, Washington, DC 20006; 202-429-9506. Classroom resource.

But Mr. Wilson . . . Why Did It Have to Be Melissa? Steven P. Lindenberg, developer. Audiocassette, 21 min. Harrisburg, PA: Professional Associates, 1982. High school senior dies of cancer. Her classmates discuss shock, fears, grief with their teacher. Insights into normal and pathological grief reactions, stages of dying, effects on religion and culture. For use in high school classrooms and counseling purposes. Ordering information: Professional Associates, P.O. Box 6254, Harrisburg, PA 17112.

Can't It Be Anyone Else? Santa Monica, CA: Pyramid Films. Color film or video, 54 min. 1980. Three youngsters (ages 10–12) with leukemia share feelings, experiences, fears with one another, family members, and filmmaker. Wisdom, courage, hope. Insight and inspiration to parents of seriously ill children and to professional caregivers. Out of print.

A Different Kind of Life. Washington, DC: PBS Video. Color, 29 min. 1980. Interviews with three cancer patients. One is a teenager named Missy. How they react to changes in lives, changed attitudes of friends, family, guilt, physical vulnerability, fear of death, trying to be normal. Missy's amputation and hair loss make her "feel like a freak." Introduction to some of the spiritual and psychosocial difficulties experienced by patients. For parents, teachers, caregivers. Out of print.

Don't Freeze Me Out. Baltimore, MD: John's Hopkins Children's Center, Adolescent Support Group. 17 min. 1988. Ordering information: The Grant-a-Wish Foundation, P.O. Box 21211, Baltimore, MD 21228; 800-933-5470 or 410-744-1032.

Jill. 26 min. Rockford, IL: Quandrus Media Ministry, 1978. Last months of young adult coming to terms with her condition through strong faith. Positive side of coping. Christian perspective.

Jocelyn. Color film or video, 28 mins. 1980. Seventeen-year-old girl dying of cancer. Tremendous spiritual strength. Good family and friends. Share with seriously ill patients who need encouragement and motivation. Ordering information: Filmmakers Library, 124th E 40th St., Suite 703A, New York, NY 10016; 212-808-4980.

Just Kids. National Film Board of Canada, 1995. 26 min. Four teens with terminal cancer. Their spirit helps them fight, endure, and celebrate life.

Lasting Impressions. 15 min. Series of vignettes depicting real-life experiences of members of support program for adolescents with cancer. How to cope with diagnosis and treatment. Patients conceived, wrote, acted in video. Ordering information: Sue Heiney, Center for Cancer Treatment and Research, Richland Memorial Hospital, Seven Richland Medical Park Drive, Columbia, SC 29203; 800-775-2287 (buy $295.00; preview $50.00—ask your social worker to buy it); http://www.rmh.edu.

The Long, Long Race. 15 min. Richmond, VA: Medical College of VA Hospitals, Department of Social Work. Interviews with 23 young adult cancer patients. Thoughts, feelings, experiences.

Princes in Exile. 1991. Rated PG-13. Out of print. Movie adaptation of novel. Gifted teen with a brain tumor spends a summer at a cancer camp.

Rising to the Challenge: Youngsters Speak Their Truth With Cancer. 15 min. Oakland, CA: Psychosocial Program, Kaiser Permenente Medical Center, 1995. Emotions of group of cancer patients (ages 10 and up), filmed during rafting adventure. Diagnosis, impact, treatment, side effects, stress, school, fear of death, siblings' concerns. Ages 12 and up. Ordering information: Aquarius Healthcare Videos, 5 Powderhouse Lane, P.O. Box 1159, Sherborn, MA 01770; 508-651-2963. ($140.00 to purchase; $50.00 to preview—ask social worker to order it).

Very Good Friends. 20 min. 1977. Thirteen-year-old girl's 11-year-old sister dies. Tortured by grief, anger, guilt. Parents help sort feelings, accept loss, rest more comfortably with memories. For classroom discussion. Out of print.

You Have Got the Power. Derry, NH: Chip Taylor Communications. 27 min. Interviews with five amputees (teenager to mature adult). At work, in rehab, sports, social life. Reactions of others, phantom pain, prostheses. Positive message. Preview free. Out of print.

PARENTS AND MATURE TEENAGERS

The Adolescent Interpretive Interview. Video and 13-page manual. Documents how team uses medical interpretive interview to help disabled or chronically ill adolescent establish competency. Ordering information: Adolescent Autonomy Program, University of VA Hospitals, 2270 Ivy Road, Charlottesville VA 22903; 804-924-2345.

Bright Beginnings. Los Angeles, CA: Braille Institute of America, 1991. For parents of children who are blind or visually impaired. Build child's interest, prepare for mainstreaming, use play as educational tool.

Coping Skills for Bone Marrow Transplantation. Karen Syrjala et al. Audiotape. 1993. Imagery and relaxation techniques developed for adults but useful for mature teenager. Ordering information: Karen Syrjala, PhD, FHCRC, 1124 Columbia Street, Seattle, WA 98104 ($10.00 payable to Fred Hutchinson Cancer Research Center).

Drying Their Tears. 1 hour. Little Rock, AR: CARTI, 1996. Video and manual to help counselors, teachers, and other professionals help children deal with grief, fear, confusion, and anger that occur after the death of a loved one. Ordering information: CARTI, P.O. Box 55050, Little Rock, AR 72215. 800-482-8561.

Family Portrait: Coping With Childhood Cancer. 1990. 25 min. Five family portraits cover guilt, sibling rivalry, maintaining discipline, divorce, adopted child, involvement of other family members. Ordering information: Films for the Humanities and Sciences, P.O. Box 253, Princeton, NJ 08543-2053; 800-257-5126 ($39.95 plus $3.95 shipping).

Gentle Fitness. Catherine MacRae. Video with natural stretches, exercises, self-massage, therapeutic breathing. Ordering information: 800-566-7780; www.gentlefitness.com.

Gentle Touch Infant Massage. Andrea Gravatt and Emma Miller. Parents demonstrate routines, and specialists explain the benefits. Communicating with, nurturing, soothing baby. Ordering information: Gentle Touch, P.O. Box 6007, Asheville, NC 28816; 888-333-3936 or 704-254-0003.

Good-bye. 27 min. 1980. Father experiences death of 12-year-old son of cancer, rethinks relationship with own father. Grieving for others part of one's own death work. Ordering information: Paulist Productions, P.O. Box 1057, Pacific Palisades, CA 90272.

Grief Comes to Class: A Teacher's Guide. Omaha, NE: Centering.

Life, Death and Baseball. Marilyn Levine. 1997. 58 min. Baseball loving sister of filmmaker died at 17 of cancer. As adult, about to become a mother she finally faces her past and how her life was affected by her sister's death. Ordering information: 212-808-4980.

No Fears, No Tears. Leora Kuttner. 27 min. Documentary of eight young children and parents as they learn how to manage pain of cancer treatment. Ordering information: Canadian Cancer Society, 265 West 10th Avenue, Vancouver, British Columbia, Canada V5Z 4J4; 604-872-4400; http://www.bc.cancer.ca/ccs/.

No Fears, No Tears—13 Years Later. 46 min. Seven survivors make sense of early traumatic experiences and demonstrate the power of mind-body pain relief. Ordering information: Fax request to 604-294-9986 or e-mail leora_kuttner@sfu.ca.

Parent-to-Parent. 12 min. Parents, children, and professionals discuss value of mutual support. Ordering information: Family Support Network of NC Campus, Box 7340, UNC, Chapel Hill, NC 27599-7340; 919-966-2841.

Parents' Responses to Their Children's Illness. Color video, 27 min. 1977. Parents of severely ill children and parents whose children have died are interviewed. Introductory. Ordering information: Universty of Michigan Medical Center, Media Library, Towsley Center for Continuing Medical Education, P.O. Box 57, Ann Arbor, MI 48109.

Siblings of Children With Cancer. 30 min. Interview with siblings. Ordering information: Biomedical Communications, University of Arizona Health Sciences Center, Tucson, AZ 85724.

A Special Love. National Cancer Institute. 18 min. Follows family through diagnosis, treatment, parent and sibling response, coping skills, support of family, parent group, treatment team.

What Do I Tell My Children: How to Help a Child Cope With the Death of a Loved One. Narrated by Joanne Woodward. Interviews with bereaved parents, children, families sharing real feelings and leading professionals in field, including Earl Grollman and Elisabeth Kübler-Ross, who offer advice for coping. Ordering information: Batesville Management Services, 1069 SR 46E, Batesville, IN 47006-9169.

When a Child Has Cancer: Helping Families Cope. Marital strain, financial crises, sibling conflicts, other situations. Video available from American Cancer Society local chapters.

Author Index

Subject Index

D

L

M

N